LIFE AFTER STROKE

A Johns Hopkins Press Health Book

To our parents, who were our first teachers,
to the doctors who taught us along the way, and
to our patients, from whom we have learned
much about healing and courage.

LIFE AFTER STROKE

The Guide to Recovering Your Health and Preventing Another Stroke

••

Joel Stein, M.D., Julie Silver, M.D., and Elizabeth Pegg Frates, M.D.

Foreword by Robert J. Wityk, M.D.

THE JOHNS HOPKINS UNIVERSITY PRESS • BALTIMORE

Note to the reader: This book is not meant to substitute for medical care of people with stroke, and treatment should not be based solely on its contents. Diet, exercise programs, and the use of medications are all matters that by their very nature vary from individual to individual. You should speak with your own doctor about your individual needs before beginning any diet or exercise program or taking any medications. It is especially important to discuss the use of medications with your doctor. These precautionary notes are most important if you are already under medical care for an illness.

The Johns Hopkins University Press
2715 North Charles Street
Baltimore, Maryland 21218-4363
www.press.jhu.edu

Library of Congress Cataloging-in-Publication Data
Stein, Joel, M.D.
    Life after stroke : the guide to recovering your health and preventing another stroke / Joel Stein, Julie Silver, Elizabeth Pegg Frates ; foreword by Robert J. Wityk.
        p. cm.
    Includes bibliographical references and index.
    ISBN 0-8018-8363-6 (hardcover : alk. paper) —
ISBN 0-8018-8364-4 (pbk. : alk. paper)
    1. Cerebrovascular disease—Patients—Rehabilitation—Popular works.
2. Cerebrovascular disease—Prevention—Popular works. I. Silver, J. K. (Julie K.),
1965– II. Frates, Elizabeth Pegg, 1967– III. Title.
RC388.5.S783 2006
616.8′1—dc22   2005028333

A catalog record for this book is available from the British Library.

Contents

Tables and Figures

Tables

Figures

Foreword

In recent years, so much has changed in medicine that the term *acute stroke* is rapidly being replaced by the term *brain attack,* to indicate that a stroke is similar to a heart attack: it is a medical emergency in which we intend to intervene to prevent and even reverse the effects of early brain damage. Modern advances in medicine have brought us to the point where we have effective treatments for many of the most feared illnesses. For example, we treat coronary heart disease by intervening during acute heart attacks, and a variety of drugs and procedures (such as bypass surgery and coronary angioplasty) alleviate persistent symptoms and prevent further cardiac injury. It is remarkable to note that as the twenty-first century progresses, each of these approaches is also being used in some form for the prevention and treatment of stroke.

We cannot treat the brain exactly the same way we treat the heart, however, even though both brain attack and heart attack are principally vascular diseases of their respective organs. Intuitively, people identify the heart as a source of strength and vitality for the body, while the brain is recognized as the repository of our conscious being and sense of self. (Among neurologists, we refer to the heart as a "dumb muscle" and the brain as "one of the most fascinating constructions of the universe.") Hence, the treatment of brain disease is a complex and delicate business. You can tinker with your car's engine, but you need to be very careful if you use a monkey wrench on your computer's motherboard.

Stroke primarily afflicts elderly people and tends not to be of interest to people unless they have had a stroke or they care for a family member with a stroke. However, 10 to 20 percent of the stroke patients I see in my specialty practice are younger than 45 years of age. In addition, pediatric stroke has just begun to be studied scientifically in the past decade. Young patients with stroke tend to have a greater recovery over a longer period of time than most people would imagine. Because, as noted above, interest in stroke generally arises only after an event, it is fitting that the authors of *Life After Stroke: The Guide to Recovering Your Health and Preventing Another Stroke* focus on helping the patient, the caretakers, and the family deal with the illness after the fact. The information about avoiding a second stroke (diet, exercise, and so on) applies to *all* of us who want to prevent stroke in the first place.

The authors have done an excellent job of explaining a complex disease in a straightforward and accurate way. The brain has many functions, with many specialized areas and connections. It is no surprise, then, that stroke is not a single disorder but an array of disorders that affect the blood vessels in the brain. Stroke due to blockage of blood vessels (ischemic stroke) is managed very differently from stroke due to bleeding of a blood vessel (hemorrhagic stroke). The medical management of stroke is usually a joint effort between the primary care physician (the internist or the family practitioner) and a consultant neurologist. Treatment after discharge from the hospital may include formal rehabilitation and the appropriate use of medications and follow-up diagnostic tests to prevent further strokes and secondary stroke complications.

The strength of this book lies in the information and guidance concerning the period of rehabilitation after stroke. For some patients this period lasts a few months, but for others it can last for years. During this time, the patient and family can participate actively in recovery and adapt to a new phase in life. Although many patients may not achieve a full recovery from neurological deficits, the aim is to recover as much as possible of the previous activities of daily life—self-care, mobility, communication, and even employment. This book is full of vignettes of patients coping with different types of stroke; I have seen similar cases in my practice as well. What makes this book unique among medical texts is the attention paid to the emotional reactions of the patient and family to the illness and its aftermath. It is vital that patient, caregiver, and physician recognize these emotions and work through them. Stroke recovery requires a significant investment of time and energy, and attitude is a very important factor in success. Some patients who seem apathetic and uninterested in working with rehabilitation therapists may have depression, a common neuropsychiatric complication of brain injury. Anxiety, denial, frustration, and fear are natural reactions to stroke that tend to arise several months later, during rehabilitation. (I like to think of the arrival of these reactions as a good thing—the brain is recovering enough complex function to recognize these "higher" emotions.)

Some researchers and other scientists predict that the real scientific advances for this century will take place in the neurosciences. The functional relationships of neurons and the ability of the brain to continue to grow and adapt to the environment (an ability called *plasticity*) are exciting concepts, particularly with the discovery of neural stem cells and the almost unbelievable possibility of brain regeneration and repair. All of these discoveries will help stroke patients someday. But we already have a wealth of information and experience to help stroke patients prevent future strokes and regain personal function right *here* and *now*.

This book will help you navigate the sometimes confusing corridors of medicine to empower you to take control of your health or that of your loved one. Read it and learn, and then discuss it with your physician. Between your involved interest, what you discover here, and your doctor's expertise, your or your loved one's recovery lies in very good hands indeed.

Robert J. Wityk, M.D.
Department of Neurology
The Johns Hopkins Hospital

Acknowledgments

We gratefully acknowledge our colleagues who are health care providers and administrators at Spaulding Rehabilitation Hospital Network and Harvard Medical School's Department of Physical Medicine and Rehabilitation. We offer a special thanks to Diana Barrett, Walter Frontera, Michael Sullivan, Steven Patrick, and Judith Waterston for their guidance and continued support of our work.

Doctors Lloyd Axelrod, Jonathan Bean, Wes Farris, Eric Isselbacher, and Jon Levinson shared their knowledge and added valuable information to this book. A special thanks goes to Dr. Philip Kistler under whose leadership the stroke program at Massachusetts General Hospital in Boston thrived for many years. Dr. Kistler was particularly generous with his time. He read the entire manuscript and offered excellent suggestions to improve it. His remarkable expertise helped to make this a better book. Terry Sutherland is a physical therapist who is knowledgeable about stroke and helped us with the chapter on exercise. Sharon Cloud Hogan's input helped to make some of the technical chapters easier and more interesting.

We would like to thank Alison Bozzi and Meaghan Muir for assistance with our research, Jessica Tyrrell, who helped with manuscript preparation, and Suzanne Lennard and Jenni Nicolla, the artists who assisted us. Our editor, Jacqueline Wehmueller, was a pleasure to work with at every stage of the publishing process.

Thank you to Donald Anderson Pegg, a stroke survivor, the father of Elizabeth Pegg Frates, and the inspiration for this book. He devoted a great deal of time and energy to proofreading various chapters and making sure they were understandable to someone who is not in the medical field.

Finally, we would like to thank our patients for showing us their grace and courage after suffering a stroke. We have shared some of their stories in this book, though we have changed names and identifying characteristics to protect their privacy.

Part I

UNDERSTANDING STROKE

Chapter 1

● ●

Understanding Stroke and Its Consequences

If you are reading this book, your life has probably been affected by stroke. Either you or someone you love has had a stroke. You are not alone. Stroke is one of the most important and difficult health challenges that we currently face worldwide. It is the leading cause of serious disability in most developed countries, including the United States and United Kingdom, and it is the third leading cause of death (heart disease and cancer are first and second, respectively).

But we know that you and your family members are not statistics. You are real people who are doing exactly what you should be doing—seeking out expert advice and researching what strokes are, why they occur, how best to recover from one, and how to prevent another one from happening. Reading this book is a good place to start on your road to recovery.

Of course, no book or other written information should take the place of your doctor's specific advice. Your doctor knows you, and he or she is able to tailor advice to meet your needs in a way that we can't. What this book can do is help you face the challenge of recovering from a stroke and avoid future problems with this disease.

We firmly believe that armed with the proper knowledge, you or your loved one can recover better from a stroke and reduce the risk of having another stroke in the future.

What Is a Stroke?

Simply stated, a stroke is local damage to the brain resulting from a malfunction in the flow of blood to the brain. To work properly, the brain needs a constant supply of oxygen and other nutrients that are carried in the blood. That means the brain needs a constant supply of blood. If there is a problem with this supply system, a stroke occurs. Usually a stroke affects only one part of the brain, but if the damage is extensive or occurs in a particularly critical area, then a stroke can be deadly.

Strokes and heart attacks are similar: both involve the blood supply to organs that keep us alive. Sometimes the problems that cause strokes and heart attacks are lumped together and called *cardiovascular disease.* Most people understand more about heart attacks than about strokes, and they know that heart attacks occur when there is a problem with the blood supply to the heart. Because the causes of heart attacks and strokes are similar, some medical professionals think it might be better to use the term *brain attack* than the term *stroke,* and the day may not be too far off when *brain attack* becomes as familiar as *heart attack.*

There are two major categories of stroke: *ischemic* (is-ᴋᴇᴇᴍ-ik) and *hemorrhagic.* Eight of ten people who suffer strokes have the ischemic type. Improper blood flow in the arteries is the cause of all strokes, but the way in which a problem occurs defines whether it is an ischemic or hemorrhagic stroke. In an ischemic stroke, a blood clot in the artery blocks the supply of blood either partially or completely. The damage done by such a blockage is called an *infarct.* If the artery is a small vessel that doesn't supply a crucial part of the brain, the problem might not be very noticeable. But if it is a large artery or one that supplies a particularly important part of the brain (like the part of the brain that controls movement or speech), then the stroke can be catastrophic. To understand an ischemic stroke, think of a garden hose that has a kink in it so that water can't get through. If a blood vessel has a clot in it, then the blood won't get through and the part of the brain that needs that blood will be injured (Figure 1.1).

In a hemorrhagic stroke, the problem with the arteries is different. There is no blood clot slowing or stopping the flow, but there is a leak in a blood vessel or a bursting of the vessel. Again, think of the garden hose analogy. If you are trying to water flowers and there is a hole in the hose, then water will spill into places where you don't want it to go. A hemorrhagic stroke happens when there is a hole in a blood vessel and the blood that is supposed to supply the brain doesn't reach it in the proper manner, instead "spilling" into other areas of the brain. This spill floods the surrounding area of the brain and causes injury to it.

Ischemic strokes are sometimes further defined by where they are located or what causes the clot. For example, the term *cardioembolic* simply means that the blood clot originally came from the heart and then traveled along the arteries until it got stuck in an artery in the brain. Although it is not always possible for doctors to figure out where the problem began,

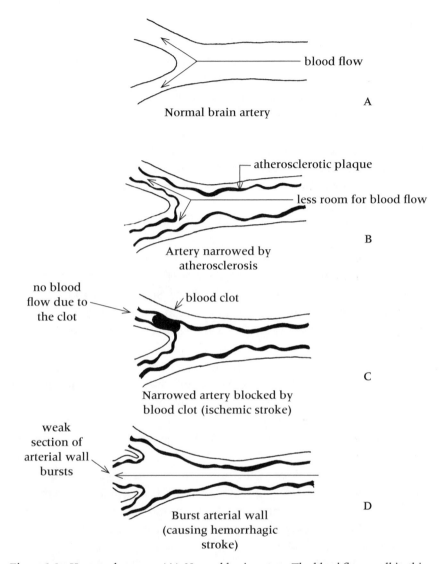

Figure 1.1. *How strokes occur.* (A) *Normal brain artery. The blood flows well in this artery because the vessel is not constricted in diameter and there is no weakness of the vessel walls.* (B) *Atherosclerotic plaque. Atherosclerosis may lead to an ischemic stroke if the diameter of the brain artery becomes so narrow that not enough blood can flow through it to supply a particular area of the brain.* (C) *Blood clot. A blood clot, usually coming from arteries in the neck or somewhere in the heart, can cause an ischemic stroke if it becomes dislodged and gets trapped in the smaller vessels of the brain.* (D) *Hemorrhagic stroke. The weak section of this arterial wall bursts and causes a hemorrhagic stroke. This kind of stroke is more common in people with high blood pressure, because of the forces their blood pressure exerts on the arterial walls.*

when they can identify the source of the clot, they are better able to treat the problem. You may hear terms like *cardioembolic, large vessel atherothrombotic,* and *lacunar,* all of which refer to ischemic strokes but offer further information about the nature of the injury.

To summarize, remember that strokes are always caused by problems with the blood vessels that supply the brain, and that strokes generally occur because either there is a clot that causes reduction or blockage of the blood flow or there is a leak in the vessel. (A small number of strokes are caused by veins that get blocked, rather than arteries.) The damage that is done depends on where the problem occurs in the brain, how extensive it is, and how long it lasts.

What Is a TIA?

A transient ischemic attack (TIA) is defined as a stroke that lasts less than twenty-four hours and has no residual effects. Some people think of a TIA as a "mini-stroke." A twenty-four-hour cutoff is an artificial concept and one that many experts have criticized in recent years. One reason it doesn't make much sense to have a timed cutoff is that studies have demonstrated that within one hour of the onset of the symptoms, up to one-third of patients will have noticeable changes on brain imaging studies that indicate injury to the brain. There is debate about whether we should be more concerned about *when* the symptoms resolve or whether there is evidence of brain injury on radiographic studies. Doctors generally are most concerned with the cause of the event, what can be done right away to lessen the damage, and what can be done in the future to prevent another event, rather than with how long the symptoms last. Still, the term *TIA* is frequently used and cited in the literature and is commonly defined as a stroke-like event that does not leave any residual symptoms after twenty-four hours have passed.

Between 200,000 and 500,000 people sustain TIAs in the United States each year, and more than 5 million Americans have been given the diagnosis of TIA in the past. Because TIAs are by definition transient (temporary) events, many people do not seek medical attention when they have symptoms, so the number of people who have TIAs is probably greatly underestimated. Some people with TIAs may be misdiagnosed as having a seizure, migraine, anxiety, or even psychosis. The diagnosis of TIA is almost always made by history alone (what the patient or family members tell the doctor), although about half of the people who have one TIA will have evidence of brain injury on a magnetic resonance imaging test (MRI, a sophisticated imaging study). Although most people with a stroke are hospitalized, many patients with TIAs are not. This practice is controversial; it is not really clear, when it comes to TIAs, who should be hospitalized and monitored closely and who does not need to be hospitalized.

Some of the controversy surrounding TIAs will be cleared up when more research has been done on this topic, but clearly TIAs are linked to more serious strokes. In one study done in Northern California, 1,707 patients with TIAs were followed for the three months immediately following their TIAs.[1] Approximately 1 in 9 of them subsequently had a stroke, and half of these strokes occurred in the first two days after the TIA.

Stroke through the Ages

Over the centuries, stroke has been known by several names. Stroke has been recognized as a distinct disease since biblical times, when the Psalmists described its symptoms: "If I forget you, O Jerusalem, let my right hand wither! Let my tongue cleave to the roof of my mouth, if I do not remember you, if I do not set Jerusalem above my highest joy!" The term *apoplexy* was used by the ancient Greek physician Hippocrates and encompassed all forms of stroke. Other terms that have been used to describe stroke include *cerebrovascular accident* (CVA) and *brain attack*. Perhaps the latter term best describes the actual event—an injury to the brain that is caused by either a hemorrhage or a blood clot and affects the nutrient supply to this vital organ. Today the commonly accepted term is simply *stroke*.

We might expect that scientists and doctors would have made tremendous gains in treating or even curing a disease with such a long history. They certainly have cured or prevented many other conditions, such as polio and smallpox. Yet even though we have known about strokes for a very long time, we still have much to learn about how to treat them. There is some wonderful news for stroke survivors, however. For thousands of years we had almost no treatments available, but in the past decade or so, our ability to treat stroke has markedly improved. And we can expect major breakthroughs in the future.

We have come to understand stroke much better since the late 1920s, when the technique for injecting dye into the neck arteries was developed. This procedure, called *cerebral angiography,* allowed doctors to visualize blood flow in vessels in the brain and to determine whether there was a blockage or severe narrowing. Although this technique helped medical scientists better understand the cause of some strokes, there was still no effective treatment. This made stroke a disease to which few doctors and researchers wanted to devote much time, because when someone had a stroke there was essentially "nothing to be done."

In 1948, a group of researchers began a study of more than 5,000 men and women in Framingham, Massachusetts. This study, widely called "The Framingham Heart Study," has become synonymous with the remarkable advances we have made in understanding the causes of heart disease. Although the initial research focused on heart disease, the research has continued to this day and has expanded to shed light on many important health concerns, including stroke.[2] The Framingham Heart Study brought attention to the need for more information about what causes strokes and how we can best treat them. Ultimately this information helped to bring about the first real treatment in the prevention of stroke—aspirin and other similar medications, which help prevent blood clots from forming. (We discuss medications that help prevent stroke in Chapter 13.)

Soon, more investigators began to study stroke, which led to worthwhile information and new treatments—much of what we present in this book. Meticulous studies of the brain and blood vessels conducted by C. Miller Fisher in the mid-twentieth century helped elucidate the mechanisms of strokes and their causes. Along with better understanding of the causes of stroke came better tools to understand what happens when someone has a stroke. In the 1970s a wonderful invention called computed tomography, or CT, scans first allowed doctors to visualize the brain. These scans helped physicians determine the location and extent of damage to the brain of someone who had a stroke. Newer imaging techniques such as MRI and ultrasound advanced our ability to find the cause of stroke in the 1980s and 1990s. We are now well into the twenty-first century and, despite a slow start, there have been marked gains in our understanding of how and why strokes occur and how to prevent them or help someone recover from one.

How Stroke Affects Us Today

More than 700,000 new strokes occur annually (500,000 are new attacks and 200,000 are recurrent strokes), and there are an estimated 5 million stroke survivors in the United States. Recent studies have suggested that the number of strokes and stroke survivors is probably *under*estimated for a variety of reasons, including that some people never seek medical attention.

The American Stroke Association notes that every 45 seconds someone in America has a stroke, and every 3.1 minutes someone dies of one. Although medical advances have reduced the death rate from stroke, the number of people who have strokes continues to increase every year. Of the individuals who survive, approximately half of them will return to work, but many will not be able to function at their previous level. Of the people who live through a serious stroke, 20 percent will need to use an assistive device such as a walker or cane and 30 percent will require help with daily tasks such as bathing and dressing.

Strokes have been called a "disease of old age" because approximately half of all strokes occur in people who are older than 75. Age is considered the most important determinant of stroke, and for every ten years after age 55, the rate of stroke more than doubles in both men and women. But although stroke becomes a much bigger risk as we age, consider that the remaining half of all strokes occur in people younger than 75 years of age. Many people think that strokes happen mostly to men, but this is not accurate. Men have a greater incidence up to age 75, but then the incidence of stroke in men and women equalizes. (Though note that more women than men have strokes after the age of 75, because women tend to live longer, so there are more women than men in this age group.) In young adults, the rate for men and women is about the same. Studies have shown that certain ethnic groups may have a higher risk of stroke and a higher risk of a stroke being deadly. The reasons for this are not entirely clear, but these groups may have less education about how to lower the risk factors for stroke and may be without access to state-of-the-art medical care if a stroke does occur.

Why Read This Book?

Before we comment on why you should *read* this book, first let us tell you why we decided to *write* this book. We decided to write this book because we had so many patients coming to us *after* they had a stroke and asking, "How can I make sure this never happens to me again?" During an office visit, most doctors, including us, cannot explain all of the different things one can do to prevent a second stroke from happening. What we do in the office (as do most doctors who treat stroke) is address the most helpful stroke prevention measures for a given individual. Still, we know that there is much more information that we simply don't have time to share, even if someone comes to see us several times.

When someone who has just had a stroke comes to see us, much of the visit might focus on helping the person recover from the effects of that stroke. This goal is incredibly important. We spend the first part of this book explaining how you or someone you love can optimally recover from a stroke. For someone who is still trying to recover from one stroke, it can be hard to take in new information about how to prevent another stroke from happening sometime in the future. Doctors want to give patients as much information as possible, but we are sensitive to the fact that overwhelming patients with too much information too soon is actually detrimental.

You and your family members can read this book at your own pace. If you want the information quickly, you can read the book in a day. If you want to take in the information in smaller bits, you can read it page-by-page or chapter-by-chapter. You can mark the information that is particularly important to you and refer back to it later. (In grade school you were probably taught not to write in books. That certainly is commendable, but feel free to write in this one. We view this as a guide to saving your life, and we want to make it as easy as possible for you to find and remember the information you need. So, if it helps you to bend the page corners, use a yellow highlighter, put stickies on important pages, whatever, go ahead and do that.) You can read this book by skipping to the chapters that interest you most or by reading it from start to finish (we recommend the latter method, since we don't want you to miss any important information).

This book can serve as an excellent resource for you, but again, it doesn't take the place of your own doctor's advice. In medicine, we often order a variety of tests. And patients frequently ask us, "Why do you need me to have this test when I just had that other one done last week?" The reason is that medical tests provide different pieces of information, and these pieces help doctors to better understand what is going on in a particular patient. Sure, a single test is helpful and there is often overlap between two tests, but sometimes two tests are much, much better than just one. They *complement* each other and allow us to understand what is happening in a way that we could not if we had results from only one test. That is how you should think of this book and your own doctor's advice. *Both* provide valuable information and complement each other, allowing you to better understand how to recover from a stroke and prevent another one from occurring.

How You Can Prevent a Stroke

We want to say a few words up front about this important topic, but much more information will come later in the book. Stroke prevention is divided into two categories, based on whether someone has had a stroke in the past. *Primary* stroke prevention focuses on preventing a stroke in someone who has never had a stroke, and *secondary* prevention is geared toward keeping someone from having another stroke.

Many of the ways to lower someone's risk of having a stroke apply whether the person has had a stroke or has never had a stroke. So, there is a lot of crossover between primary and secondary stroke prevention. Secondary stroke prevention, however, involves more medical interventions and options, because we know that someone who has already had a stroke or TIA is more likely to have a recurrent problem than someone who has never had a stroke. If the cause of the first stroke is known, secondary stroke prevention can also be more personalized than primary stroke prevention. In this book we focus on *secondary* stroke prevention, but much of our advice helps prevent a first stroke as well as recurrent strokes.

To help protect yourself from having a stroke, you need to know why you might be at risk to have one. The risk factors for stroke are divided into three categories:

1. Things you can change through lifestyle modifications
2. Things you can change with the help of your doctor
3. Things you cannot change

Tables 1.1, 1.2, and 1.3 provide more information about risk factors and how you and your doctor can work together to lower your chances of having a stroke.

This book is divided into five parts. In Part I (Chapters 1–3) we explain what a stroke is, how it occurs, and what kinds of injuries it can cause. In Part II (Chapters 4–6), we discuss stroke recovery. In Part III (Chapters 7–14) we focus on how you can work with your doctor to lower your risk of a future stroke. In Part IV (Chapters 15–17), we describe how you can alter your habits and lifestyle to reduce your risk of having a stroke or recurrent stroke. Finally, in Part V (Chapters 18–19), we take a look at stroke research that will provide us with better treatment options, and we offer a relatively simple plan for taking control in preventing another stroke. Knowing what to do and actually making these changes are two different

Table 1.1. Changing Your Habits to Help Prevent Another Stroke

If you smoke, stop smoking.
Don't drink alcohol, or if you do, drink only in small quantities.
If you are overweight, lose weight.
Exercise regularly.
Take every dose of your medications without fail.
Consult with your doctor regularly and keep all of your appointments.

Table 1.2. How Your Doctor Can Help You Lower Your Risk of Having Another Stroke

By helping to keep your blood sugar in good control if you have diabetes
By helping to keep your blood pressure in good range if you have hypertension
By helping you to stop smoking if you smoke
By helping to keep the triglyceride and cholesterol levels in your blood in a safe range

Table 1.3. Things You Cannot Change That May Affect Your Risk of Having a Stroke

Your age
Your ethnic background
Your sex

things, however. We understand this, and we have a lot of experience helping people not only learn what they need to do but also acquire additional information that can help them follow through with the actions that will reduce their risk of having a stroke.

As physicians who treat people who have had strokes, we know what will make a difference medically, and we want you to understand how you can best help yourself and your loved ones. Published research studies have shown that many people do not know what they can do to prevent a stroke from occurring or, if one does occur, how they should react—or even that they should be concerned and educated about stroke. For example, in one study only 8 percent of the women surveyed identified heart disease and stroke as their greatest health concern, despite the fact that cardiovascular disease, which includes both heart attack and stroke, is the leading cause of death in men and women in the United States.[3] Also, while 9 of 10 women surveyed reported that they would like to talk to their doctors about how they can reduce their risk of having a stroke or heart attack, 7 of 10 of these women said that they had not done this.

Researchers have also looked at whether adults in the general population are able to correctly identify the symptoms of stroke and the risk factors associated with having a stroke. These studies have shown that the vast majority of people do not recognize the major symptoms of stroke and that they also don't know what they can do to lower their risk of having a stroke. For example, in one study nearly 40 percent of people who were admitted to the hospital with a suspected stroke were not able to identify a single sign or symptom of this condition. This situation is slowly changing, as stroke education is becoming an important public health issue. Still, many lives are lost or irreparably harmed because people simply are not educated enough about what causes a stroke, what a stroke looks like when it is happening, and how to respond when someone is having a stroke.

In writing this book, we had four straightforward goals that may help you or someone you love avoid the tragic results of a serious stroke:

1. We want you to understand the risk factors for having a stroke (or recurrent stroke) and how you can reduce them with medical help from your doctor and through your own efforts with simple lifestyle changes.
2. We want you to be able to quickly recognize the signs and symptoms of a stroke, so you can take immediate lifesaving action.
3. We want you to know that it is important to call 9-1-1 the instant you suspect that someone is having a stroke.
4. We want you to be aware of how doctors and other health care providers can help you or someone you love optimally recover from a stroke.

••

Chapter 2

How Strokes Affect Our Brains and Bodies

Our brains are very complex organs. The *right* side of the brain is responsible for movement and feeling on the *left* side of the body. A stroke on the right side of the brain may cause paralysis on the left side of the body and problems with visual-spatial relationships. Problems with visual-spatial relationships mean that someone might find it hard to evaluate where things are located in relation to his own body; someone with this problem might not be aware of an object or person on his left side, for example. People who have right-brain strokes may also have difficulty with judgment and may be impulsive and quick to react without thinking. Strokes on the *left* side of the brain may affect movement on the *right* side of the body and cause injury to the speech center. Thus, many people with a left-brain stroke have right-sided paralysis and problems with speech. Strokes in the back of the brain often lead to complications with vision and balance.

In this chapter we describe how strokes can affect the brain and the body. We also describe the importance of early medical treatment and the use of clot-busting drugs. We investigate the relationships between stroke and dementia and stroke and the emotions. And we describe the signs of stroke, which everyone should learn to recognize.

Anatomy of a Stroke

The brain is composed of many parts. The first major division is between the upper brain (called the *cerebral cortex*) and the lower brain (*cerebellum* and *brainstem*). In general, the cerebral cortex controls how we think, speak, move, and see, and the cerebellum controls balance and coordination. The brainstem controls many of the body functions that we take for granted, such as heart rate, body temperature, breathing, sleep cycles, and the regulation of some hormones (see Figure 2.1).

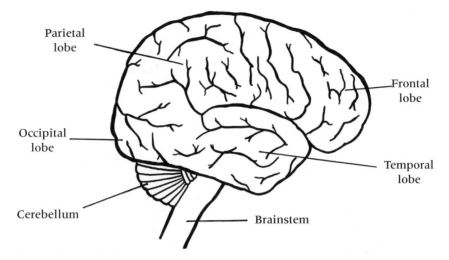

Figure 2.1. Strokes can occur anywhere in the brain. The region of the brain that is injured in a stroke determines what kind of problems the person will encounter.

Looking at the top of the brain, it appears to be split down the center. We call each side a *hemisphere*. Each hemisphere has four separate regions, or *lobes,* each of which performs important functions. Someone who has had a stroke will encounter different problems depending on which lobe of the brain is affected and how seriously the stroke damaged the surrounding brain tissue. The four lobes of each hemisphere perform the following functions:

Frontal lobes (located in the front of the brain) control setting goals, behavioral and social graces, and body movement.
Parietal lobes (located in the upper middle section) are involved with sensation, mathematical abilities, abstract thinking, our sense of the space around us, and language.
Temporal lobes (located in the lower middle section) control emotions and memory as well as some language functions.
Occipital lobes (located in the back of the brain) interpret what we see.

Our brains' two hemispheres may look similar, but the individual lobes on each side control different functions. For example, your left frontal lobe controls body movement on the right side of your body, and vice versa. You may have heard that right-handed people have a "dominant" left brain and left-handed people have a "dominant" right brain. In fact, the side that is primarily responsible for language is considered the dominant side. In most people language is primarily a left-brain function (including most left-handed people). The point here is to understand that the brain consists of many "crossed connections," and this means that an injury to one side of your brain may affect your body on the opposite side. For example, if you have a stroke on the right side of your brain, the left side typically will be affected. One important exception is strokes affecting the cerebellum, because each side of the cerebellum controls balance and coordination on the same side of the body. Of note is the connection between the two sides of the brain called the *corpus callosum,* which is important for exchanging information between the right and left hemispheres.

In Chapter 1 we described *how* strokes occur: because of problems in the blood supply to the brain. We also described the two basic kinds of stroke: ischemic and hemorrhagic. In this section we describe the effects of stroke according to *where* in the brain it occurs. For example, you might hear someone refer to a stroke's location using the side on which it occurred (such as a right-hemisphere stroke). There are four primary "blood-flow" areas of the brain that can be affected by stroke. These areas are delineated by the arterial supply to the region. The terms we use to describe strokes typically include the name of the blood vessel involved. The main types of strokes (based on anatomical location) are *anterior cerebral artery stroke, middle cerebral artery stroke, posterior cerebral artery stroke,* and *brain-stem stroke.* The arteries involved in a brain-stem stroke are usually either the vertebral arteries or the basilar arteries. Table 2.1 lists the most common deficits that someone might have if their stroke occurs in one of these four areas.

Some Strokes Can Be Reversed

One notion that many people believe and that is simply not true is that strokes are irreversible—that there is nothing someone can do to lessen the injury once it has begun. A stroke is an event that evolves over a period of time, and the amount of injury to the brain is strongly related to how long it takes to get the blood flowing through the blood vessel again. This fact has important implications for medical therapy, because restoring blood flow as quickly as possible generally helps salvage brain tissue. This translates into one simple concept that everyone should remember: *the damage from a stroke occasionally can be reversed and frequently can be reduced if the patient gets to the hospital right away.*

Table 2.1. Types of Strokes by Anatomical Location

Anterior Cerebral Artery Stroke

Weakness or paralysis on the side of the body opposite the side where the stroke occurred

Leg usually weaker than arm

Unusually strong grasp reflex that makes it difficult to let go of objects

Inability to perform tasks when asked but ability to perform them spontaneously at other times (*apraxia*)

Loss of sensation on the side of the body opposite where the stroke occurred

Repetitive thoughts and speech

Disorientation, confusion, and memory problems

Problems with bowel and bladder control

Middle Cerebral Artery Stroke

Weakness or paralysis on the side of the body opposite the side where the stroke occurred

Arm usually weaker than leg

Drooping of the lower half of the face and drooling

Blind spots or loss of vision

Difficulty producing and understanding language

Inability to differentiate between right and left

Posterior Cerebral Artery Stroke

Weakness and involuntary movements

Loss of coordination (*ataxia*)

Loss of sensation

Blind spots on the side opposite where the brain injury occurred

Inability to interpret what the eyes are seeing (*cortical blindness*)

Burning sensation in the extremities (*thalamic pain syndrome*)

Memory problems and difficulty reading

Brainstem Stroke

Weakness on one side of the body and poor coordination

Sensory loss

Swallowing problems

Slurred speech

Visual problems including double vision

Emotionally inappropriate behavior or speech

Dizziness (*vertigo*)

Headaches

Note: Strokes generally do not cause *all* of the problems listed for an area of the brain, but they often cause some combination of the difficulties listed in a category.

It's true that in the recent past nothing could be done to help someone who was having a stroke. In 1986, however, a lifesaving medication became available that is able to dissolve clots that cause stroke. (Though the medication became available in 1986, it wasn't until nearly a decade later that the research showing its benefit for stroke was compelling enough for doctors to use it regularly.) This drug, *tissue plasminogen activator,* or *tPA* for short, represents a major advance in helping someone live through a stroke with as little injury as possible. (Other "clot-busting" drugs are now being developed for treating strokes in the very early stages.) Because treatment with tPA is so important, you need to understand how it is used, when it is used, and when it should *not* be used.

A person who is having an *ischemic* stroke, which is the most common type of stroke, is a candidate to receive tPA. But there is a catch—you have to get to the hospital right away, because tPA must be given within three hours of the onset of stroke symptoms. If you think about the garden hose analogy, this makes sense. Flowers need water to survive, but they can live a short time, perhaps a few days at most, without water. Even if there is a kink in the hose and the flowers aren't getting the water they need, if you fix the kink before they die, they will survive. Even if they've begun to droop, they usually revive with proper nutrition. The same is true for your brain cells. Without blood they die but not immediately—it usually takes a few hours. So, if you are in the middle of having an ischemic stroke and you rush to the hospital where they can give you medicine to help dissolve the clot, then chances are the damage to your brain will be limited.

Although tPA (and other clot-busting medications) can be a wonder drug for someone suffering from an ischemic stroke, it can be dangerous and even deadly for some people, particularly for someone having a hemorrhagic stroke, because it can cause more hemorrhaging at the injury site in the brain. It is essential that this drug be administered by experienced doctors who can quickly assess whether someone is a good candidate for it. The primary method of assessment is an imaging study of the brain (such as CT or MRI), which can quickly show whether there is an area of blood pooled in the brain (signifying a hemorrhagic stroke) or whether the injury appears to be due to a lack of blood flow to a given area (signifying an ischemic stroke). *Note that it is always important to get medical care right away if you are having a stroke.*

What can you do to make sure that you or a family member is able to properly receive tPA or other lifesaving medications? You need to make sure that when there is an emergency, the sick person is taken to a major medical center or hospital where the staff is able to handle life-threatening emergencies with state-of-the-art medical interventions. Don't wait until an emergency situation to call the administration office of the hospital where you would go in the event of a stroke and ask these questions:

1. Are you able to obtain imaging studies such as CT and MRI scans twenty-four hours a day and seven days a week?
2. Is there a doctor on duty at all times who can read these studies?
3. Is your hospital staff trained to give tPA (or other lifesaving stroke medications), and is a doctor always available to give it?

The good news is that some strokes are *reversible,* and many others cause only limited injury if treated promptly. The bad news is that most people don't know the importance of early treatment and don't get to the hospital in time. Some experts estimate that 90 percent or more of the people who *could* receive tPA don't get it—usually because there is a delay in getting to the hospital. This happened to Sally.

When the right side of her body suddenly felt weak, Sally, who is the mother of eight children and is a calm woman not given to complaining, simply sat down in a chair and waited for her husband, Joe, to return home from the grocery store. When Joe walked in two hours later, he and Sally argued about whether she should go to the hospital (Joe wanted her to go, but Sally refused). Neither recognized that Sally was having a stroke. After thirty minutes of arguing, Sally's speech began to slur, and Joe finally called 9-1-1. The ambulance arrived and took Sally to the nearest medical center, which was twenty minutes from her home. The doctors and nurses started treating her right away and took a CT scan of her brain to identify what kind of stroke she was having. (Again, since tPA makes hemorrhagic strokes worse, it is essential that an imaging study of the brain confirms ischemic stroke before this medication is given.) By this time, Sally had had symptoms for nearly four hours. She did not receive tPA, and although she survived, she is unable to speak clearly and she walks with a brace and a cane. While tPA doesn't work in every instance, when it is given within three hours to someone who is having an ischemic stroke, it often will reduce tremendously the amount of brain damage that occurs. Sally never had the chance to find out if it would work because neither she nor her husband understood the symptoms of stroke or that at the first suspicion that someone is having a stroke, the most important thing to do is immediately call 9-1-1 to have them rushed to the hospital.

The Relationship between Stroke and Dementia

It is well established that stroke and dementia are related, and that multiple strokes can affect a person's personality, memory, and ability to process information. Strokes have the potential to make someone more impulsive and less aware of how their actions affect others. An extreme example of the effects of stroke is Joseph Stalin.

Stalin, a brilliant but ruthless and paranoid dictator under whose rule approximately 23 million Soviets perished, died at age 73 from a hemorrhagic stroke on March 5, 1953. His death ended a reign of terror unsurpassed to date in sheer numbers of victims. Whether he had multiple small strokes and how they affected him (for example, making him more paranoid of people—even his closest advisors and his wife, whose deaths came at his hand) is the subject of much debate. In an article titled "Stalin's Last Years: Delusions or Dementia?" Vladimir Hachinski writes: "Stalin suffered at least one stroke prior to his fatal intracerebral haemorrhage in 1953. Given his untreated hypertension and the autopsy report, it is probable that he had a number of lacunar strokes. These tend to predominate in the fronto-basal areas, and disconnect the circuits that underpin cognition and behaviour. The most plausible explanation of Stalin's late behaviour is the dimming of a superior intellect and the unleashing of a paranoid personality by a multi-infarct state."[1]

How Joseph Stalin was affected by his strokes will never truly be known. We use this example because it is fascinating to consider how Stalin's strokes affected his judgment, memory, and underlying paranoid personality—perhaps intensifying a long and brutal reign of terror. Even as a healthy young man, however, Stalin seemed evil and paranoid and appeared to have no remorse for his vicious actions. The strokes that he may have suffered are not what caused him to become a megalomaniac with a "persecution complex," but they may have increased his disregard for human life and the values that most of us embrace.[2] We include this example not to suggest that most strokes cause negative effects on personality, but to illustrate that a stroke, or series of strokes, can exacerbate already existing problems. We also include this example to show that strokes can happen to anyone, regardless of their wealth or access to medical care, and that strokes in world leaders have affected the course of history.

Because strokes sometimes cause memory problems and potentially may cause personality changes, many people who have had a stroke (or a series of small strokes or TIAs) and their families wonder whether the person with stroke is developing dementia. While stroke can cause problems with memory, these problems are not the same as Alzheimer's disease, which is the disease that most people think of when the word *dementia* is used. On the other hand, stroke *can* cause dementia because it interferes with blood flow to the brain.

Vascular dementia is typically caused by multiple strokes or mini-strokes (which is why it is sometimes called *multi-infarct dementia*) and is the second leading cause of dementia after Alzheimer's.

Dementia due to problems with blood flow to the brain (such as multiple TIAs or a stroke) is often subtle. Someone with this problem may have only minor or vague difficulties, such as trouble coming up with the right word. Memory and concentration can certainly be affected by stroke, as can mood and personality. In general, vascular dementia is characterized by stepwise (progressive) deterioration of intellectual ability. The good news is that this type of dementia, if caught early, may respond to treatments aimed at keeping a proper blood supply to the brain.

How You Can Quickly Recognize Stroke Symptoms

When former president Gerald Ford had a stroke in August 2000, he went to the emergency room of Philadelphia's well-respected Hahnemann University Hospital complaining of an earache and dizziness. The doctors who treated him diagnosed an inner ear infection and sent him off with antibiotics. Ford returned to the hospital shortly thereafter with more classic stroke symptoms of slurred speech, shaky balance, and weakness in his left arm. An article in *Time* magazine commented, "How could a team of specially trained physicians initially misdiagnose a stroke, especially in a former President, who, one assumes, always receives the very best medical care?"[3]

The answer is that even the best doctors can be fooled by stroke symptoms at times, because the symptoms often mimic a variety of other conditions.

Lorna's husband was "always ailing from something or other." He had a long list of medical problems, including high blood pressure and diabetes, and he relied on Lorna to do all of the household chores as well as assist him when necessary. One day Lorna's husband began to act a little odd. He was forgetful and withdrawn. Lorna took him to the emergency room, and he was admitted to the hospital. Lorna was exhausted from caring for him at home, and she hoped the doctors would be able to "tune him up." When she arrived at his room, however, she was shocked to see that he had been admitted to the psychiatric floor. Within twenty-four hours it became clear that her husband was not psychotic or severely depressed as the doctors had initially surmised, but rather that he had suffered a stroke. Lorna is still angry that the doctors "assumed the problem was psychological."

It is essential for everyone to learn to identify the symptoms of stroke so that they can act quickly to help themselves or others. The classic symptoms of stroke are:

• Sudden weakness or paralysis

The weakness or paralysis may appear as difficulty walking, trouble moving an arm or leg, or lurching to one side. Paralysis of the face can cause one side of the face to droop, along with drooling or slurred speech. Numbness in part of the body or dizziness may also be symptoms of stroke—particularly if they come on quickly.

• Sudden confusion or disorientation

Loved ones often don't act quickly when someone appears just a little confused or disoriented. Keep in mind that *any* change in someone's behavior that is sudden and out of character can signal the start of a stroke or TIA.

• Sudden problems with speech

Slurred speech, inability to talk at all, incoherent speech that doesn't make sense, difficulty finding the correct word to name an object—all are examples of speech problems. Any sudden new speech problem may indicate that someone is having a stroke.

• Sudden loss of vision in one or both eyes

This impaired vision can be a total or a partial loss of vision in one or both eyes. Sometimes people who are having a stroke will suddenly complain of double vision. Other times, an individual is not able to explain what is happening to his vision, but he just doesn't seem to recognize familiar objects or people. This difficulty can be due to problems with vision or comprehension, depending on which area of the brain is affected. Any new changes in vision that happen over a short period of time should be immediately investigated.

Of course, it's easy to know to dial 9-1-1 when someone appears to be terribly ill and is not able to walk or talk. But what happens when you or someone you love has subtle symptoms? Or if he or she demands to be left alone and won't go to the hospital? There are many times when loved ones aren't sure what to do. You are doing exactly the right thing by reading this book. You are educating yourself and you can help to educate your family members about what to look for and how to respond quickly when someone is having a stroke. Reading this book and sharing it with others is a critical first step in saving a life—maybe even your own.

Taking Control after a Stroke

In her book *Illness as Metaphor,* Susan Sontag writes, "Illness is the nightside of life, a more onerous citizenship. Everyone who is born holds dual citizenship, in the kingdom of the well and in the kingdom of the sick. Although we all prefer to use only the good passport, sooner or later each of us is obliged, at least for a spell, to identify ourselves as citizens of that other place."[4] Regardless of whether it was you or your loved one who suffered a stroke, you may have been surprised and even alarmed by the suddenness and unexpectedness of the event. You may be devastated by its physical consequences. Or, you may be grateful that you have minimal or no lasting effects, but at the same time worried and anxious as you wait to see if it will happen again—possibly with far more serious consequences. Stroke is a sudden and sometimes catastrophic illness that leaves in its wake tremendous fear and anxiety.

After a stroke, many people feel powerless and nervous about the future—a very normal reaction. There are ways to deal with this post-stroke anxiousness. The best antidote to feeling out of control and on pins and needles is to take action to prevent another stroke. There are good ways to do just that. For example, many people believe that strokes are entirely random, unpredictable, and meteoric events. This is not true. Research shows that there are ways to predict who is at risk for having a stroke and who is at risk for having a recurrent stroke. People often ignore the early warning signals that devastating and even deadly strokes can give. But if your worst fears come true and you or your loved one has another stroke, there are steps you can take to limit the damage and permanent injury.

We explore all of these issues in the chapters that follow.

Chapter 3

• •

Tests Your Doctor May Order

It often seems that modern doctors are obsessed with tests. CT scans, MRIs, Holter monitors, and blood tests galore await many stroke survivors. Yet these tests are ordered for a very important reason: to identify what caused your stroke and to determine the best way to prevent another stroke from occurring. In this chapter we discuss many of the most common tests performed for stroke survivors and explain how the studies are done, what the risks are (if any), and what information they provide. Understanding these tests may help you accept the need for them and avoid the misperception that the testing process is pointless. The medical care of a stroke patient must be individualized, however, so while a chapter such as this provides a basis for understanding what tests you or your loved one *might* undergo, we are not attempting to suggest that these are all tests you *should* have done. Our explanations are not a substitute for the explanations of your doctor.

The tests you need to have done will depend on your current situation, what has been done for you in the past, and what future problems the doctors are concerned about. It is important to do some studies quickly. If your doctor suggests that a test needs to be done right away, there is probably a good reason, and he should be able to tell you that reason. If your doctor is not available to discuss it with you, try to find out as much as possible about the study but don't delay it. Any delay may have serious implications for the validity of the evaluation or the usefulness of the test results. The bottom line is this: *during the first few hours and days after a stroke, some tests likely will need to be done quickly in order to make the best decisions for care and maybe even to save someone's life. We encourage patients and families to be as informed as possible but not to delay diagnostic testing and treatment.*

The tests doctors order to assess stroke patients can be broken down into several categories (see Table 3.1). The first and often most important category contains brain imaging studies. Since a stroke by definition is an

Table 3.1. **Tests Doctors Frequently Order to Diagnose and Assess Stroke**

Studies That Image the Brain
Computerized tomography (CT)
Magnetic resonance imaging (MRI)

Studies That Provide Information on Blood Flow
Blood pressure monitoring
Carotid artery ultrasound/Doppler
Magnetic resonance angiogram
Computerized tomography angiography
Angiography

Studies That Test the Heart
Electrocardiogram (EKG)
Holter monitor
Echocardiogram

Studies of the Blood
Blood glucose level
Complete blood count (CBC), which includes hemoglobin level
Lipid profile (cholesterol)
Homocysteine level
C-reactive protein
Hypercoagulable test

injury to the brain, it makes sense that it is incredibly helpful to have some type of image, or picture, of the brain. A *computerized tomography scan* is a brain imaging study that is very commonly done when someone has a stroke. Computerized tomography, or CT, is sometimes called a "CAT" scan but is more properly pronounced "see-tea." This study may reveal a number of things, including where the stroke occurred in the brain, how extensive it is, and whether it is an ischemic or hemorrhagic type of stroke.

The second category of tests is imaging tests of the blood vessels. These tests are extremely important too, because the blood vessels are often the *cause* of a stroke. One test that images the blood vessels is the *carotid artery ultrasound* (an ultrasound of the neck arteries). This study can help determine whether there is a significant narrowing of the carotid arteries in the neck. Arteries that are very narrow may not allow the blood to sufficiently pass through them, which can lead to a stroke.

A third category of tests look at heart function. An *echocardiogram* (sometimes called an "echo"), for example, is an ultrasound that can show many of the heart structures as they operate. An echocardiogram can reveal whether there is a blood clot sitting in the heart. A blood clot in the heart can break off and become an *embolus* (or loose clot) that travels to the brain. In the brain it may get stuck in a smaller blood vessel and shut off the blood supply in that vessel. Using the garden hose analogy from Chapter 1, if the hose starts out big but narrows as it goes along, then a marble could easily pass through the first part of the hose but might get stuck later on where the hose circumference is much smaller. This is how it works in the body, too. A blood clot doesn't usually cause problems unless it gets stuck somewhere and begins to impede the flow of blood to vital organs like the brain.

A fourth category is blood tests. Many types of blood tests can be done, and which ones are recommended will depend on a variety of factors. For example, it would be important to check someone's blood sugar level if diabetes were suspected (strokes occur more commonly in people with diabetes). Oxygen is essential for all of our organs, so checking the hemoglobin level (one way to measure blood levels, which gives indirect information about oxygen) is important. These are just a couple of examples of useful blood tests.

Other tests (a spinal tap, for example) may also be necessary. If you or someone you love is scheduled for a test, feel free to ask the doctor why it was ordered, what the study is like, how it will help, whether there are any potential side effects or complications of having it done, and when you will find out the results.

All stroke patients also have their vital signs (blood pressure, heart rate, temperature, and respiratory rate) closely monitored in the hospital. These signs really are "vital" to check and to keep within an appropriate range. Any abnormalities may signify problems or potential problems. An increased respiratory rate may be due to undetected pneumonia (one possible early post-stroke complication). Elevated blood pressure that is not controlled may lead to a second stroke. For these and other reasons, vital signs are usually vigorously monitored in the hospital (to the point of having someone wake you up in the middle of the night to measure them). Researchers have found that minimizing fever and (in people with diabetes) controlling elevated blood sugars can help reduce the negative impact of a stroke.

We will now get to the heart of this chapter, the tests themselves. Table 3.1 gives a quick overview of the tests we will discuss in this chapter. Virtually all of these studies (with the exception of angiograms) are considered *noninvasive*; that is, they are done without requiring any procedures that physically penetrate or "invade" the body. Noninvasive tests are usually easier to conduct and less time-consuming than invasive studies, and generally involve a low level of risk. Doctors typically perform noninvasive tests first. Only when the noninvasive tests do not provide enough information will doctors recommend more invasive studies to complete the evaluation.

Brain Imaging Tests

Imaging tests have revolutionized the way we practice medicine. In the nineteenth century, the concept of physical examination became accepted in medicine and doctors became extremely skilled at palpating (touching) with their hands, observing with their eyes, and auscultating (listening) with their ears. In general, the only options for diagnosing medical problems inside the human body were the physical exam and, in some cases, exploratory surgery. Few tests were available during most of the 1800s, and certainly no imaging studies had yet been invented. This would change as the century came to a close. In 1895, the physicist Wilhelm Roentgen discovered that by passing a high voltage through a vacuum tube he could generate electromagnetic waves capable of penetrating the human body. This process would then leave an imprint on a photographic plate. These were the first x-rays, initially called Roentgengrams, and in the twentieth century they dramatically changed how medicine was practiced. Now when a doctor listened with his stethoscope to someone's chest, if he heard dullness in a certain region, he could order an x-ray and see whether there was an infection or a tumor. X-rays became the primary tool used by orthopedists to diagnose and treat fractures and other injuries. So popular and important was this discovery that by the 1950s almost half of American general practitioners had an x-ray machine in their offices.

Today doctors still rely on physical examination, but imaging studies often supersede all other methods of reaching a diagnosis. This is certainly true in diagnosing stroke, where imaging studies are of utmost importance in determining where the stroke occurred and whether it is of the ischemic or hemorrhagic variety.

CT Scans

CT (computerized tomography) scans were a major advance in *visual diagnostics*, the growing field of imaging parts of the body in order to see them and make a diagnosis. Godfrey Newbold Hounsfield, a British electri-

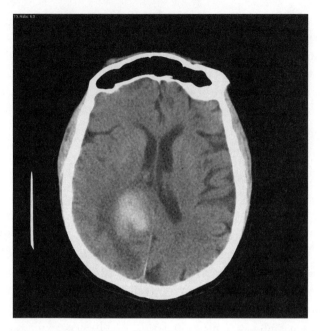

Figure 3.1. Computerized tomography (CT) scan showing a hemorrhagic stroke. The bleeding appears lighter than the surrounding brain tissue.

cal engineer, developed a system in the 1970s in which x-ray beams could be resolved with computer assistance to produce a cross-sectional picture of the human body. The CT scan was a major breakthrough in our ability to diagnose diseases noninvasively (without such measures as exploratory surgery). For this discovery, Hounsfield won the Nobel Prize for medicine in 1979. He shared this prize with his colleague Allan M. Cormack, a physicist who established the mathematical principles behind the CT scan. Today, this test remains widely available and useful for evaluating stroke. CT scans use x-rays, just like a standard chest or dental x-ray, but the x-rays are obtained using a computerized scanner that assembles a much more detailed image than could be obtained using a regular x-ray machine. These images are like cross-sectional slices of the body, and they show the body (or brain) as a series of pictures from bottom to top.

With modern CT machines, scans can be obtained very quickly and are relatively easily interpreted. They are often used in hospital emergency departments for this reason. CT scans can clearly show whether a stroke is due to bleeding within the brain (a cerebral hemorrhage; Figure 3.1), or due to a blockage in an artery (an infarct; Figure 3.2). Since treatment for

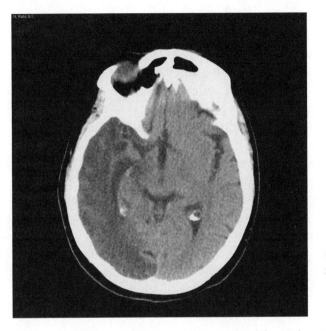

Figure 3.2. CT scan showing an ischemic stroke. The area of the stroke appears darker than the surrounding brain tissue.

these two conditions is dramatically different (in fact, treatments may literally be the opposite for the two types of stroke), CT scans are very helpful when decisions need to be made quickly.

CT scans are usually very safe and easily tolerated. The amount of radiation exposure is relatively low and is not a health risk for most people. Pregnant women should alert their physician, however, since even small amounts of radiation may be harmful to an unborn child. CT scans do not interact with any medical equipment (such as pacemakers), so almost anyone can safely have a CT scan performed. Scanners are a little confining and occasionally someone experiences claustrophobia, but much less frequently than with the more confining MRI scanners. The machine is donut shaped, and you lie on a table. You are not enclosed in the scanner the way you are for an MRI. The CT scan images are obtained quickly (within a matter of minutes), so claustrophobia is not a common problem.

Sometimes a medication known as *intravenous contrast* (or IV contrast) is administered before or during a CT scan. This medication, which acts as a dye, makes it easier to distinguish between certain structures in the brain, providing the physician with additional information. IV contrast is most useful when performing a CT angiogram (we describe this test later in the chapter), or when a tumor, infection, or other non-stroke diagnosis is being considered. Occasionally people will have allergic reactions to the IV contrast.

In addition to determining whether a stroke is due to bleeding or to a blood vessel blockage, CT scans can show physicians where the stroke is and how large it is. This provides clues as to the cause of the stroke and helps the doctor determine the best treatment for prevention of another stroke. For example, a large stroke in the area of the brain that receives its blood from the left carotid artery suggests that there might be a blockage in this artery. Further tests may be needed to make a final diagnosis, but the CT scan points the doctor in the right direction. Occasionally, a bright spot (technically known as a "high intensity signal") is seen within one of the major blood vessels in the brain on a CT scan. This spot may represent the actual blood clot blocking the blood vessel, since blood clots are brighter on CT scans than the blood and blood vessel. This information, too, is useful for the physician, and may help him select the best treatment for the current stroke and for prevention of a future stroke.

MRI Scans

Magnetic resonance imaging (MRI) uses powerful magnets and radio waves to obtain images of the brain (Figure 3.3). Unlike CT scans, MRIs do not require the use of radiation. They are generally considered harmless to the patient. MRIs take longer than CT scans and may last forty-five minutes in some cases, as compared with several minutes for a CT scan. This is a disadvantage in emergency situations, such as when a person comes to the emergency room with symptoms of a stroke and a decision needs to be made immediately whether or not to use a clot-dissolving medication. For this reason, even in hospitals well equipped with MRI scanners, CT scans are usually the first test done in the emergency room for suspected stroke.

MRIs provide a wealth of information that CT cannot provide, however, including more detailed images that are able to give information about the "age" of a stroke (how long ago it occurred), and identify smaller strokes and even brain tissue affected by the stroke but not necessarily permanently damaged. Newer MRI scanners are able to collect certain images more quickly than older models and are being used in some hospitals in place of or in addition to CT scans in emergency situations.

Still, the downside of MRI scans is that they can take a long time and are difficult for some people to tolerate. The patient is placed inside of a long, narrow tube for the duration of the test. This is confining, and it is often

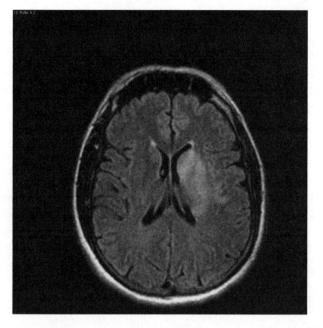

Figure 3.3. Magnetic resonance imaging (MRI) showing a stroke. On this type of MRI image, the stroke appears lighter than the surrounding brain tissue.

hard even for people who are not terribly claustrophobic to tolerate being motionless inside of the scanner for the duration of the test. Claustrophobia is a fairly common problem and may affect some people who didn't realize that they were claustrophobic before the scan. If you are going to have an MRI and feel as though you may not tolerate it, ask your doctor to prescribe a medication such as diazepam (Valium) to help alleviate anxiety. Wearing a mask over your eyes can help too, because you cannot see how confining the space is. At the very least, close your eyes before you enter the tube and don't open them until you get out. MRI scanners make loud "knocking" noises during the scan. Earplugs are generally provided to help block out the noises, but the sound can be another anxiety-provoking aspect of these scans.

Almost anyone can undergo a CT scan (pregnant women being one important exception). MRI, however, can be a problem for anyone with metal in his body, because the powerful magnets used for MRI can cause metal within the body to shift position and cause damage. There is a long list of metal items that may be found in people, not all of which would come to mind for the average person. These include metal shrapnel from war injuries, metal fragments from people who grind metals for a living (especially since these can get into the eye), and various medical implants such as insulin pumps and orthopedic hardware. Many medical device manufacturers have deliberately created devices that use metals that are not affected by MRI scans and do not pose any risk. The person who schedules your MRI should be able to tell you whether any metal in your body may be problematic. If there is any question of a reaction, the radiologist can offer advice. If you have any possible complicating factors, you should not have an MRI.

Vascular Tests

The humoral theory of medicine developed by the ancient Greeks placed great importance on our bodies' fluids. They believed there were four main fluids, or *humors*: black bile, yellow bile, phlegm, and blood. The underlying theory was that these four humors needed to be in balance and that illness occurred when there was imbalance. Although this theory has long since been discarded, it cannot be disputed that illness occurs when there is a problem with our blood supply. Stroke is a prime example of how important blood is for a properly functioning body. When the blood supply to the brain is disrupted, either from a blockage or from a hemorrhage, a stroke occurs. It is probably not surprising, then, that some of the most important tests we give stroke survivors investigate blood flows through the vessels from the heart to the brain. In the next section we describe the tests commonly used to visualize the arteries and the flow of blood through them.

Blood Pressure Monitoring

Elevated blood pressure is a well known and extremely common cause of stroke. In most cases, simply checking your blood pressure at home and in the doctor's office can determine whether you have high blood pressure. In some cases, however, blood pressure seems to "bounce around," with fluctuating readings that may be different at the physician's office than at home. Some people get nervous when a doctor or nurse takes their blood pressure, and as a consequence their pressure suddenly becomes elevated—a phenomenon known as "white coat" hypertension (because of the white coats worn by health care workers). One way to sort out fluctuating blood pressure readings is to use a blood pressure monitor that is worn throughout the day, so blood pressure can be checked and recorded during a person's usual daytime activities. Known as *ambulatory blood pressure monitoring*, this technique may clarify whether someone needs treatment for elevated blood pressure.

Carotid Noninvasive Tests and Transcranial Dopplers

These tests, often known as *carotid duplex ultrasound exams,* use specialized ultrasound equipment to evaluate blood flow and produce images of arteries within the neck and head. They use very high frequency sound waves (beyond humans' ability to hear), and bounce these sound waves off the body part that is being examined. Like MRI, these tests do not involve any radiation and are considered harmless, even during pregnancy. Duplex ultrasonography can estimate the velocity of blood flowing through an artery as well as the amount of blockage in an artery. Most often it is used to evaluate the large carotid arteries in the neck, but it can also be used to look at the smaller vertebral arteries located at the base of the head in the back of the neck, and even the blood flow in arteries within the head (*transcranial doppler* studies). With this study, a doctor can visualize the opening of the arteries to estimate the amount of cholesterol plaque and determine how much of the artery is blocked by the plaque. This amount is referred to as the percentage of *occlusion* (blockage) for the artery. For the carotids, the percentage of occlusion dictates treatment options. Surgery may be appropriate if the blockage is severe. (Details of surgical treatment options are provided in Chapter 14.)

The carotid duplex ultrasound study is a painless test that requires no preparation on the part of the patient and takes less than an hour to complete. It is performed in a dark room by an *ultrasonographer* (technician trained in ultrasound), radiologist, or neurologist. First the person performing the test exposes the patient's neck area and applies a gel to it. Gel is also applied to the *transducer* (also known as a probe), a small, hand-held instrument that both generates the sound waves and picks them up after they "bounce" off structures within the body. The person performing the test gently moves this small hand-held device over the patient's neck and the base of her head. High frequency sound waves are sent into the neck and head and bounce off the blood vessel walls as well as the blood cells traveling inside arteries and veins. The echoes of the sound waves are transformed by a computer into pictures of arteries and veins that can be seen on the computer screen, as well as information on how fast the blood is flowing through the blood vessels.

MRI and CT Angiograms

Both CT and MRI scanners can be used to obtain images of blood vessels, as well as the body and brain. Obtaining images of the vessels generally requires the injection of a material into the bloodstream to help the

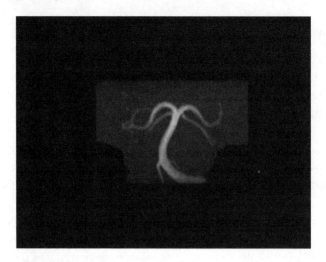

Figure 3.4. MRA of the normal vertebrobasilar arteries of the brain.

blood "stand out" on these images. These injectable materials, known as intravenous contrast (or IV contrast) materials, are usually well tolerated, though allergic reactions can occur. In a small number of people, generally those with diabetes or kidney problems, contrast can adversely affect kidney function. Use of newer, low-risk contrast materials and pretreatment medication can reduce the risk of this complication.

These images show the blood flowing within the blood vessel rather than the walls of the blood vessel tube (Figure 3.4), so the images provide information needed by physicians to help determine the cause of a stroke and devise an appropriate prevention strategy. The actual scans produced by CT and MRI angiography are similar in nature to regular CTs and MRIs.

Angiograms

Angiograms are x-rays of the blood vessels of the head and neck. This test is performed by threading a thin flexible tube (known as a catheter) through the blood vessels and then injecting contrast material that shows up on x-rays to outline the inside of the blood vessel (Figure 3.5). The catheter usually is threaded through a blood vessel in the groin or the arm and into the neck by a radiologist who is an expert in this type of procedure. Angiograms give the most detailed and precise pictures of the blood vessels in the head and neck, but they are also the most risky of the procedures described in this chapter. Because the catheter is threaded through the blood vessels, it can accidentally dislodge a clot or damage a blood vessel wall and cause a

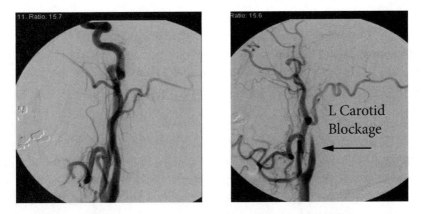

Figure 3.5. Angiograms of the carotid artery. (A) *The normal right carotid artery.* (B) *Tapering of the left internal carotid artery, with a complete blockage due to a carotid artery dissection.*

stroke. The risk for this occurring is generally estimated at about 1 in 1,000 cases. The contrast material can also cause allergic reactions or kidney damage (though this damage is usually temporary). As noted in the discussion of CT angiography, there are now ways to reduce, though not eliminate, the risk of the kidney complications from contrast.

Because of the highly detailed pictures that angiograms provide, they are often used before a possible operation to confirm that surgery is the appropriate treatment for a narrowed blood vessel and to help the surgeon visualize exactly where the problem lies.

Tests of the Heart

Though we have known for centuries that the heart is a critical organ, tests of the heart have only been developed over the past two hundred years or so. In September of 1816, a buxom young woman went to a French physician, René Laennec, who was unmarried at the time. Convinced that the woman had heart problems, the doctor fretted over how he would listen to her heart. The morals of the day prevented him from evaluating her heartbeat the way he would a man's, by simply putting his ear to the patient's chest. Also, because she had an ample bosom, he knew that even if he put his ear to her chest it would be difficult to hear her heart. Doctor Laennec, who was also a musician, decided to roll a piece of paper into a tube, like a flute. He placed one end of the tube on her chest and the other end at his ear. This was the first stethoscope.

In 1903, the Dutch physiologist Willem Einthoven published details of the first electrocardiograph, which recorded electrical activity from the heart. Unlike the x-ray, it took many years for what we now commonly call an electrocardiogram (also known as an EKG or ECG) to become popular in medical diagnostics. James Mackenzie, a brilliant physician who pioneered the use of the polygraph for recording the pulse and its relationship to heart disease, did not include details of how to use an EKG in his popular 1908 medical textbook, *Diseases of the Heart,* even though these details were first published five years earlier. It took many years before doctors and scientists mastered EKG technology. Today, we consider this test extremely important in detecting such electrical problems with the heart as atrial fibrillation, which can lead to stroke.

Electrocardiogram (EKG)

An EKG is done using small skin sensors, and it takes only a minute to obtain results. This study shows a tracing of the heart's electrical activity rather than an image of the body such as a CT or MRI would show. It is a completely noninvasive and safe test, though it provides only a snapshot of the heart's electrical activity. While this snapshot can often identify an abnormal heart rhythm that may have led to a stroke, it can also miss abnormal heart rhythms that come and go. If there are significant concerns about whether an abnormal heart rhythm is the cause of a stroke, then a Holter monitor is generally required. It is also important to realize that EKG and Holter monitor testing only provide information about the electrical activity of the heart. Some causes of stroke that originate from the heart do not show up on this type of study.

Holter Monitor

A *Holter monitor* is a device that is worn for twenty-four hours (or sometimes longer) in order to record the electrical activity of the heart, like a prolonged EKG. Portable recorders are used to collect data that is analyzed after completion of the recording. The equipment is similar in size to a cell phone and has sticky skin sensors that attach to the chest. The patient also records any possible heart-related symptoms, such as fluttering in the chest, chest pain, or shortness of breath, in a written log. Holter monitors are generally good at identifying intermittent heart rhythm problems, but some people have such occasional abnormal rhythms that the problems may be missed on a twenty-hour Holter monitor. If your doctor has a particular concern that this may be the case, she may ask you to use a specialized "event monitor" at home over an extended period of time to capture a recording of an infrequent heart rhythm problem.

Echocardiogram

An echocardiogram, sometimes referred to as an "echo" for short, consists of images of the heart obtained using *ultrasound* (very high-pitched sound waves which are beyond human hearing). Echocardiograms are usually obtained by a technician using a hand-held ultrasound probe in a safe, non-painful, and relatively quick process.

These images are used to form a video of the heart's functioning, which allows the physician to learn about the heart's size, how well its chambers are emptying themselves, and whether its valves are functioning normally. Echocardiograms can also be used to test for abnormal openings between the two sides of the heart (see the discussion of patent foramen ovale in Chapter 9 for more information). Because it can sometimes reveal blood clots within the heart, this test may be decisive in determining the cause of a stroke and helping to identify the best treatment to prevent another stroke.

Blood Tests

The most common surgical procedure during the 1800s was bloodletting, also called *venesection* or *phlebotomy,* and often performed at the patient's request. The usual procedure involved a surgeon tying a bandage around a patient's arm in order to engorge the veins and then slicing the exposed vein with a lancet. This process was popularly called "breathing a vein." Bloodletting was supported by the beliefs of that time, which included the belief that many diseases were caused by a buildup of blood. (Some experts believe that George Washington's death, on December 13, 1799, was caused by bloodletting during his final illness.)

Fortunately, today we have discarded the practice of bloodletting. We have not discarded the idea that obtaining blood is extremely useful, however. We now have many diagnostic tests that can be performed on a sample of blood. When someone has had a stroke, the following tests are often quite helpful.

Cholesterol and Lipid Profile

The human body contains a number of fats and related substances that are critical to normal functioning. Everyone needs some cholesterol and triglycerides, for example. In some individuals, however, due to a combination of factors including genes, poor diet, and physical inactivity, these materials may reach dangerous levels in the blood and contribute to the risk of stroke.

Blood is normally drawn for tests for cholesterol and other fatty substances in the blood (*lipids*) in the morning, before breakfast. A number of lipid tests (typically total cholesterol, LDL and HDL cholesterol, and triglycerides) are usually obtained at the same time and together are known as a *lipid profile*. Having even a cup of coffee in the morning before having the blood drawn for this test can temporarily affect the blood levels and lead to misinterpretation of the results. This blood test poses no risks except for those who have a fear of needles. (Consider asking the phlebotomist—the person who draws the blood—to use a "butterfly," a device that puts the collection tubes far away from the vein and allows for a more gentle insertion of the needle.)

There are several different components of cholesterol, some of which are actually good for you and help prevent stroke or heart disease. The "bad" cholesterol is known as LDL cholesterol (low density lipoprotein), and the higher the level of LDL, the higher the risk of stroke and heart disease. Generally speaking, a level of 130 or higher may be cause for concern. On the other hand, HDL cholesterol (high density lipoprotein) protects against stroke and heart disease. The higher the HDL level, the better off you are. HDL levels between 40 and 60 are generally considered normal. Higher levels of HDL help protect against blood vessel blockage, whereas levels below 40 are associated with an increased risk of blockage. Another way of interpreting cholesterol values is to use the ratio of total cholesterol divided by HDL. The higher this ratio, the higher the risk of developing heart disease or stroke. A ratio above 5 or 6 is generally considered elevated and may require treatment with lifestyle changes and medication.

Triglycerides are another fatty material found in the blood, though they aren't as important a risk factor for heart disease and stroke. High triglyceride levels are undesirable—there is no "good" triglyceride comparable to HDL cholesterol (these issues are discussed in greater detail in Chapter 15).

Again, eating can temporarily affect the results of these tests. Illness and malnutrition can also reduce LDL cholesterol and triglycerides, so someone who has a severe stroke and spends several weeks in the hospital might have a low cholesterol level when checked immediately after discharge. This test should be performed again once someone has had some time to resume their usual diet and activity level, since this reading will be a more accurate indicator of possible future risks and the need for treatment.

Homocysteine

Checking *homocysteine* levels is a relatively new concept in stroke prevention. Homocysteine is a chemical found in the blood that is formed by the body naturally. High levels of homocysteine have been found in some people who have had a stroke. Whether lowering homocysteine reduces the risk of stroke remains uncertain. Homocysteine can be lowered by taking certain vitamins, including folate, pyridoxine, and vitamin B_{12}. For this reason, levels of folate and B_{12} are often checked if homocysteine levels are high. The role of vitamin levels and homocysteine levels in determining treatment for stroke prevention remains unclear at present.

C-Reactive Protein

C-reactive protein (*CRP*) is normally found in the body in small amounts and is used by doctors as an indicator of inflammation within the body. While scientists are still working to understand the role of inflammation and learn how to use CRP to direct treatment, some physicians now check CRP levels in patients who have had a stroke as another tool to understand their risk of having another stroke. Higher levels of CRP indicate a somewhat higher risk of stroke. No specific treatment to lower CRP is available at this time, and this information is mostly used to help physicians make decisions about treating other risk factors for stroke that may respond to treatment. For example, if someone has a borderline abnormal lipid profile but has a high CRP level, the physician might decide to prescribe medications to lower the cholesterol level.

Hypercoagulable Tests

A number of chemicals normally present in the blood are important for forming blood clots and preventing bleeding in normal people. Due to genetics, some people may have higher levels of certain blood clotting factors (substances in the blood that make it more or less likely to form clots), or lower levels of other factors that normally help "balance" the clotting system by preventing blood clots. Some blood tests can determine if blood clotting factors are out of balance, and can help determine if medication to reduce blood clotting, such as warfarin (Coumadin), is needed.

Sometimes the body forms antibodies that attack healthy components of the body—a condition known as an autoimmune disorder. Certain abnormal antibodies can stimulate the blood to form blood clots and lead to stroke. These antibodies can be detected by appropriate blood tests, and treatment can be given to help reduce the risk of abnormal blood clots. As with other blood tests, there is practically no risk to having these studies performed. These tests are not affected by diet or time of day, and can be obtained at any time.

Testing Strategies

Doctors vary in their approach to testing after stroke, but they typically follow a similar overall strategy. The goal is always the same: to determine the cause of the stroke, allowing the physician to prescribe the most effective treatments to limit damage from the stroke and prevent a future stroke.

Once someone has been tentatively diagnosed with a stroke based on her medical history, symptoms, and examination, her doctor orders an initial battery of basic tests. These tests search for the most common causes of stroke and determine initial treatment. In most cases, this initial battery of tests will include a CT scan, an EKG, and some basic blood tests to exclude other medical conditions that might mimic a stroke (such as a very low blood sugar in someone who takes insulin).

In some cases, these initial studies may be the only tests required to determine the cause of the stroke; in other cases, further evaluations may be necessary. For example, if a person with a history of severe, poorly controlled high blood pressure is found to have a hemorrhage deep within the brain, a diagnosis of a hypertensive hemorrhage can generally be made using these tests, without further investigation. For other people, the initial tests will need to be supplemented promptly by more tests to fully determine the cause of the stroke. For example, if a CT scan reveals that the likely culprit is a blocked left carotid artery, the doctor will typically order a second test (perhaps a carotid ultrasound or a magnetic resonance angiogram) to further evaluate the carotid arteries. The treating physician will then be able to make recommendations about the most appropriate course of action, which in this case might be surgery to remove a partial blockage.

In some patients, the diagnosis remains elusive, and multiple tests are required. A common example of this is a stroke that occurs suddenly and blocks one of the major arteries to the brain (most usually the middle cerebral artery). This type of stroke appears to be due to an embolism (a blood clot traveling from another part of the body to block the blood vessel), but the source of the embolism may not be obvious. Testing might involve a Holter monitor to exclude atrial fibrillation (an abnormal heart rhythm) and an echocardiogram to examine the heart for any valve abnormalities, enlarged heart chambers, or *patent foramen ovale* (a small hole in the heart).

Despite the best efforts of doctors, sometimes no explanation for a stroke can be found. These strokes are known as *cryptogenic*—that is, the cause of the stroke is hidden. The most common treatment to try and prevent these strokes is aspirin or Plavix, although other treatments are sometimes used.

Effective stroke prevention begins with an accurate diagnosis. A targeted and thorough evaluation is the key element in arriving at this diagnosis. Ask your doctor to explain to you the purpose of each test you are undergoing and how it will help her determine the cause of your stroke and the best preventive treatment. With this information in hand you can take charge of your stroke prevention program and reduce your risk of another stroke.

Part II

STROKE RECOVERY

• •

Chapter 4

Minimizing Early Post-Stroke Disability and Complications

Helen Keller once noted that "although the world is full of suffering, it is full also of overcoming it." Of course, if you have had a stroke, the less you have to overcome, the better. It is important to avoid or to minimize early post-stroke complications whenever possible. The good news is that stroke care is getting better all the time. Health care providers are learning more about what stroke patients need from the start and throughout their care. Many hospitals have established specialized stroke teams or units to provide stroke care in an efficient and coordinated manner, in an effort to minimize the impact of stroke.

By definition, the symptoms of a stroke occur *suddenly* and usually without warning. Your life is irrevocably altered in an instant. The suddenness of the event can catapult you into a position in which you know very little about what is happening and what to expect, even if you are an intelligent and well-informed person. That is why we are including this chapter in *Life After Stroke.* We want you to understand what kind of medical care you can expect, how to try to avoid unnecessary complications, and what to do if they occur.

The Worst Comes First

Unless the person has major medical complications from stroke (which often, but not always, can be avoided with proper care), the first few days or even weeks after someone has a stroke are usually the worst. One of the positive things about the aftermath of stroke is that most people who survive the initial few days can expect some improvement in their condition over a period of weeks to months. If you or a member of your family has just had a stroke, it can be encouraging to know that the next few weeks and months will probably bring some recovery.

Even if there is good news on the way, you must deal with whatever is happening *now*, on this particular day. You live in the present, not the future. If you or someone you love has recently had a stroke, it is natural for you to experience loss and to grieve. In her book *When Life Becomes Precious*, Elise NeeDell Babcock encourages us to grieve when we experience a negative change in our health status. She writes, "From the moment this disease storms in and turns your world upside down, you experience losses. You experience some losses right away and others later on, as the illness progresses. . . . Grief is the natural way to respond to loss. Suppressing or denying grief is not only abnormal, it will have a detrimental effect on your well-being."[1]

You must also deal with a certain amount of uncertainty. This perhaps may be the hardest part of the first few days and weeks. After a stroke, uncertainty looms over us, challenging our long-held beliefs about the paths our lives will take. It destroys our dreams and forces us to create new ones at a time when we are most vulnerable. The famous mythologist Joseph Campbell wrote, "We must be willing to get rid of the life we have planned, so as to have the life that is waiting for us." But, in the first few days and weeks after a stroke, most people are not willing or able to think about a new life. Most will need time to come to grips with the fact that their old life has been irrevocably altered.

Television personality and award-winning author Betty Rollin wrote that during the initial phases after being diagnosed with breast cancer all she could do was "bear it." She wrote in her memoir *First, You Cry*: "You bear it, because not to bear is to crack or to kill yourself. One can't choose to crack—you do or you don't—so that is not an alternative. To kill yourself is, but who would be crazy enough to do that?"[2] During the first few awful days and weeks after a stroke, the most you can really expect of yourself and your loved ones is to bear it. There will be time later to develop the coping skills you all will need for the rest of this journey.

For some individuals, the effects of a stroke will resolve very quickly and completely, requiring minimal coping skills. This is obviously a best-case scenario—one that we wish for all of our patients. Even if you or your loved one don't experience dramatic improvement in the first few days or weeks, keep in mind that recovery can take months or even a year or more. No matter how long the recovery process takes, the first few days can be terribly frightening as you struggle to deal with an event that you neither planned nor expected.

If your stroke symptoms do improve rapidly, remember that there is still the need to protect against *another* stroke. In *The Alchemy of Illness*, Kat Duff, who has chronic fatigue syndrome, writes, "Memories of illness fade quickly under the glare and hubris of health, dropping into the background of life, only to rise to the forefront with the onset of yet another illness."[3] While we want everyone to recover as fully and optimally as possible after a stroke, we also want people to staunchly defend against having a second stroke. This defense will begin almost immediately after the first stroke occurs as the medical team works to discover what caused the initial stroke and how they can help to prevent a recurrence. There are things that stroke survivors can do to protect themselves, as well, but the acute phase of a stroke, while someone is in the hospital, is not the time to institute lifestyle changes that may reduce the future risk of stroke—that will come later, after discharge from the hospital.

Problems Directly Related to Stroke

The treatment of stroke depends on what problems someone is experiencing. Since strokes can occur in different parts of the brain, they may cause a variety of injuries that can affect how the body functions. Some of the more common problems include paralysis on one side of the body, difficulty with talking and swallowing, urinary and sometimes bowel incontinence, sexual dysfunction, problems with memory and concentration, intellectual deficits, visual disturbances, and anxiety and depression. Perhaps the most classic and obvious stroke-related problems are leg or arm paralysis or weakness and difficulty with speaking. The rehabilitation team often spends the most time and attention addressing these issues because they are so important to people's quality of life.

We assume that your doctors and therapists will discuss paralysis (especially as it relates to mobility) and speech (including both understanding and speaking words) in depth with you and your family. We will not spend an extensive amount of time on these issues. Rather, we will mention the "usual" post-stroke complications here and then move on to other topics such as early post-stroke problems that survivors and family members may help to prevent. In Chapter 6 we also discuss a number of stroke-related medical and social issues that you may not yet have discussed with your doctor. Nevertheless, no stroke book would be complete without mentioning the most important stroke-related consequences that may occur. We

Table 4.1. **Problems That May Occur after a Stroke**

Right-Brain Strokes
Numbness or weakness on left side
Difficulty performing daily tasks
Perception problems
Neglect of left side
Excessive talking
Visual memory problems
Short attention span
Poor judgment
Time disorientation
Loss of left visual field
Confusion between left and right
Impaired abstract thinking
Emotional lability—extreme highs and lows of mood
Lethargy
Impulsiveness

Left-Brain Strokes
Numbness or weakness on right side
Partial or complete loss of speaking or understanding language
Impaired thought processing, including decreased problem-solving ability,
    poor judgment, and an inability to see errors
Lack of insight
Loss of right visual field
Decreased memory
Depression

Brainstem Strokes
Ataxia (lack of muscular coordination)
Impaired swallowing
Coma or low-level consciousness
Loss of balance
Unstable blood pressure
Double vision
Paralysis on both sides of the body
Difficulty breathing
Nausea and vomiting

(continued)

Table 4.1. **Problems That May Occur after a Stroke,** *continued*

Cerebellar Strokes
Slurred speech
Abnormal movements or tremors
Ataxia or lack of muscle coordination
Imbalance
Dizziness
Queasiness and nausea
Uncontrollable vomiting

---

have listed these in Table 4.1 (according to which part of the brain is affected). Table 4.2 lists some of the speech and swallowing problems that may occur after a stroke.

With stroke, disability can be extremely mild and even imperceptible, very severe, or anywhere in between. As we said earlier, if you or a loved one has had a stroke recently, the likelihood for some improvement is quite high. The problem is that doctors are not able to reliably tell patients and family members how much return of previous function will occur. This

Table 4.2. **Stroke-Related Speech and Swallowing Problems**

Aphasia is a general term for any problem with spoken language processing in the brain. *Receptive aphasia* (also known as *fluent aphasia*) refers primarily to difficulty with understanding, and *expressive aphasia* (also known as *nonfluent aphasia*) refers to difficulty with speaking, but with relative preservation of understanding speech. *Global aphasia* (also known as *total aphasia*) is severe loss of both expression and comprehension. There are several other types of aphasias as well.

Apraxia is lack of coordination of the muscles that form the sounds of speech. It results in effortful and halting speech. Language comprehension is not affected.

Dysarthria is weakness of the muscles that form the sounds of speech, causing the speech to sound slurred or unintelligible. The ability to comprehend and to produce language is not affected in pure dysarthria.

Dysphagia is weakness of the mouth and throat muscles, causing difficulty with swallowing.

---

information is simply beyond what we are able to predict in most cases. Although there have been numerous studies looking at how to predict how well an individual will do, we still haven't found surefire methods for understanding what the future holds for someone who has recently had a stroke. It does appear that people who have only mild weakness (or partial paralysis, which is also called *paresis*) initially, or whose paralysis improves very quickly, tend to have a good prognosis. However, optimism early in the recovery process is certainly warranted in most stroke situations. As time passes, someone's ability to regain function will become increasingly clear.

Achieving Medical Stability Soon after a Stroke

In the first few days after someone has a stroke, the main goal is to make sure that the person is medically stable. This means that the hospital team, which usually consists mostly of doctors and nurses in the first few days, is vigilant about trying to ensure that a patient's blood pressure is not too high or too low, a second stroke doesn't occur, pneumonia or other breathing problems are prevented, heart irregularities are identified, and so on.

In order to achieve medical stability, most patients will have a battery of tests that help the doctors to identify and treat the cause of the stroke. Identifying the cause of stroke is essential in trying to prevent a second stroke. These tests can be a particularly dehumanizing part of the stroke experience, as you or your loved one is shuttled off to various hospital departments with technicians and orderlies who don't know you and who are most concerned with simply getting the study completed. While they might be efficient, they can also seem unfriendly and unconcerned. Keep in mind that these people are not really the ones who are caring for you—they are foot soldiers carrying out your doctors' orders. Their jobs are incredibly important and they do wonderful work, but they might not be very nurturing. So, if the experience of getting tests is uncomfortable and impersonal, it might help to know that these studies will almost certainly help the doctors take better care of you.

Achieving medical stability is of utmost importance in the first few days or even weeks after a stroke. The flurry of hospital activity and all of the tests and monitoring of vital signs are truly essential to help ensure that you or your loved one will not only survive, but also avoid as many potential post-stroke complications as possible. Finally, this is the time when doctors will first assess ways to prevent a *second* stroke.

Avoiding Early Post-Stroke Complications

One of the primary concerns that doctors have during the first few days and even weeks of caring for someone after a stroke is to prevent complications that are not specifically related to the actual problem in the brain. These complications are varied, but include such things as pneumonia or other infections, blood clots that can develop in the legs, seizures, and bedsores. In one study, more than half of all stroke patients developed at least one medical complication. Not surprisingly, the more severe the stroke is, the more likely someone is to develop medical complications. Since not every complication can be prevented, we are going to review the most common or worrisome problems. Early detection usually means that the treatment for the complication will be very effective. If you notice symptoms of any of the complications we describe, be sure to alert the health care team immediately.

Deep Vein Thrombosis

Deep vein thrombosis (or *DVT* for short) is the medical term for a blood clot that forms in a vein in the leg (or less commonly in the arm). In stroke patients DVT is quite common (some studies suggest that clots form in up to half or even more of all people who have significant paralysis, though these clots commonly do not cause symptoms). Inactivity, whether due to paralysis or bed rest or a combination of both, makes it more likely that someone will get a blood clot. Symptoms of a blood clot in the leg include swelling, redness, increased warmth, and sensitivity to touch. If any of these symptoms are present, let the doctor in charge know right away.

Blood clots in the leg (or elsewhere) have the potential to break away and travel to the lungs. This event is called a *pulmonary embolism* and it can cause tremendous injury to the lungs by cutting off the blood supply to portions of them. Stroke teams usually employ preventive treatments to try to avoid DVTs. These methods may include air-filled sequential compression boots (to help the blood flow better) and low doses of anti-clotting medications such as subcutaneous (injected under the skin) heparin. Compression boots may be particularly appropriate early after a hemorrhagic stroke, when your physician may wish to avoid using anti-clotting medications because of the risk of causing additional bleeding in the brain. DVTs can usually be effectively treated if they do form, and the most common treatment is anti-clotting medications.

Falls

Falls are relatively common complications of stroke and can occur at any time during the recovery course and beyond. In one study, more than one-third of the inpatients on a stroke unit fell at least once. Of these, about half had injuries—mostly skin abrasions. Falls are a concern primarily because they may result in serious injury. Especially in the early recovery period when a person has not had much time to practice standing and walking, it is important that a staff person is there to help during every attempt to be mobile (to move around out of bed).

Infection

Pneumonia is an infection (bacterial or viral) that causes inflammation in the lungs. Symptoms of pneumonia include coughing, sputum production, fever, shortness of breath, and lethargy. Pneumonia is not as common as some of the other complications (it occurs in about 1 in 20 hospitalized stroke patients), but it can be a major problem if it occurs. In one study, more than half of the pneumonias that occurred were due to dysphagia (swallowing problems). Dysphagia, which has been found to be present in as many as 45 percent of all stroke patients admitted to a hospital, can lead to food or liquids passing into the wrong tube (the trachea instead of the esophagus) which is called aspiration. Aspiration can lead to choking or infections such as pneumonia.

In order to prevent pneumonia, it is important not to feed someone by mouth before he is ready. The person must be in proper position, sitting erect so that food and drink go down the esophagus. If choking or other signs (such as excessive clearing of the throat, coughing, or gagging) occur, then chances are the patient is not yet ready to eat by mouth. Some people have difficulty swallowing safely but may not have obvious symptoms such as choking or gagging. If there is any question about swallowing, ask to have a consultation with a speech and language pathologist. (Speech therapists focus not only on speech, but also on swallowing problems.)

Bacterial pneumonia is treated with antibiotics, and early recognition and treatment help resolve this infection promptly. (Most post-stroke pneumonia is caused by aspiration of bacteria from bacteria in the mouth.)

Urinary tract infections (*UTIs*) are another common complication in the early post-stroke phase, occurring in 15 percent or more of patients. Many urinary tract infections are due to urinary catheters that may have been put in place in the emergency room to help drain the bladder. These catheters, while often necessary, can certainly lead to infections in the bladder. Retention of urine (inability to void completely) can also lead to infections. The symptoms of a UTI include painful urination, blood in the urine, fever, and lethargy. Antibiotics usually will clear up the infection—especially if urinary catheters have been removed.

Malnutrition

Malnutrition is caused by an unbalanced or insufficient diet. It is common in stroke patients and can be detected very early. In up to 30 percent of patients, malnutrition is seen within one week after a stroke. Addressing or preventing malnutrition involves determining what someone is able and willing to eat.

The first step is usually to have a consultation with a hospital dietician, who will assess the situation and make appropriate recommendations. He or she may suggest supplements rich in protein.

If difficulty swallowing (*dysphagia*) is present, a speech therapist may provide instruction in special ways of helping someone to eat (turning the head a particular direction, for example, or modifying the diet by avoiding textures that are difficult to swallow). If they detect swallowing problems, the doctors and a speech and swallowing therapist may recommend feeding someone in a way that bypasses the mouth. Alternate methods of feeding include feeding through a tube that goes from the nose to the stomach (*nasogastric tube*) or temporarily through an intravenous line (IV in the arm or elsewhere). If feeding and swallowing is going to be a long-term problem, then doctors usually recommend that a feeding tube be placed in the stomach or upper intestines (*G-tube* or *J-tube*). Placing the G- or J-tube is a minor surgical procedure that is commonly performed within several days or a week after a stroke when it becomes clear that a patient will have ongoing nutritional needs that can't be met through the oral intake of food and liquids. These tubes have an opening on the outside of the belly that allows liquid nutrition to be fed into them.

Pressure Sores

Skin abrasions and pressure sores (sometimes called bedsores) are a relatively common and usually preventable early post-stroke complication. In one study, just over 20 percent of stroke patients had some type of skin break. Skin breaks that become infected or deep wounds that occur due to prolonged pressure in one position are relatively uncommon—particularly on stroke units where the nursing staff is vigilant about helping patients to move about in bed and not stay too long in one position.

Seizures

Fewer than 1 in 10 patients will have a seizure after a stroke (some studies report that as few as 3 percent of stroke survivors will have a seizure). Most seizures occur within two weeks of having a stroke. The risk of recurrent seizure after the first one is about 55 percent. After one seizure the patient is usually placed on medication to prevent future seizures.

How You Can Advocate for Yourself or a Loved One

The worst part of a stroke is usually over in the first few days and weeks. There may still be a very difficult journey ahead, however. Arm yourself and your loved ones with information. By reading this book you are already doing a great job as an advocate. (As you continue reading this book, feel free to mark important pages and share the information with your loved ones. All advocates need to have the proper information.) Early on, you may feel overwhelmed. Even if that happens, be sure to ask questions of all of the health care providers involved. If you can't remember what someone said, don't be embarrassed to ask again; you have a lot going on and you will almost certainly need to hear some of the information more than once. It might help to take notes during your visits with your doctor, if you are able to. Feel free to ask him to spell any words that are unfamiliar to you.

This book is a source of *credible* information, but it is not the only source. Seek out other legitimate sources of information, too. Talk to the doctors and therapists involved in treating the stroke survivor. Contact the American Stroke Association or some of the other groups listed in the Resources section of this book. Include your primary care physician in the communication loop. At the same time, be wary of information that is *not* credible. This includes tips from well-meaning friends and neighbors. Also, keep in mind that anyone with a serious illness is vulnerable and can be a target for quacks and charlatans. There is a story that goes something like this: there were two men sitting on a porch and one man said, "Life is like a fountain." The other man, intrigued, asked, "How is life like a fountain?" A few minutes later the first man replied, "Well, maybe life isn't like a fountain, after all." The point here is to talk to people who are experts. Read printed materials that offer sound medical advice. Don't rely on information that is not credible.

●●●

Chapter 5

Maximizing Recovery from a Stroke

In April of 1945, only three months into his fourth term, President Franklin Delano Roosevelt died of a hemorrhagic stroke. Although his death was unexpected, it was the culmination of years of living with severe hypertension—a condition we can now usually manage quite well with medications but for which at that time there were no effective treatments. During the last year of his life, Roosevelt's doctor prescribed a variety of therapies, including bed rest (which was highly impractical for him—especially during World War II), weight reduction, and multiple medications that did little to lower his blood pressure. According to one published report, "In retrospect, there is little doubt that FDR's heart failure and terminal stroke could have been prevented had effective antihypertensive therapy been available."[1] Roosevelt's stroke was devastating, and he did not live long enough to undergo any rehabilitation. It is now more than half a century since FDR died, and we have made remarkable progress in treating hypertension and addressing other risk factors for a first or a recurrent stroke. Moreover, we have made significant gains in helping people *recover* from a stroke.

If you or a loved one has had a stroke, then you probably already know or at least suspect that the recovery process will likely be long and possibly fraught with complications and potential setbacks. Although recovering from a stroke is often difficult, there are more therapies and treatments available today than ever before. Of course, it is always best to get expert assistance with your recovery right from the start, but even if your stroke happened months or even years ago, there still may be things you can do to more fully recover and maximize your ability to function.

The Process of Stroke Recovery

Stroke recovery is often divided into two categories: *neurological recovery* and *functional recovery.* Neurological recovery has to do with how much the brain is able to regain lost abilities. This depends on many factors, including the extent of injury to the brain, the location of the injury, whether any treatment was initiated early on to help facilitate returning blood flow to the injured area (in an ischemic stroke), and the individual's pre-stroke health and intellectual status.

Part of neurological recovery also depends on something doctors and scientists call brain "plasticity." The concept of plasticity involves the brain making connections that are new or different from the connections that existed before an injury occurred. A neurologist colleague of ours has a series of slides that explain plasticity metaphorically. The first slide shows a room filled with various electronic equipment and many, many cords that are correctly plugged in to various sockets (the room is the brain and the cords are the nerve connections that help the different areas of the brain to function). In the next slide a number of the cords are unplugged (this is the slide that symbolizes someone having a stroke), and it is obvious that some of the equipment won't work because it isn't connected to a power source. In the third slide, many of the remaining (undamaged) cords are plugged in to new locations (demonstrating how a brain can heal after a stroke). This third slide represents plasticity, the process by which our brains can make allowances and can reconfigure in order to compensate for an injury such as a stroke.

Functional recovery takes into account how much someone can improve in day-to-day activities. These activities include bathing, dressing, walking, and talking. They may also include higher level physical activities such as golfing or playing tennis. What is hopeful about functional recovery is that people can continue to improve their ability to perform a variety of tasks long after neurologic recovery has ceased.

Rosie had a stroke when she was in her late forties. Initially her left side was paralyzed and she had some difficulty with talking, though she understood what people were saying to her. Eight months after her stroke, Rosie's speech was almost back to the way it had been before the stroke, but she continued to have some difficulty with walking—especially on uneven terrain and on stairs. She met with her doctor, who told her that although her neurologic recovery was essentially complete, there was still the possibility that her walking would improve with more therapy. Rosie and her family were delighted to hear this, because they had been trying to decide whether to sell their two-level family home and move into a single-level home. Moving would mean a major adjustment for Rosie's young children, who would have to go to a new school.

Rosie and her husband had been considering putting in a stair lift, but after their visit to the doctor, they decided to see how she progressed in therapy over the next few months. Rosie worked hard in physical therapy and each week she saw a little bit of improvement. These small gains added up and a little over a year after her stroke, she was able to climb stairs easily, though she had learned to take her time and not rush. For Rosie and her family, the functional recovery in what we would call higher-level walking skills, several months after her stroke and also after neurological recovery had ceased, was of paramount importance.

For specialists in rehabilitation medicine, the concepts of neurological and functional recovery are essential. We have found that explaining the two categories of recovery to patients and their families helps them to feel more secure with this recovery process. It is reassuring for you and your loved ones to know that stroke recovery may continue for many months after the initial event. You and your family should have realistic expectations about the recovery process, however. Healing from a stroke and predicting when recovery will stop are not perfect sciences. There is no way to say exactly when someone has finished the neurological or functional recovery process. We do know that neurological recovery occurs in the first few months after a stroke and could possibly take up to one year. Functional recovery also begins immediately after a stroke and usually outlasts neurological recovery by several months. Both processes are essential during the recovery phase, and the greater the neurological and functional recovery, the better the prognosis for someone who has had a stroke.

Physiatrists (doctors who specialize in physical medicine and rehabilitation, also known as PM&R) and other health care providers who are knowledgeable about stroke recovery can also help improve your ability to function by prescribing specialized equipment such as a properly fitted cane or a brace that helps stabilize the foot and ankle when walking.

Finding and Selecting a Rehabilitation Team

If you or a family member have recently had a stroke, then you are likely in the process of searching for the right rehabilitation team to help you on your road to recovery. This can be a confusing time and there are a number of options to choose from. As physiatrists, we thoroughly understand this process but also recognize that it is not intuitive or familiar to people who don't work in a rehabilitation environment. We will begin with the basic general choices for rehabilitation and then move on to explain more specific issues that can affect rehabilitation care. Rehabilitation from a stroke (or any other serious medical condition) works best when different specialists treat someone over the same time period—usually on the same day, several times a week for several weeks. This is the true multidisciplinary structure that is the basis for nearly all successful rehabilitation programs, regardless of where you go for treatment.

You and your family and the doctors involved with your care at the beginning stages of stroke recovery will decide together, first, *where* to go to get rehabilitation treatment. The varieties of types of facilities might seem too numerous initially, but the general categories of rehabilitation care are actually straightforward. There are guidelines to help you choose the right one at any given time during the recovery process. (Please keep in mind that these are general guidelines and that you should always discuss all of the treatment options with your doctor before deciding how to proceed.)

Acute Inpatient Rehabilitation

This kind of care involves a team of rehabilitation professionals (listed in Table 5.1) who help an individual to recover either in a freestanding rehabilitation hospital or on a rehabilitation stroke unit in an acute care hospital. This option is usually available to people who have just sustained a stroke and are currently hospitalized and need a substantial amount of care before returning home (or in some cases going to a nursing home). To receive this kind of care you usually need to meet three criteria:

1. You need to have had a stroke recently and still be hospitalized (insurers generally pay for this level of care only if a patient is transferred from an acute care hospital shortly after having had a stroke).
2. You need to have problems from the stroke that are serious enough to require remaining in a hospital setting (qualifying problems include difficulty with dressing, walking, talking, and swallowing).
3. You should both require and be able to participate in at least three hours per day of therapy (most health insurers enforce this requirement in determining whether to pay for the care of someone in an acute rehabilitation setting). Three hours per day of therapy may include occupational therapy, in which the therapist comes to your bedside to help you relearn how to dress, bathe, shave, and so on. It also includes working with the physical therapist on some exercises or walking, and having speech or swallowing therapy.

Table 5.1. Members of a Stroke Rehabilitation Team

Medical doctor. This is usually a neurologist (a doctor specializing in the care of people with neurological disorders) or a physiatrist (a doctor specializing in *physical medicine and rehabilitation,* or PM&R). The medical doctor leads the team and orders appropriate treatment for the stroke survivor.

Physical therapist. The physical therapist is primarily involved in helping someone recover strength, flexibility, and the ability to move about, either by walking or in a wheelchair. Because of their focus on improving mobility, physical therapists tend to devote much of their effort to improving leg function, though they work on arm activities as well.

Occupational therapist. Many people don't understand what an occupational therapist does. The primary goal of occupational therapy is to help someone resume doing her usual daily activities such as bathing and dressing. As a result, occupational therapists devote considerable effort to improving the functional use of the arm, including helping to improve arm strength, coordination, and range of motion. Occupational therapists help people to regain the use of their arms after stroke, and they are also instrumental in assessing things like the ability to return to driving and prescribing adaptive equipment such as a one-handed computer keyboard that may assist with returning to work.

Speech and language pathologist. This type of therapist concentrates on problems that have to do with language comprehension or expression and with swallowing issues. A speech and language pathologist is often able to offer someone very simple strategies that will help with speaking and swallowing. Sophisticated speech and language therapists will work with a stroke survivor on many "higher-level" cognitive activities such as memory, concentration, planning, abstract reasoning, and decision making.

Rehabilitation nurse. These health care specialists are always available in inpatient rehabilitation settings. They often work in outpatient settings as well. Rehabilitation nurses perform all of the usual nursing functions but also focus on helping patients with bowel and bladder function, sexuality issues, and providing education and support for the family. Good rehab nurses will help a stroke survivor learn to regain the ability to move, speak, swallow, and so on, reinforcing what the therapy team is working on through practice of functional tasks.

(continued)

Table 5.1. **Members of a Stroke Rehabilitation Team,** *continued*

Vocational specialist. This individual provides stroke survivors with an initial vocational assessment: Can she return to her former job? Will she need any special equipment (such as a one-handed computer keyboard)? If not, is she a candidate to be retrained for work in a different type of job? A vocational specialist attempts to answer all of these questions in the evaluation process. This specialist then moves on to helping someone obtain and learn to use special equipment and/or retrain in a different occupation.

Therapeutic recreational therapist. These therapists are not always found in rehabilitation settings, but the most comprehensive hospitals have at least one therapeutic recreational therapist on staff. This specialist helps a stroke survivor embrace leisure and educational activities that are both therapeutic and part of having a good quality of life. These activities may include cooking, gardening, and playing sports.

Mental health counselor. Most rehabilitation settings will have some type of mental health counseling available. The counseling might include a consultation with a medical doctor who specializes in psychiatry (and can prescribe medications if needed) or perhaps visits with a psychologist or clinical social worker. Adjusting to having a stroke is often a difficult process, and these experienced specialists help people adjust psychologically to a life that is likely different than what they had before the stroke.

Neuropsychologist. This is a specific type of mental health specialist who is responsible for initial formal testing and identification of cognitive deficits in a stroke survivor. The results from these tests can be very helpful to the staff and the patient, who can focus on how best to overcome or accommodate these weaknesses.

Clinical dietician. Sometimes after a stroke a person is not able to eat the types of foods he is accustomed to, or is able to eat but is disinterested in food. Whatever the reason for the change in eating habits, the clinical dietician is responsible for helping a stroke survivor maintain the best possible nutritional health. A dietician can also offer guidance as to how to lose or gain weight, lower cholesterol levels, improve the control of diabetes, and reduce salt in the diet.

(continued)

Table 5.1. **Members of a Stroke Rehabilitation Team,** *continued*

Orthotist. This is someone who has training in how to fit and make braces. Not everyone will need a brace after a stroke, but for those who have a paralyzed or weak arm or leg, a brace can sometimes be extremely beneficial in resuming physical activity such as walking.

Case manager. This is someone you really want to make contact with early after a stroke—especially if you or a loved one is in the hospital. Case managers also sometimes work in outpatient settings. This person acts as a liaison between the rehabilitation team, the insurance company, the patient, and the family. This can be a tricky job—especially if an insurance company is not willing to pay for a certain treatment. Usually case managers are very helpful in answering your questions and assisting with getting the best possible care. You should always ask who the case manager works for (the insurance company or the hospital, typically), so you know where his primary allegiance is. This doesn't mean that he won't be a strong advocate for you, but if issues come up that make you feel uncomfortable, or if the case manager does not seem to be a strong advocate for you, you may need to be more assertive. Most people really appreciate their case managers, who are accomplished at assisting people through a complicated stroke rehabilitation process.

After a stroke some people are not able to participate in a rehabilitation program of this intensity; in that case, other options are available. However, if you have just had a stroke and you are able to actively participate in three hours a day of treatment, then acute inpatient rehabilitation is an excellent option to help you with your recovery. Before being discharged from a rehabilitation hospital, you can request a home visit from your occupational and/or physical therapists, who will visit your home and make recommendations about how to make it safer and more accessible. If this visit cannot be arranged prior to discharge from the rehabilitation hospital, a similar evaluation can be performed by the home care therapists.

Subacute Nursing Facilities

SNFs (pronounced "sniffs") are a good option for people who have recently had a stroke and are unable to go directly home but cannot tolerate a full three hours of daily therapy. At a subacute rehabilitation facility, you would still be in a supportive, medically supervised environment but you would

not have to participate in as much therapy as you would in an acute rehabilitation hospital or ward. This option allows a slower pace for recovery
but still offers rehabilitation care and medical services.

Home Therapy

Home therapy or Visiting Nurses' Association (VNA) services are reserved
for stroke survivors who are discharged to their home but can't easily leave
to receive therapy at an outpatient facility. This type of rehabilitation is
often part of a transition from a hospital or a SNF to an outpatient facility.
You want to use these services for only a short time, if possible, to reaccli-
mate to home and to your usual routine. Outpatient services provide more
equipment and opportunities for you to advance in your recovery once you
are able to travel to a nearby facility.

You may never want or need home services, but they are a wonderful
option for some people immediately after their hospital discharge, because
they help them to feel comfortable and safe moving about their home and
returning to doing some of the things they usually do. These services can
involve having a physical or occupational therapist come to your home
several times a week to help you relearn how to use your body safely and
efficiently. Speech therapists are available to help you with speech or swallowing, social workers can assist with arranging services in the community
(such as a service to provide meals) and emotional adjustment, nurses can
come to take your blood pressure and help with other medical issues, and
home health aides are available to do some shopping, cooking, and cleaning, and to help with bathing and dressing.

Outpatient Therapy

The majority of stroke survivors will receive treatment in an outpatient rehabilitation facility, either at the local hospital or in a freestanding therapy
center, once they are medically stable and able to drive (or be driven) to
treatment. These centers vary in terms of the extent of services offered. The
more comprehensive facilities offer most of the services listed in Table 5.2.
An outpatient center is usually your "last stop" on the road to stroke recovery, and the intensity and length of treatment will depend on your specific
needs. Typically a stroke survivor receives a couple of hours of therapy,
two to three days a week for weeks or months, in an outpatient setting. At
the conclusion of outpatient therapy, patients are given a home exercise
program specifically designed to help them progress and remain physically
active.

Table 5.2. Services Provided in a Rehabilitation Setting

Medical evaluation and follow up	Sexuality counseling
Physical therapy	Driving evaluations
Occupational therapy	Spasticity clinic or treatment
Speech and swallowing therapy	Bracing clinic
Vocational therapy	Wheelchair and scooter clinic
Recreational therapy	Assistive technology
Mental health counseling	Clinical dietician

The Goals of Rehabilitation

The major goal of rehabilitation treatment is *to assist someone in reaching his or her full potential.* What that potential is will certainly vary depending on many factors, such as pre-stroke physical activity level, pre-stroke intellect, and the severity of the stroke and subsequent disability.

Rehabilitation treatment is exceedingly goal oriented. You will hear this statement time and again as you go through the rehabilitation process. Those of us who are health care providers in this field focus on both short-term goals (usually, what someone can accomplish in a matter of days or a couple of weeks) and long-term goals (those activities that someone can accomplish over the time frame of weeks to months). Insurance companies require that we document both short- and long-term goals, and how successful someone is in reaching those goals, in our medical notes. Usually insurers will continue to pay for treatment as long as a stroke survivor is making progress. Once someone has reached a plateau, though, and is no longer able to achieve success in reaching either short- or long-term goals, treatment is generally discontinued.

The concept of goal-oriented rehabilitation treatment is an important one. It doesn't make much sense to keep treating someone who is not improving. Doing so is hard for the stroke survivor and very discouraging. Insurers understandably are unwilling to pay for treatment unless that treatment is going to be beneficial to the recipient. Thus, when patients or family members ask how long someone will be in treatment, the usual response is, "As long as he or she is making progress." This is not an attempt to be indirect, but rather a genuine response that takes into account that in most instances we are unable to predict either exactly how much someone will improve after a stroke or the time frame for that improvement.

Table 5.3. **Information to Tell Your Rehabilitation Specialists**

Write this information down (or, even better, type it up) and make several copies to bring with you to the initial medical and therapy appointments.

History of Present Illness
Your name (including any nickname that you like to go by)
Your date of birth
Your age (they can do the math, but it is better if you just write it down for them)
Whether you are right-handed or left-handed
The date of your stroke
Where you were hospitalized after your stroke (include dates and the name of each hospital)
The medical problems you are having now that are related to the stroke

Medications
Your current medications (include the dose and how often you take them)

Allergies
Allergies to medications (write down what happened when you took them in the past)

Past Medical History
Medical problems that you have had in the past or ongoing medical problems (not related to the stroke)
Surgeries you have had for any condition (include the year you had them if possible)

Family History
Medical conditions that run in your family (including your parents, siblings, and children)

Social History
Tell about your home life (Who do you live with? Does your home have stairs?)
Write about your work life (What is your vocation? Are you retired?)
Describe your habits (especially how much alcohol you drink and whether you smoke now or have in the past)

Tests
If you are able to remember the tests you had after your stroke, make a note of them. Providing written reports from these studies is ideal. Some doctors will want to see the actual films from imaging tests, so you might want to inquire about obtaining copies of these films to take with you or having them sent before your appointment.

Meeting with a New Doctor or Therapist

Meeting with a new doctor or therapist can be stressful. No one wants to be ill, and a new health care provider is just one more reminder that you are going through a difficult time. It is the rare person who goes to see the doctor for treatment of a serious medical problem without any angst at all. And if you or a loved one has had a stroke, you will be in the position of meeting a new health care provider on a number of occasions—whether he or she is a doctor, therapist, or other rehabilitation specialist. In order to make this difficult process as smooth as possible for you, we have made a list of what health care providers typically ask at a first visit (Table 5.3).

Doctors and therapists are trained to ask questions in a specific order, and it is incredibly helpful to them when a patient arrives with written answers to their questions. This allows them to get to know you very quickly and to spend the majority of the visit on the essential aspects of your care rather than the mundane task of gathering information about such things as your medication allergies. Write this information down (or, even better, type it up) and make several copies to bring with you to the initial medical and therapy appointments. Although it may seem bothersome to do so, it will almost certainly save you time and energy when you meet with different members of your rehabilitation team. There is a good chance that the time you put into preparing for these visits will help facilitate your care.

You only have to write or type this information out once (with periodic updates if things change) and then give a copy to each new person with whom you meet. (In an ideal world, of course, you would just need to bring one copy and the members of your team would share it with each other. However, rehabilitation specialists are busy people, and they may not have the opportunity to make copies of your list or to share the one copy you bring with each other. So, just in case, bring several copies and be sure to give each person their own copy.) If more than one person asks you the same question or series of questions (for example, whether you have any allergies to medications), try to be patient and respond each time you are asked. Again, in an ideal world, you would only have to answer each question one time; unfortunately, we are not at the point where all of the information you provide to us is promptly shared with everyone who needs it.

How the Family Can Help

In Betty Rollin's memoir *Last Wish*, about her mother's struggle with poor health, she wrote of how illness affects the entire family. Rollin poignantly summed it up this way, "Disease may score a direct hit on only one member of a family, but shrapnel tears the flesh of the others."[2] Whether it is you or a loved one who has had a stroke, this difficult disease has affected you all. It is important to note that you can control only how *you* react and behave throughout this ordeal. While you can be supportive and encouraging to your loved ones, you can't control how they feel or what they do. Presenting as a "unified family," whose members are all in agreement and in sync with one another, can be an onerous burden and nearly impossible to achieve. Instead, focus on what *you* are able to do to improve this situation and on how *you* can support your loved ones so that they can better cope.

As rehabilitation physicians who have been in medicine for many years, we have seen many families that are appropriately supportive, as well as some who are uninvolved or inattentive, and those who smother a loved one with too much attention. If you or someone you love has just had a stroke, of course you want to fall into the first group, but it is difficult when your world is turned upside down to do and say all the right things. And you may not do so. There is no way that you or your loved ones can be perfect, even under the best of circumstances—and these certainly are not the best of circumstances. So, go easy on yourself and your loved ones and just try to do the best job you can.

You should be commended already for doing a good job, just by reading this book. You are gathering information that will undoubtedly help you and those you care most about. You are obviously thinking about how best to handle this difficult situation, and that is excellent. Sharing this book with your family and friends will help them to understand more about strokes and the recovery process as well as how to prevent a stroke in the future. The more your friends and family understand about this disease, the more helpful they can be to you and to each other.

Besides reading this book and sharing it with others, there are some other helpful things that you can consider doing for yourself and those you love:

1. Many people think they should give up everything they enjoy doing to help an ill family member or to focus on their own condition. Inevitably this does not work well. You and your family members will have a much better quality of life if you continue to do things

that you enjoy while at the same time being a loving and considerate person.

2. Most people are independent by nature and not entirely comfortable with asking others for help. If you have a loved one who has had a stroke, you want to offer your support in a loving and helpful manner. Assisting your loved one will also help you to cope with what is a difficult situation. At the same time, there are others who probably want to help *you* and your family in this crisis. Consider what you need and how they can help. When they ask what they can do, give them concrete answers that will be meaningful to you and your family.

3. Be truthful about how you are feeling. Of course there is a balance between letting others know your every thought and emotion and sealing yourself off emotionally from those you care about. In general, the truth is a powerful aid in healing. Just saying out loud, "I am afraid," or "I am anxious," or "I am sad," lessens the power these feelings have over you.

4. Take an interest in the post-stroke treatment plan. Understanding what the plan is and how you or your loved one will improve over time can be very helpful in establishing realistic expectations for the future.

5. Stay involved. This one is really important. Too often we see families rush in and offer to help right after someone has a stroke. Usually there is little they can do initially, so they send flowers and then go on with their own lives. Stroke survivors will greatly benefit from the continued interest and support of their loved ones for weeks, months, and even years after the stroke has passed. Even if there is not much you can do, a simple phone call, card, or personal visit done as regularly as you can manage is extremely meaningful to your loved ones.

Help for the Family

If someone you love has had a stroke, you may be in the role of a caregiver. When this happens, your relationship with your loved one often changes. Caregivers face both physical and emotional hardships after a stroke in the family. Although this is definitely an extreme example, we wanted to share a letter with you that was published in the *Boston Globe* in January 2004 in a column called "Annie's Mailbox." This letter from a reader sums up how difficult post-stroke care can be on a spouse or other family member:

Dear Annie:

My husband, "Todd," had a stroke at the age of 38. He is now blind, nearly deaf, has seizures, severe short-term memory problems, mood swings and needs care 24/7. He's also selfish, self-centered, and can be physically, verbally, mentally and emotionally abusive.

Todd never leaves me alone. I can't eat a relaxed meal and haven't had a full night's sleep since his stroke. He wants me to be the only one who takes care of him. Frankly, I'm at the end of my rope. . . . (Signed, Nothing Left in Illinois).

We hope your situation is better than this Illinois caregiver's; however, there is no doubt that strokes often leave people with significant impairments and the need to rely heavily on loved ones for help. Strokes can also significantly negatively affect someone's mood, attitude, and behavior. No matter what your situation is, there are many resources to help you and your family as you go through the post-stroke rehabilitation process. We have found that many people find enormous support from friends, colleagues, and clergy with whom they have established relationships but from whom in the past they may not have required much support. These people are usually anxious to help, and they frequently are your best source of help, because they know you and care about you.

Even with assistance, though, you may feel "burned out," lonely, and confused. In *Staying Sane: When You Care for Someone with Chronic Illness,* Drs. Melvin Pohl and Deniston Kay describe burnout as not just one feeling but a combination of feelings:

Stressed much of the time
Worthless
Tired and out of energy
Out of shape
Emotionally out of control
Constantly in the grip of negative thoughts
Out of time
Out of money
Alone and disconnected
Depressed
Anxious about the future
Used up

Professionals who specialize in helping patients and families through the difficult post-stroke period may also be a source of wonderful support. Research has shown that caregivers who have support from professionals are better prepared for their roles and have better problem-solving skills and less depression. It has been estimated that 1 out of 3 caregivers suffers from "poor psychological health." It makes sense that a caregiver, whose quality of life has been reduced when a family member has had a serious stroke, is under a lot of stress and might be prone to depression and anxiety.

If you are a caregiver and the stress seems overwhelming or you are anxious or depressed, ask your doctor for a referral to a clinical social worker, psychologist, or psychiatrist. You deserve some help and attention. Remember that both your quality of life and the quality of life of the person you are trying to help will be improved if you take care of yourself, too.

Finally, there are a number of excellent organizations that provide useful information and support for stroke survivors and their families. These organizations are listed in the Resources.

Whether you or a loved one has had a stroke, there are people who can help. But they can only help if you let them know that you are interested in their support. Now is a good time to reach out to others. Just as you would reach out to them if they were struggling, let them assist you during this difficult time. Having people involved in your life who are supportive and helpful greatly enhances your quality of life—regardless of the physical stroke recovery process. As Saint Francis of Assisi said, "It is in giving that we receive." It makes others feel good to help you, so let them.

Chapter 6

● ●

Post-Stroke Medical and Social Issues

If you have had a stroke, you may have medical problems related to the stroke for months or even years afterward. You may also have social and work difficulties due to stroke-related disability. In this chapter, we focus on bladder and bowel problems, mood disorders, pain, and spasticity—difficulties that are encountered by many stroke survivors. Where in the brain the stroke occurred and how much injury it caused to the surrounding tissues determines whether these troubles arise and how severe they are. These post-stroke medical issues often resolve on their own over time; nevertheless, proper intervention and treatment can make a world of difference for some stroke survivors. Social and employment-related issues include resuming intimacy with a spouse or partner and returning to driving and work. These important quality-of-life issues can be dramatically altered by a stroke. In this chapter we offer suggestions for how to tackle these problems and provide insight about what you might expect in the future.

Bladder Problems

Urinary incontinence is very common for stroke patients when they are first hospitalized. For the majority of people who have had a stroke, this incontinence will clear up before they are discharged from the hospital. Approximately one-fourth of stroke survivors will experience urinary incontinence for some period of time after they return home. Incontinence is an embarrassing problem; people are usually mortified when they can't control their bladders. If they can't get the incontinence under control, they may avoid social situations and become reclusive. The symptoms most commonly associated with post-stroke bladder problems, such as feeling an urgent need to urinate, can also cause people to rush to get to the bathroom and risk having a fall.

To better understand post-stroke urinary issues, it is helpful to review how the urinary system works. Our urinary systems are designed to help maintain proper salt and water balance throughout our body. The kidneys begin the process by producing urine by filtering our blood. The urine then flows through two long tubes called *ureters* into the organ called the *bladder*. The bladder is a muscular sack that stores the urine until it leaves our body through a single tube called the *urethra*. The two phases in normal urination are the filling and storage phase, which consists of producing urine and storing it in the bladder, and the emptying phase, which consists of *voiding*, or releasing the urine.

The bladder has a valve-like structure known as the *sphincter* that controls the flow of urine. The activity of the sphincter is closely integrated with bladder contraction. Normally, when the bladder fills with urine, a bladder contraction occurs and the sphincter opens, allowing urine to flow out of the bladder. This process is controlled by the brain, which can keep a damper on the process until the right time (a convenient bathroom, for example).

Normal urination can be affected by a stroke in a number of ways. We will discuss the most common problem, which is called *detrusor hyperreflexia*. Normally, when it is time to void, the muscle surrounding the bladder (called the detrusor) contracts while the muscles in the bladder outlet (sphincters) relax. Think of a tube of toothpaste, with your hand as the detrusor muscle that surrounds the bladder and the cap on the toothpaste as the sphincter that either keeps the material in or lets it out. You squeeze the tube from one end, and the toothpaste comes out if the cap is released. This is what normally happens in the bladder. The detrusor muscle contracts and the sphincters relax in a coordinated manner.

After a stroke, however, the neurological signaling systems between the bladder and the brain may not work properly. When this happens, the most common problem is that the detrusor muscle contracts either too often or at inappropriate times, or both. When this occurs, the stroke survivor may have trouble keeping the bladder from contracting as it fills up, and keeping the sphincters closed. This leads to a sense of urgency when the bladder fills, since the system begins working automatically rather than being delayed until a convenient time by the brain. This is why detrusor hyperreflexia is sometimes called a "hyperactive" or "irritable" bladder.

Several other factors may influence someone's ability to be continent after a stroke. These factors include urinary tract infection, excess fluid intake, constipation, lack of motivation caused by a mood disturbance such as depression, medication side effects, use of caffeine or alcohol, and

Table 6.1. **Urinary Information to Tell Your Doctor**

What problem you are having
When the problem began
How often you urinate
How often and how much urine you are leaking
Whether your bladder feels empty after urinating
How forceful your urine stream is
Whether there is blood or an unusual color or odor in your urine
Whether you have a burning sensation or other symptoms when you
    urinate
What medications you currently take
Amount of fluid you drink daily
How much alcohol and caffeine you consume

---

difficulty walking or moving around. Someone with pre-existing problems with urination (such as a man with an enlarged prostate or a woman who has had urinary issues after having a hysterectomy) may be more vulnerable to voiding problems after experiencing a stroke. The most common post-stroke urinary symptom is feeling the need to urinate frequently, with subsequent leakage. Total incontinence results if the person is unaware of the urge to urinate, unmotivated to respond to the urge, or unable to respond due to mobility problems.

Fortunately for most stroke survivors, urinary problems often improve greatly over time. If you or your loved one are currently experiencing urinary issues, you need to discuss this problem with a knowledgeable stroke doctor or urologist. The doctor will want to know a number of things, which are listed in Table 6.1. You might want to keep a log for a few days. Write down what is happening and then show the urinary log to the doctor.

Treatment for urinary system problems vary widely and are based on what exactly the problem is, how severe it is, what has been tried in the past, and what the patient is interested in trying now. There are three general approaches: (1) behavioral (see Table 6.2 for behavioral approaches to try), (2) medications, and (3) medical procedures. Anyone who is experiencing incontinence can and should try behavioral approaches because they are simple and have no risk of side effects. Medications often can be helpful; which one to use will depend on what the problem is and what the doctor thinks will best treat it. There are numerous surgical procedures to treat urinary incontinence, although the majority of stroke patients will *not*

Table 6.2. **Behavioral Treatment Approaches for Urinary Incontinence**

Set up a schedule where you go to the bathroom once every hour, and gradually increase this to the point where you are going every 3 to 4 hours.

Avoid drinking alcoholic beverages.

Avoid caffeine in foods and drinks.

Don't severely limit your fluid intake; instead aim for drinking 2 to 3 quarts per day.

Stop drinking liquids 2 to 4 hours before bedtime.

Drink cranberry juice, which may help prevent urinary tract infections. (Low-calorie options are available.)

Eat foods rich in fiber, because constipation can make symptoms of urinary incontinence worse.

require any type of procedure. Procedures are reserved for people with severe bladder problems that do not respond to behavior modification methods or medications.

Bowel Problems

Normal defecation requires the action of four major mechanisms working in concert. They are (1) an urge to go to the bathroom, (2) relaxation of the anal sphincters, (3) propulsion of the stool by the colon, and (4) an increase in intra-abdominal pressure by "bearing down" or "pushing." After a stroke, one or more of these factors may be affected for various reasons, and constipation or stool incontinence may result. Constipation can be a result of reduced physical mobility or a change in diet (perhaps as a consequence of swallowing problems). It can also occur if bowel motility (the propulsion of stool in the intestine) is decreased due to a disruption in nerve signals from the brain. Some medications cause constipation. Finally, stroke can affect a person's motivation to defecate (they may not want to make the effort) or their ability to sense the need to defecate (and failing to defecate regularly can lead to drying of stool and constipation).

Incontinence of stool (stool "accidents" or soiling) may result from the same factors: medication side effects, reduced mobility, changes in diet, and changes in sensation or motivation. Stool incontinence may also be a direct result of constipation, when dry, hard feces in the intestine cause a blockage and only liquid stool is able to flow around the obstruction.

If you are experiencing constipation or incontinence or any problems with your bowels, report your symptoms to your doctor so she can evaluate what might be causing your problem. The good news is that bowel problems are typically fairly easy to identify and treat. Comfort is an issue, of course, but there are other, more serious, health reasons to address bowel problems. The most troubling problem occurs in extreme cases of constipation, when the stool causes a major blockage in the intestines. This blockage can severely distend the intestinal wall and even cause it to rupture. This problem is rare but can be serious. Again, seek out medical intervention whenever there is a post-stroke bowel problem.

Symptoms of stool incontinence (very loose or leaking stool, possibly staining the underwear) are fairly straightforward and recognizable. As noted above, leaking stool may actually be a sign of constipation. Other symptoms of constipation can be subtler. Often the only complaint is, "I feel constipated." What this means varies depending on the individual and their perception. For example, someone who reports that they are constipated may actually be having regular bowel movements every third day but are accustomed to having daily bowel movements. Other symptoms of constipation include straining to defecate, passage of firm or small-volume fecal material, blood on the toilet paper due to passing hard stools, pain with defecation, and abdominal fullness, bloating, or cramping. Your doctor may want to order tests to identify the cause of the problem. For example, a simple x-ray of the abdomen will show how much stool is being held in the colon and whether it is causing distension and potential blockage. Tests are not usually necessary, however, and your doctor may simply proceed with treatment suggestions. Treatment will vary depending on what your doctor identifies or suspects as the cause of the problem.

Although, as we mentioned, you should report any bowel problems to your doctor, there are some remedies you can try at home to help prevent or alleviate symptoms of constipation. First, you should increase the amount of fiber in your diet. High-fiber foods include raw vegetables and fruits and whole grains. You may wish to discuss these dietary changes with a nutritionist, especially if you are on a restricted diet due to swallowing difficulties. Second, you can eat a warm meal or drink warm fluids after rising in the morning. Following this meal you can try to move your bowels by sitting on the toilet and bearing down intermittently for 5 to 10 seconds. If these methods don't work, talk to your doctor about what medications you are currently taking to determine whether these might be causing bowel problems as a side effect. Your doctor will also likely offer you advice about what medications you might want to take to help with your bowel problem. Fiber supplements, laxatives, stool softeners, suppositories, and other prescription and over-the-counter treatments are usually effective.

Changes in Mood

Depression is very common for people who have experienced a major health problem, but it seems to be particularly prevalent among stroke survivors. It is estimated that approximately half of all stroke survivors experience depression within one year after their injury. The reasons for this high incidence of depression are not entirely clear but may be related to the injury to the brain, the level of disability following a stroke, lack of a strong family and social support network, and potential side effects of medications. Depression after a stroke can make someone more disabled in the short term and may indirectly contribute to a higher risk of another stroke in the long term. The higher future risk of stroke may be related to a number of factors, including that someone who is depressed might not be able to make the lifestyle changes necessary to reduce the risk of recurrent stroke or might not take his medications regularly.

Untreated depression greatly impacts one's quality of life. The obvious effect is that it makes someone unhappy and unable to enjoy any of life's pleasures. Other effects might not be so obvious. For example, people who are depressed experience more pain, and more severe pain, than nondepressed people do. Depression also leads to fatigue, which can affect the ability of a stroke survivor to think clearly. Treating stroke survivors' depression can markedly improve their ability to process new information and express themselves.

On the other hand, sometimes family members and health care providers attribute too many symptoms to depression. For example, a stroke survivor with fatigue may actually have sleep apnea, a condition that involves not getting enough oxygen when sleeping. True cognitive deficits such as inattention may be a result of the injury to the brain and not due to depression. Cardiac deconditioning or congestive heart failure can also make someone appear tired and depressed. For all of these reasons, it is important for readers to review the symptoms of depression listed in Table 6.3 and then to pursue any concerns with a knowledgeable medical doctor. Note that anxiety can occur after stroke and may be present alone or in combination with depression. The symptoms of anxiety are listed in Table 6.4. Both anxiety and depression are highly treatable in most individuals.

Table 6.3. **Symptoms of Depression**

Losing interest in usual activities and pastimes
Feeling irritable
Crying frequently
Feeling sad
Feeling hopeless
Having a poor appetite or significant weight loss
Having an increased appetite or significant weight gain
Sleeping poorly
Sleeping too much
Feeling agitated or restless
Feeling unusually fatigued
Having difficulty concentrating
Having difficulty making decisions
Feeling self-critical
Feeling excessively guilty
Feeling worthless
Having recurrent thoughts of dying or suicidal thoughts

Source: Reprinted with permission from Julie K. Silver, *Post-Polio Syndrome: A Guide for Polio Survivors and Their Families* (Yale University Press, 2001).

Treating underlying problems with mood will not only improve your quality of life but also may improve your physical health and make it less likely that you will have a stroke in the future.

Pain

After a stroke, there are three primary reasons why someone might experience pain. The first reason is by far the most common and has to do with arm weakness or paralysis, which causes shoulder pain in many stroke survivors. The pain occurs because the top of the arm, the *humeral head,* is not very well supported by the surrounding muscles. This results in what we call *shoulder subluxation.* In shoulder subluxation, the shoulder becomes partially dislocated because the paralyzed or weak muscles can't hold it in place. How displaced the shoulder joint is depends on the amount of weakness and whether there is significant spasticity. For people who have very weak arms, spasticity may actually help to keep the shoulder somewhat in place. Shoulder subluxation is usually treated with physical interventions

Table 6.4. **Symptoms of Anxiety**

Feeling tense or nervous

Feeling jittery or jumpy

Having difficulty relaxing

Feeling fatigued

Having muscle aches

Feeling restless

Feeling apprehensive

Feeling fearful or anticipating misfortune

Feeling sweaty or having clammy hands

Feeling chest palpitations or heart racing

Having a stomachache

Feeling light-headed or dizzy

Having difficulty sleeping

Feeling "on edge"

Feeling terrified without apparent reason

Anticipating impending doom

Feeling short of breath

Experiencing a choking or smothering sensation

Feeling faint

Trembling or shaking

Source: Reprinted with permission from Julie K. Silver, *Post-Polio Syndrome: A Guide for Polio Survivors and Their Families* (Yale University Press, 2001).

such as proper positioning of the arm on some type of armrest or other support, use of a sling, and gentle range-of-motion exercises. Some doctors recommend using medications such as acetaminophen (Tylenol) or anti-inflammatories (such as ibuprofen or naproxen) to help lessen the pain. To help with severe refractory pain (*refractory pain* is pain that does not improve with oral or intravenous pain medication), *transcutaneous electrical nerve stimulation (TENS)* or *functional electrical stimulation (FES)* are sometimes used, though their use remains somewhat controversial. TENS machines produce non-painful electrical signals on the skin, which are transmitted to the brain and may decrease pain by not allowing so many pain signals to reach the brain. A TENS unit is about as big as a cell phone and can hook onto slacks in the same manner as a cell phone. Small electrodes that stick to the skin are attached to the unit. A TENS unit can be worn intermittently or all day.

A second reason why someone might experience pain after a stroke is *reflex sympathetic dystrophy (RSD)* or what is now called *complex regional pain syndrome (CRPS) type I*. This type of pain usually involves the affected arm and/or hand. We don't know why or exactly how CRPS occurs after a stroke, but it usually starts with noticeable and sometimes quite severe pain in the arm or hand and swelling of the hand, which becomes either warm or cool to the touch. The treatment for CRPS can be very involved and generally includes oral medications and/or injections. Physical or occupational therapy may also improve symptoms and can involve gentle massage, hot and cold baths, warm paraffin wax baths, and trying a TENS unit or FES.

A third possible cause of pain in stroke survivors is what we used to call a *thalamic pain syndrome*, because it seemed to occur primarily in people who had an injury to the part of the brain called the *thalamus*. We now know that it can occur in stroke survivors who had injuries in other brain locations, so we now call it *central post-stroke pain syndrome*. Most patients who have this condition experience pain on one side of the body that may affect the arm, trunk, and leg. The pain may be worse with external stimuli such as heat or cold. Many people with this syndrome complain of feeling uncomfortably cold on one side of their body. This type of pain can be quite severe and often does not respond very well to medications, which are the primary source of treatment. Fortunately, it is not very common, affecting perhaps 2 to 3 percent of stroke survivors. If you think you may be suffering from central post-stroke pain syndrome, talk to your doctor about treatment options. Even though this type of pain can be difficult to treat, many people find relief from a variety of different medications.

Spasticity

Spasticity is often defined as an abnormal increase in muscle tone. This means that the muscles feel stiff and don't move fluidly as they normally would. For instance, if someone has spasticity in his leg, the leg will feel stiff and he will have to fight against this stiffness to bend the knee or to lift the foot off the ground when walking. Spasticity frequently occurs after a stroke. It can range in severity from subtle to profound. Sometimes spasms and pain are associated with spasticity, but more often the primary symptom of spasticity after stroke is simply that the affected arm or leg is not moving as easily as it once did.

Spasticity is a problem when it interferes with someone's ability to do everyday activities such as walking, dressing, or having sexual relations. On the other hand, if an individual has a lot of leg weakness after a stroke,

Table 6.5. Oral Medications for Spasticity

Lioresal (baclofen)

Benzodiazepines, such as Valium (diazepam)

Zanaflex (tizanidine)

Dantrium (dantrolene)

Note: In addition to other potential side effects, all of these medications may cause sedation and a change in cognitive ability. Usually this is a dose-dependent effect, and sedation is minimized with a lower dose.

spasticity can actually help them walk better. If the leg weren't stiff from the increased spasticity, it would not be able to hold the person upright.

There are no special tests to diagnose spasticity. Rather, a doctor diagnoses the condition by physical examination. Stroke alone is the underlying *cause* of the spasticity, but the spasticity can be increased by extreme heat or cold, anxiety, infections, and pain (even something as seemingly benign as an ingrown toenail can make it worse). The first attempt to treat spasticity involves removing anything that could possibly cause it to be more pronounced. Treatment is then directed at reducing the amount of stiffness without causing intolerable side effects. Unfortunately, many oral medications used to treat spasticity are limited in their usefulness because they cause severe fatigue. (The oral medications used to treat spasticity are listed in Table 6.5.) Injections are sometimes helpful to treat spasticity; the two main types of injections used are botulinum toxin and phenol blocks. Both types can be very useful in certain situations, and botulinum toxin injections in particular are very well tolerated. Gentle stretching is an important part of managing spasticity, and sometimes splints or even temporary casts may also be needed to help with positioning. In extreme cases, surgical procedures can be beneficial; however, in most patients, spasticity is managed with stretching, positioning, and medications.

Driving

Driving gives people a lot of independence and greatly adds to their quality of life. It is also inherently dangerous—even under the best of circumstances. If you or someone you love has had a stroke, getting right back into the driver's seat is probably not a wise move. After a stroke, there are many things that can interfere with someone's ability to drive safely. These problems include, but are not limited to, seizures, difficulty with vision (including depth perception), inability to correctly take in all of the surroundings (often found with stroke-related "neglect syndromes," which can cause someone to not be aware of certain things in the environment or even of parts of their own body), partial paralysis of extremities, and cognitive issues such as impulsivity, slowed reactions, indecisiveness, distractibility, and poor judgment.

Despite all of these potential problems, many stroke survivors do return to driving. If you have had a stroke, we recommend checking with your doctor before you resume driving—to protect yourself and others. Many doctors will order a computer-simulated driving evaluation that can be done at a rehabilitation facility with a therapist who is skilled in assessing things like reaction time, visual acuity, and so on. If you pass this test, you may also be referred to a driving instructor for an "on the road" assessment. You may also need to take a formal driving road test from your local motor vehicle agency. If you pass these tests, it is safe to assume that you are ready to get behind the steering wheel. If you are excessively nervous about taking these tests, you should stop and consider whether it is truly safe for you to drive. Although driving allows people a great deal of independence, it can be a very dangerous activity for someone who has had a stroke. Formal testing is the best way there is of assessing whether someone is competent to drive. This type of testing is designed to protect the stroke survivor as well as innocent passengers, pedestrians, and other drivers.

We understand that the loss of the ability to drive can be devastating, but it is essential to note that many people have happy and productive lives without ever driving. For example, people with unpredictable seizure disorders are restricted from driving. Most people have numerous options for travel within their community without driving themselves, such as public transportation, taxis, van services, and buses that cater to individuals with disabilities. These services are often subsidized so that the cost to the user who is unable to drive for medical reasons is minimal or even free. If you are unable to drive, consider trying other means of getting around. Ask your rehabilitation team about services in your community. You can contact the local hospital social work department for this information. Boredom leads to depression after a stroke, and for most people, the ability to go places is what matters—the process of driving is not usually essential to happiness.

Before we leave the topic of going places, we want to mention that handicapped plates or placards are available to people who have had a stroke—whether they drive or are a passenger. These notices allow people to park in specific areas located close to entrances, limiting the distance they have to move from their vehicle. Applying for a handicapped plate does not mean that you can't drive. Simply contact your local motor vehicle registry and ask for the application. This simple form contains a section for you to fill out and a section for your doctor to complete, and takes about five minutes. We routinely encourage people who have had a stroke to obtain a handicapped plate or placard if they have any mobility issues at all. If you have had a stroke but are not inclined to use the handicapped license plate, then consider obtaining the placard, which you can put in your window only when you need it. Some people just use it in inclement weather or when they have to walk a long distance (such as at a stadium or amusement park, where the entrance can be quite a hike from the parking), so they don't risk falling or becoming excessively tired.

Work

Billions of dollars are lost each year due to employment issues (including direct health care costs and lost productivity) stemming from chronic illness. Although statistics can be impressive, they cannot express the real suffering that occurs when someone who provides financial support to their family is affected by a stroke or any other medical condition. Work is valued in society and has been for centuries—the Bible says, "There is nothing better for a man than to rejoice in his work" (Ecclesiastes 3:22). After a stroke, many people simply can't work—their injuries are too severe. Others are able to return to work with some adaptations such as working shorter hours or typing using voice-activated computer software instead of a keyboard. Still others are able to return to their regular jobs without any significant accommodations.

A few years ago, a study titled "The Impact of Stroke on World Leaders" was published.[1] In this study, the authors identified twenty world leaders who had suffered strokes during a thirty-year period beginning in 1970. Although half of the affected leaders lost their political power immediately or shortly after their injury, the other half remained in power for three or more years after their strokes. The study does not give any details on the severity of the strokes or on rehabilitation treatment efforts for any of the leaders, but it is probably safe to assume that they all had access to state-of-the-art medical care. However, state-of-the-art medical care in 1970 was certainly not the same as it is now. It is likely that with the treatments currently available, even more of these leaders would have been able to remain in power if they had a stroke while in office today.

Research on stroke survivors returning to work has given varied results, but it seems that 60 percent or more of previously employed stroke survivors do return to some type of gainful employment. Whether to return to work is a complicated decision that affects many members of the family, who may rely on the income of the stroke survivor. The loss of previous financial status can be devastating for the entire family. When Maggie Strong's husband became ill with a stroke, she wrote about her family's ordeal and coined the term "downwardly mobile" to describe the effect his loss of income had on her and her children.

> Jeremy had a stroke when he was 40 years old. Jeremy was a self-employed computer consultant, and he and his family accumulated more than $50,000 in debt during the time that he was out of work due to his stroke. Although he recovered quickly and well (his recovery was nearly complete after the first three months), he was out of work for four months and then worked part time for the next twelve months. Of course, both Jeremy and his wife were delighted with how well he recovered; however, their entire family struggled financially for the next few years as Jeremy worked to repay the debt.

Many stroke survivors do not recover as well as Jeremy and may have ongoing health problems that make returning to work difficult or even impossible.

There are many useful types of adaptive equipment that may help someone who has had a stroke return to work, including computer keyboards designed to be used with just one hand and voice-activated word processing programs that are becoming increasingly easy to use. In fact, there are so many types of equipment that may be helpful that there isn't space here to describe them all. And though the examples given are for office workers, there is adaptive equipment to help people in nearly all professions. If you or a loved one needs assistance returning to work, the ideal place to find help is a rehabilitation facility that has occupational therapists, vocational rehabilitation professionals, and perhaps even an assistive technology department (usually located in a rehabilitation hospital) specializing in prescribing adaptive equipment.

In 1990, the Americans with Disabilities Act (ADA) made it illegal for employers to discriminate against individuals with disabilities, including stroke, as long as they could perform the *essential functions of their jobs with or without reasonable accommodations*. The heart of the ADA is that employers must provide "reasonable accommodations" for employees who have a disability and require some type of assistance or special equipment in order to continue working. The law was designed to try to level the playing field a little bit, and in fact, the ADA defines reasonable accommodations as "changes to the work environment or the way in which tasks are customarily performed to enable an individual with a disability to enjoy equal employment opportunities." Reasonable accommodations can vary greatly. They might be a reduced workload or a special piece of equipment. We generally recommend that people who have had a stroke use the term "reasonable accommodation" in any written communications with their employers about making changes to their work environment.

In some instances, there are no reasonable accommodations that will allow someone to resume the job they had before a stroke. In this case, there are two choices: either retrain in another vocation or discontinue working. We generally encourage stroke survivors who are not near retirement age to seek vocational retraining whenever possible. Most people in this society see work as an important part of who they are and how they view themselves. People who become totally disabled and don't return to work often lose their sense of self-esteem and their social support system and face serious financial hardship. Not only does financial hardship affect the entire family, but family members will also be affected if a parent or partner loses their sense of purpose and self-esteem.

The cost of meeting with a vocational counselor and undergoing retraining will usually be paid by either your health or disability insurer or by a government agency dedicated to providing vocational guidance and counseling. Most vocational services are funded by the federal government (through the United States Department of Health and Human Services) and channeled to state vocational agencies. For more information, contact the Council of State Administrators of Vocational Rehabilitation (see Resources). The agency names vary from state to state, but they are similar in their mission, which is to restore individuals with disabilities to the highest level of employment of which they are capable.

The second option is to stop working. Retirement may be an option for some people. Others can apply for "total disability" benefits (meaning that they are completely disabled—usually for life) through a private disability insurance policy (if they have one) or through the government's Social Security Disability Insurance or Social Security Income programs. The difference between the two government-supported disability programs is, in part, that to qualify for Social Security Disability Insurance you must have contributed to this fund through taxes.

Intimacy and Sex

The majority of stroke survivors and spouses report a change in intimacy and sexual intercourse after a stroke. In one study, more than half the men surveyed reported difficulty having an erection at all, and 1 of 3 men complained of having difficulty with erections and ejaculation. There are many reasons for a decrease in intimacy, including that one or both partners becomes less interested. This lack of interest might be due to injury to the brain from the stroke, side effects of medications, concern about having another stroke, or depression in either partner. The partner may not want to engage in sexual activity for fear of hurting the person who has had a stroke or because the partner is depressed. Some partners might also be concerned about having sex with a "sick person" and may believe that physical intimacy is only for healthy people and might cause harm or even another stroke. If the person who has had a stroke requires a lot of care, especially with bathing and other hygiene issues, this can change the nature of the relationship and affect intimacy.

If you or your loved one has had a negative change in your sexual life because of a stroke, you are not alone. However, there may be help. Talking to a doctor knowledgeable about intimacy issues is a good place to start. She can review medications that might cause sexual side effects and consider the possibility of untreated depression in either partner. Clinical social workers and psychiatrists may also be able to offer counseling on intimacy issues as they relate to disability.

Intimacy involves many facets of a relationship, and love can be communicated in many ways, including a gentle voice or a soft caress.

In this chapter we have described some of the more common medical and social post-stroke issues that you or a loved one may be facing. Your doctor should be able to provide you with more specific information and help. In the Resources section of this book, we list some additional resources that may assist you.

••

Part III

PREVENTING STROKE: MEDICAL ISSUES

•••

Chapter 7

Risk Factors for Having a Stroke: An Introduction

In Part I we discussed what a stroke is and how it can affect our bodies and our brains. In Part II, we described the process of recovering from a stroke. Now we are ready to move on to what we consider the heart of this book: *how to prevent another stroke from occurring.* This chapter is a short overview of what you can do to protect yourself from having another stroke. Of course, no one can guarantee that you won't have another stroke, but what we *can* tell you is that there are a number of proven ways to reduce your chance of having a stroke.

In Parts III and IV we break these approaches down into discussions of medical issues and lifestyle issues. We know that it is unlikely that anyone reading this book will have all of the medical problems that we review; however, even if you don't have a particular medical condition, such as diabetes, you may find some of the information in that chapter helpful. This is also true for the lifestyle issues.

Our goal is to provide you with a general overview of the most common medical conditions and lifestyle factors that can contribute to having a stroke. We firmly believe that the better informed you are, the healthier you can become. However, this book can in no way replace good advice from your doctor about the exact steps you should take to minimize your risk of having a stroke in the future. For example, in Chapter 16 we discuss the tremendous benefits of exercise for stroke prevention. Yet, we know that some people who read this book will not be able to exercise sufficiently to reduce their stroke risk. In fact, for a few people (such as those with severe heart valve problems), exercise may be downright dangerous. As you read the next two sections, we encourage you to take in as much of the information as possible, but when it comes time to incorporate our suggestions into your life, we ask that you consult with your doctor, who will be best able to give you advice about your health.

Table 7.1. **Stroke Risk Factors You Can Change**

Smoking
Excessive alcohol use
Illicit drug use
Obesity
Physical inactivity

Table 7.2. **Stroke Risk Factors You Can Influence**

History of diabetes
History of high cholesterol
History of high blood pressure
History of heart conditions (such as atrial fibrillation)
History of narrowing of the arteries (such as carotid stenosis)

Table 7.3. **Stroke Risk Factors You Cannot Change**

Age
Race
Sex
Family history of medical conditions related to stroke

When we talk about someone's risk of having another stroke, we are analyzing those factors that make it more or less likely for a stroke to occur. You can change some risk factors, such as your diet. The risk factors you can change are listed in Table 7.1. Other risk factors you can't entirely change, but you can modify to some degree (Table 7.2). For example, if you have hypertension, you may not be able to change the fact that you have this condition, but you certainly can lower your blood pressure by eating a diet low in salt and taking medications that your doctor prescribes. And finally, there are some risk factors that you can't do anything about (Table 7.3). For instance, your age. If you are 80 years old, you are certainly at higher risk for a stroke than if you are 40, but you can't do anything to change that.

Table 7.4. **The Top Ten Stroke Prevention Guidelines**

---

1. Know your blood pressure. Have it checked at least once a year. If it is elevated, work with your doctor to keep it under control.
2. If you smoke, stop.
3. Find out if you have atrial fibrillation.
4. If you drink alcohol, do so in moderation.
5. Find out if you have high cholesterol, and if so, work with your doctor to control it.
6. If you are diabetic, follow your doctor's recommendations carefully to control your diabetes.
7. Include exercise in the activities you enjoy in your daily routine.
8. Enjoy a lower-sodium (salt), lower-fat diet.
9. Ask your doctor if you have circulation problems that increase your risk for stroke.
10. If you experience any stroke symptoms, seek immediate medical attention.

Source: Adapted from the National Stroke Association.

When we assess someone's risk of having another stroke, we think about all of these factors, whether they can be changed or not. Being aware of any risk factors you may have for stroke that can't be changed (such as a family history of stroke) may help you focus your efforts on fixing the other risk factors that you can impact (such as your diet). In this book we pay most attention to the risk factors that you can either change or at least influence in your favor. In the next few chapters, we will discuss these risk factors in greater detail.

If you have had a stroke, now is a good time to make some changes in your life. You may already have started. If so, you are ahead of the game, and making a few more changes will be easier. If not, then there are likely many things that you can do to help yourself. Either way, think of this in a positive way: there are things that you can do to help yourself, so read about them and then put them into practice. Your doctor can assist you by providing good medical information and by prescribing appropriate treatments based on your particular needs. You will likely have to make several appointments with your physician over the next few weeks or months to attend to all of the various issues that we discuss in the next two sections. Your family and friends can help you by encouraging you to make healthy lifestyle changes. Perhaps they can even make these healthy lifestyle changes, too.

While we certainly recognize that there is often a period of grief mixed with anxiety after someone has had a stroke, we also know that people who "take charge" and begin to make positive changes will feel empowered. As well they should, because the truth is that there are a number of steps you can take to lower your risk of having another stroke. To begin, take a look at Table 7.4, which is a good summary of the top ten things you can do to prevent another stroke.

• •

Chapter 8

Heart and Blood Vessel Conditions and Stroke

The heart and the brain work together, so it's easy to see how certain conditions of the heart and the blood vessels can lead to stroke. The heart pumps blood that contains oxygen and nutrients through the arteries to the brain. As we discussed in earlier chapters, the brain is like a garden that needs regular infusions from a garden hose (the arteries) in order to thrive. The brain is very sensitive to the availability of oxygen and nutrients and requires an uninterrupted supply of fresh blood.

What can go wrong? Even a brief interruption of the blood supply, lasting less than a minute, can cause part of the brain to temporarily stop functioning. If the interruption lasts long enough, permanent damage to the brain can result—a stroke. One cause of an interruption in the blood supply is a buildup of fatty material in the blood vessels that carry blood from the heart to the brain; this condition is called *atherosclerosis*. Problems with the heart's rhythm, efficiency of pumping, or anatomical structure also can cause a stroke. Let's look at each of these situations in more detail.

Atherosclerosis and Stroke

In Greek, the word *atheroma* means porridge, or gruel. That's an easy way to remember that *atherosclerosis* means blockage of the medium-sized and large arteries due to a buildup of gunky, fatty material called *cholesterol plaque* (Figure 8.1). Atherosclerosis is also sometimes called *hardening of the arteries*. Although atherosclerosis doesn't usually cause symptoms until middle or old age, the process of atherosclerosis appears to start in young adulthood.

The Layers of the Artery

Looking at an artery under a microscope, one sees three distinct layers that are normally neat and organized.

1. The first, innermost, layer of the artery is called the *intima*. It makes direct contact with the circulating blood, which does not normally make contact with the other blood vessel layers. This layer is mostly made up of specialized, relatively flat cells called *endothelial cells.*

2. The next (middle) layer of the artery is known as the *media.* This layer, which is thicker than the intima, is made up of smooth muscle cells. These muscle cells can contract or relax; they help to regulate the blood flow through the blood vessel by controlling the diameter of the blood vessel.

3. The outermost layer of the artery is called the *adventitia*. The adventitia provides structural support for the blood vessels. It is made up of a fibrous substance called connective tissue.

Cholesterol and the Artery

Think about your arteries as hosting a wild party. The arteries are a great location for this party because a lot of partiers can get there easily. When they arrive at the party, the guests must enter through a door. They must make their way between and past some cells that serve as "bouncers." The bouncers are the *endothelial (E) cells* in the intima layer of the blood vessels. Normally, the E cells work hard to maintain the organization and the integrity of the arteries. This job involves being selective about which cells gain entrance into the artery wall. E cells also send substances into the blood to prevent the formation of blood clots.

Any damage to the E cells disrupts their ability to perform their bouncer duties. Atherosclerosis begins when these E cells are damaged because of any of the following conditions:

1. Turbulent blood flow through the arteries, which occurs in parts of the arteries where smaller blood vessels branch off
2. High blood pressure (hypertension) in the arteries
3. Too much cholesterol in the blood
4. Too much sugar in the blood (diabetes)
5. Toxic chemicals in the blood (such as those from cigarette smoking)

Damage to the E cells can make them less effective in protecting the artery wall; in other words, they open more doors and they open them wider to allow additional cells to exit the blood and enter the arterial walls. When the E cells are damaged, more cells can join the party.

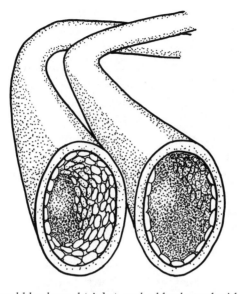

Figure 8.1. *A normal blood vessel* (right) *and a blood vessel with atherosclerosis and plaque formation* (left). *Atherosclerosis is a condition that gets worse over time. As the plaque in the arteries builds up along the walls, the diameter of the blood vessel gets smaller. In come cases, the diameter becomes narrow enough that blood flow is restricted. This restriction of blood flow can lead to stroke.*

What's being served at the party? The answer is lots of cholesterol, mostly low density lipoprotein (LDL) cholesterol. Once in the arteries, LDL can be modified or changed. For the sake of our analogy, we will say the change adds salt to them. Regular LDL is like potato chips without salt, and modified LDL is like potato chips with salt. The partiers love the potato chips with salt and can't stop eating them.

Who are the partiers? Who is entering through the spaces in between the damaged bouncers—the E cells—and eating all the modified LDL (the salted potato chips)? The answer is white blood cells (cells that usually fight infections) called *monocytes* (*M cells*). These M cells love potato chips with salt. In fact, they fill up on the salty chips. They are so excited about the party that the M cells send out invitations to their friends, the *smooth muscle (SM) cells*. The SM cells receive these invitations to join the party. They move from their middle layer of the artery into the inside layer of the artery to join the M cells. They surround the M cells and eat some salted potato chips (modified LDL) as well.

As with every party, there is a mess at the end. In this case, the mess is a clump of partiers: the filled-up M cells and their friends, the SM cells. The nice, neat, normal artery wall is now completely disrupted. A clump of cells protrudes from the artery wall into the hole of the artery where the blood flows. This clump of cells is called a *plaque*. Plaques are made up primarily of the M and SM cells that have eaten modified LDL. The clumps can get large and clog or block the artery. No one is left to clean up the mess. A cholesterol party in an artery leading to the brain could create such a large mess (plaque) that the artery might be clogged and a stroke might occur. Likewise, a cholesterol party in an artery inside the brain itself might cause a stroke.

The cholesterol party in the artery is a simple analogy for a very complex process. The important things to remember about the analogy are:

1. Damage to the E cells is necessary to start the party, because the damage disrupts the function of the bouncers, who then become much less selective about which cells and how many cells they allow into the arterial wall. Damage is created by the stress of high blood pressure, high cholesterol, high blood sugar, and toxins (from cigarette smoking, for example).
2. Cholesterol is necessary for the party. The more cholesterol you eat, the more food you are supplying for the M cells. The more the M cells eat at the party, the more plaque they will make.
3. If the plaque is large enough, it may block blood flow in the artery. That's why you should watch the amount of cholesterol in your diet. Just think of the M cells getting fatter and fatter inside your arteries and making a bigger and bigger mess.

Again, the condition in which fatty buildup blocks blood flow is called *atherosclerosis*; it is also sometimes called *hardening of the arteries.*

How Atherosclerosis Causes Stroke

Sometimes a cholesterol plaque grows large enough to block the entire opening within the artery, and blood flow will no longer be possible. If this artery is located within the heart, the blockage may cause a heart attack. If the blocked artery supplies blood to the brain, the blockage may cause a stroke. A complete blockage of a blood vessel doesn't always result in a stroke, though. In fact, if the blood vessel blockage proceeds slowly, the body will often recruit nearby blood vessels to help out. These helper blood vessels, known as *collateral blood vessels,* are the body's own natural way of bypassing the blockage. If these collaterals are sufficient in size and number, enough blood may flow through them to prevent a stroke by supplying the area beyond the blood vessel blockage, even if the blockage of the main artery to this area is complete. In other cases, the collaterals do not prevent the stroke, but they do reduce the extent of the damage. It takes time for collaterals to develop, so a sudden blockage of a blood vessel may cause more severe damage than a blockage that develops gradually.

Blockages of the arteries can cause stroke in several different ways. In some cases, the plaque first partially blocks the artery, and then a blood clot forms on top of the plaque, causing a complete blockage of the blood vessel. This type of stroke is known as *thrombosis* or *thrombotic stroke* (a blood clot is a *thrombus*). In other cases, a piece of the plaque breaks off and blocks blood flow downstream; the mass is known as an *embolus,* and if an embolus causes a stroke, it is said to be an *embolic stroke.* A piece of plaque from a larger artery such as the carotid artery (located in the neck) can break off and end up in a smaller artery, such as the middle cerebral artery in the brain. When this happens, the plaque can block blood flow and cause a stroke. There are other causes of embolic stroke, as well, such as a blood clot developing in the heart and breaking off (these will be discussed in the next section). Sometimes doctors have difficulty determining whether a stroke resulted from a thrombus or an embolus, because the result is the same.

Symptoms of Atherosclerosis

The symptoms of atherosclerosis depend on the location of the cholesterol buildup. If the plaques are in the arteries in the heart (known as the *coronary arteries*), then the symptoms will be related to the heart and the person will develop coronary artery disease. Symptoms do not usually appear until the disease is in the advanced stages, with plaque blocking 70 percent of the opening in the artery. The first symptom may be chest pain or even a heart attack. If the buildup of cholesterol is in the cerebral arteries (the arteries in the brain), the person may experience a stroke or transient ischemic attack as the first symptom of atherosclerosis. Another common area for cholesterol buildup is the arteries that supply the legs. When people have a buildup of plaque there, they experience pain in their legs after walking. This condition is called *claudication.*

Diagnosing Atherosclerosis

There are several ways to obtain images of the blood vessels to make a definitive diagnosis of atherosclerosis in the cerebral vessels. The most detailed images are obtained through a test called an *angiogram,* or *angiography.* In an angiogram, a special dye (contrast material) is injected into the blood vessels, and then x-rays are taken of the blood vessels. This dye shows up on x-rays, so the outline of the vessels can be clearly visualized. Angiograms can be taken of the arteries in the brain, heart, or legs. Similar images can now be obtained using CT scans with a less invasive technique (known as *CT angiography*), as well as using MRI (*MR angiography*). These tests allow physicians to look at the arteries to see if there are blockages. For more information on these tests, please refer to Chapter 3.

There is a simple, painless test to evaluate for atherosclerosis in the carotid arteries of the neck that send blood to the brain. This test is known as the *carotid duplex ultrasound study.* The carotid duplex ultrasound study uses high frequency sound waves to demonstrate blood flow in the large arteries and veins of the head and neck. (Details of carotid duplex ultrasound tests are provided in Chapter 3.)

Again, individuals who have high cholesterol are more likely to have atherosclerosis. A simple blood test can reveal your cholesterol level. All it takes is about five milliliters of blood, which equals one teaspoonful. A fasting cholesterol test is the most helpful type, because it does not allow your last meal to heavily influence your results, and it allows you to check your low density lipoprotein (LDL) and high density lipoprotein (HDL) levels as well as your total cholesterol. From the cholesterol party analogy, you know that the LDL is the "bad" cholesterol, the kind that the M cells eat at the party. There is also "good" cholesterol, the HDL, whose job it is to take the cholesterol out of the bloodstream and return it to the liver. HDL helps to decrease the chance that a cholesterol party will form.

Check Tables 8.1, 8.2, and 8.3 to determine whether your cholesterol levels are desirable. This categorization system is the one used by the American Heart Association. If you have high total cholesterol with a value of 240 mg/dL or greater, then you have more than twice the risk of heart disease compared to someone whose cholesterol is below 200 mg/dL. If your HDL is equal to or greater than 60 mg/dL, then your HDL is considered protective against heart disease. However, if your HDL is less than 40 mg/dL, then your HDL is considered a risk factor for heart disease.

Table 8.1. Interpreting Total Cholesterol Levels

Cholesterol value mg/dL	
<200	Normal
200–239	Borderline high
≥240	High

Table 8.2. Interpreting LDL Cholesterol Levels

LDL mg/dL	
<100	Optimal
100–129	Near optimal
130–159	Borderline high
160–189	High
>190	Very high

Table 8.3. Interpreting HDL Cholesterol Levels

HDL mg/dL	
<40	Risk factor for heart disease
>60	Protective against heart disease

Preventing Atherosclerosis

Prevention is the optimal approach to reducing the risk of stroke from atherosclerosis, just as it is for many other causes of stroke. Thankfully, effective treatments for atherosclerosis now exist even for individuals who have already had a stroke due to atherosclerosis. If your first stroke was caused by atherosclerosis, or if your doctor tells you that you have this condition, there are some steps you can take.

In his book *I Am What I Ate . . . and I'm Frightened!!!*, comedian Bill Cosby describes how he reacted when his doctor told him that with his high cholesterol level he might have some blockage in his carotid artery: "Now generally, you can wish things away. But carotid artery! Blockage! These are words one doesn't want to hear in the same sentence. . . . And there is no carotid artery floss. Not even if you're the grand master of yoga. You can't put a string in your nose and floss. . . . So this stuff, this plaque, is stuck. And I thought to myself, Oh my God! I am what I ate. And I'm frightened."[1]

You needn't panic like Bill Cosby did if your doctor tells you that your cholesterol level is too high. Remember, knowledge is power, so first learn what you can about what cholesterol is and how you can get your total cholesterol level down. The lower the level of LDL (the "bad cholesterol"), the better. The higher the level of HDL (the "good cholesterol"), the lower the risk of atherosclerosis.

The first step in controlling elevated cholesterol is improving your diet and increasing your exercise level. If we are beginning to sound redundant, it is because diet and exercise are incredibly important in preventing recurrent stroke. We can't emphasize this truth enough, though we do advise you to use caution when changing your diet or exercise regimen. Consult a physician before planning any drastic changes in diet. Paying attention to these two areas can help alleviate medical problems and reduce your risk of stroke in multiple ways. Diets lower in fat and higher in fruits, vegetables, and whole grains are important in reducing your level of LDL ("bad") cholesterol and raising your level of HDL ("good") cholesterol. Exercise simultaneously lowers LDL and raises HDL cholesterol.

For many individuals, exercise and diet are enough to bring cholesterol levels into the healthy range, and they do not need to take cholesterol-lowering medications. For others, exercise and diet help reduce the dose of medication needed and contribute to overall control of high cholesterol. In someone who has already had a stroke, the goal should be to lower the cholesterol level to a safe range through an aggressive regimen that often contains all three elements: diet, exercise, and prescription medications. If you have had a stroke or are at risk of having a stroke, your doctor may have a low threshold for starting you on a cholesterol-lowering medication and may not think it is advisable to wait several months to see if diet and exercise alone will work.

While several classes of medication are available for reducing high cholesterol, the most widely used are the "statin" medications. These include atorvastatin (Lipitor), pravastatin (Pravachol), fluvastatin (Lescol), simvastatin (Zocor), rosuvastatin (Crestor), and lovastatin (Mevacor). While all of these medications are effective in lowering cholesterol, some of them are more powerful than others, with Lipitor and Crestor the most potent available in the United States. These medications are generally well tolerated (they produce few side effects) and can result in cholesterol reductions ranging from 20 to 60 percent. The most common side effect of these medications is muscle inflammation, which can make the muscles weak and painful and make it necessary to stop taking the medication. Some individuals are able to tolerate an alternative statin, though some need to switch to other, non-statin, cholesterol-lowering medications.

Alternative medications include bile acid binding medications, such as cholestyramine (Questran) or colestipol (Colestid). These medications can cause gastrointestinal side effects, such as constipation and flatulence. Nicotinic acid is effective for reducing LDL cholesterol and increasing HDL but can cause a flushing sensation and is not tolerated by many people.

Fibrate medications, which include gemfibrozol (Lopid) and fenofibrate (Triglide, Tricor), help to elevate HDL cholesterol levels but have less effect on LDL cholesterol. These medications can also cause gastrointestinal side effects, such as abdominal discomfort or diarrhea. When used in conjunction with statins, they increase the risk of muscle inflammation as well.

Ezetimibe (Zetia) is a newer and easier to take non-statin drug that reduces cholesterol absorption in the intestine, resulting in a reduction in LDL cholesterol. It may be particularly useful when taken in combination with a statin. A combination tablet containing both ezetimibe and simvistatin is now available (Vytorin).

Coronary Artery Disease and Stroke

Atherosclerosis in the coronary arteries—the blood vessels supplying blood to the heart—is known as *coronary artery disease,* or CAD. Many people know CAD simply as *heart disease,* but heart disease actually encompasses CAD and many other conditions that can affect the heart. CAD is a dangerous disease because it can lead to a heart attack (*myocardial infarction*) and sudden death from cardiac arrest. According to the American Heart Association, 13 million Americans have coronary artery disease. In the United States, 7.1 million people who are still living have had a heart attack. Coronary artery disease is the number one killer in the United States, causing about 500,000 deaths each year.

Risk Factors for Coronary Artery Disease

Of the many risk factors for coronary artery disease, some are within our control and some are beyond our control. These risk factors are listed in Table 8.4.

Although coronary artery disease is often thought of as a disease of men, and more men than women experience heart attacks before the age of 55, women are also at risk for this disease. In fact, by the age of 65, women

Table 8.4. Risk Factors for Coronary Artery Disease

Risk Factors You Can Change or Influence
Elevated cholesterol
High blood pressure
Obesity (>30 percent over ideal body weight)
Smoking
Diabetes
Sedentary lifestyle

Risk Factors You Cannot Change
Male sex
Age (55 years or older)
A family history of a father who had a heart attack before age 55 or a
    mother who had a heart attack before age 65
A disorder known as *familial hypercholesterolemia* (unusually high choles-
    terol levels from a very early age)

---

catch up to men as their incidence of heart attacks increases. We don't
know why CAD develops at different ages in men and women. In the past,
it was thought that estrogen played a role in this difference between the
sexes. (We discuss estrogen in Chapter 11.)

The Association between Coronary Artery Disease and Stroke

There is a strong connection between CAD and stroke. When atherosclerosis develops in the arteries of the heart, it often develops elsewhere in the
body at the same time, such as in the blood vessels that supply the brain
with blood. In fact, the most common cause of death in stroke survivors is
CAD, not a second stroke. Conversely, a person who has just had a large
heart attack is at risk for suffering from a stroke because her heart may not
be pumping efficiently, allowing blood to pool in the heart. This pooled
blood can clot and act as a source for an embolus (a piece of clot that breaks
off and travels to a smaller vessel).

Symptoms of Coronary Artery Disease

Atherosclerosis does not cause CAD symptoms until a cholesterol plaque
blocks about 70 percent of the blood flow to an area of the heart. At this point,
the heart cells no longer receive enough blood to keep them supplied with
oxygen and other nutrients, and they send out pain signals to the brain.

When the heart works harder during exercise, it requires more blood and oxygen. For this reason, the first symptom of coronary artery disease is typically chest pain (*angina pectoris*) that occur during exertion such as exercise. As CAD progresses and plaque blocks more of the blood vessel or vessels, people also notice angina when they are resting. The symptoms of angina are often described as a pressure, heaviness, or tightness in the chest, but it can also be a sharp or gassy-feeling pain. Some people describe it as "heartburn" or feeling like "an elephant is sitting on my chest." Along with the angina, some people experience pain or numbness and tingling in the left arm, shortness of breath, nausea, and sweating. It is important to know that heart attacks can occur without chest or arm pain. People with diabetes are particularly prone to having advanced CAD without chest pain; this condition is known as *silent ischemia*.

Don, a 51-year-old New York businessman, was running to catch an 11:00 p.m. train home when he experienced a "pressure in his chest." He described the pain as feeling as though someone were sitting on top of his chest. The chest pressure was accompanied by tingling in his left arm and difficulty breathing. When Don arrived home half an hour later, his wife immediately took him to the hospital. The doctors in the emergency room quickly diagnosed a heart attack and admitted him to the hospital. The next morning, he collapsed when trying to walk to the bathroom. After performing several tests, the doctors discovered that Don had suffered a stroke.

Don had no idea that he had coronary artery disease. Despite the absence of warning symptoms, a large cholesterol plaque was now blocking one of his coronary arteries and cutting off the blood supply to a large part of his heart. This loss of blood supply resulted in the death of heart muscle cells. When the heart muscle is significantly injured, it does not pump efficiently, and blood may pool inside the heart. If blood sits still, it can gel together and form a blood clot. This is exactly what happened in Don's heart. A blood clot developed within his heart because of stagnant blood flow in the area of the heart muscle damage.

Don's stroke occurred because a small piece of the blood clot in his heart broke off and traveled to his brain. This fragment, known as an embolus, entered the bloodstream through the arteries and traveled as far as it could go until it got stuck. It happened to get stuck in the right middle cerebral artery that supplies blood to the brain.

Don's story illustrates how a heart attack can lead to a stroke. Of course, not every heart attack causes a stroke. In fact, when a patient is admitted to the hospital with a heart attack, doctors often immediately prescribe a blood thinner to prevent a clot from forming in the heart or its arteries. In particular, a blood thinner called heparin is often given intravenously to these patients. By the time the patient is discharged, the heparin can be discontinued unless a thrombus has formed in the heart. In some circumstances, a blood thinner may be inappropriate, such as for a person with recent abnormal bleeding from the stomach or in the brain.

Diagnosing Coronary Artery Disease

If you have chest pain or have had a heart attack, a cardiologist can examine your coronary arteries in several different ways: a stress test, a radioisotope stress test, or an angiogram. Each method has some degree of risk and each method has its limitations.

The least invasive of the tests is the exercise stress test. During this test, a person exercises on a treadmill or on a stationary bicycle. Prior to the exercise, a nurse places EKG leads (small, sticky patches) directly on the person's skin in specific positions on the chest. Attaching the sticky patches to the skin is painless but removing them can be slightly uncomfortable, similar to removing a Band-Aid. The test starts when the EKG leads are in place and the person starts exercising. The EKG leads record the electrical activity of the heart, which gives the cardiologist an idea of how the heart is functioning. The exercise stresses the heart and makes it pump harder and more frequently. Blockages in the coronary arteries that are not evident at rest may become clear during exercise when the heart is stressed. Certain patterns on the EKG tracing are considered normal, and other patterns demonstrate that the heart is not functioning properly. There are specific patterns that reveal *ischemia* (lack of blood supply to the heart). If one of the coronary arteries has a buildup of cholesterol plaque that is not allowing an adequate blood supply to the heart during exercise, this will show up on the EKG. It tells the cardiologist that there is evidence of coronary artery disease in that heart.

During a stress test, a doctor carefully monitors the EKG tracing, blood pressure, heart rate, and a person's symptoms. The treadmill increases its grade and speed as the test continues. The doctor stops the test if the EKG reveals any ischemia, the blood pressure changes dramatically, or the person experiences any chest pain. Once the person reaches a certain exercise intensity or target heart rate, the test is over. The test usually provides a great deal of information to the cardiologist with minimal pain on the part of the patient. Risks of the procedure include abnormal heart rhythm (arrhythmia) and heart attack (which is rare because doctors closely monitor the person for changes in the EKG and stop the test at the first sign that the heart is not getting adequate oxygen).

If a person cannot exercise, a "chemical" stress test can be conducted. In a chemical stress test, the cardiologist prescribes the medication dipyridamole or adenosine to the person who cannot exercise. These medications have the same effect on the heart as exercise would, including increasing the workload of the heart, the heart rate, and the force of the heart's contractions. The patient is monitored the same way as in an exercise stress test, with EKG leads and blood pressure monitoring. The same information can be gathered from a chemical stress test as from an exercise stress test.

If a *radioisotope* (radioactive tracer) is added to the exercise stress test, more information can be obtained. This type of stress test is called a thallium stress test because the radioactive tracer used is thallium. This type of stress test is similar to the exercise stress test discussed above. However, in this test, thallium is injected into the bloodstream through the veins (intravenously) when the person reaches his maximum level of exercise. After the injection, the person lies down under a *gamma* camera, which detects the radioactive tracer. The gamma camera takes a number of pictures right after exercise. After the person rests for two to three hours, more pictures are taken by the gamma camera to get an idea of what the heart looks like at rest.

Both the after-exercise pictures and the rest pictures of the heart are informative. Examining these pictures is critical. After the thallium is injected into the bloodstream, it enters the heart muscle. In a normal heart, after exercise the radioactive tracer will be present throughout the entire heart muscle. In an abnormal heart with blockages in the coronary arteries, the radioactive tracer will not make it to certain areas of the heart muscle because the blood vessels to that area are blocked. If the area of the heart that did not pick up the radioisotope during exercise also does not pick it up at rest, this indicates there is scar tissue in the heart, most likely from an old heart attack. If the area lacking radioactive tracer after exercise picks up radioactive tracer after a period of rest, this indicates that there is some blockage in the artery supplying that part of the heart, but that part of the heart is still viable. Reading the pictures created from the thallium stress test can tell the story of the arteries without the doctor actually seeing them directly.

To see the arteries directly, a more invasive test is required—an *angiogram*. With this test, doctors get a good look at the outline of the actual arteries. With an angiogram, doctors can examine the arteries and get a sense of the amount of plaque that has built up in them, and they can estimate the amount of blood that is able to pass through the artery. How can it do all this? It uses contrast dye and x-ray pictures.

For the patient, an angiogram is not very uncomfortable. The patient lies on a table similar to an operating table throughout the procedure. Before the procedure begins, a nurse cleans the patient's groin and numbs the area with a local anesthetic. The nurse also administers intravenous pain medicine as well as medicine that will help to relax the patient. When the doctor and nurse are ready to begin, the cardiologist inserts a catheter (a tiny hollow tube that is 2 to 3 mm in size) into the groin. The catheter passes through the artery in the groin and follows the path of arteries up the body until it reaches the heart. With the help of an x-ray technology called *fluoroscopy*, the cardiologist can watch the catheter advancing through the body. When the catheter is in the heart, the cardiologist will inject a contrast dye into the catheter, which may create a momentary hot sensation in the patient's body. Contrast may need to be used multiple times. The contrast allows the doctors to see the outlines of the arteries. When the doctors have seen all the different pictures of the heart and the coronary arteries that they need, the procedure is over. A routine angiogram takes about a half an hour. However, each case is treated individually and the time could vary. At the end of the procedure, the catheter is removed and a nurse applies pressure to the site of insertion in order to stop the bleeding. In some cases, the doctor sutures the insertion site, where the catheter was placed, to keep it closed. It is generally a small open area requiring only a few stitches.

An angiogram provides the best picture of the coronary arteries and the blood flowing through them. It can also help with treatment decisions. If a person has had severe chest pain, a heart attack, or a significantly abnormal stress test, then the angiogram can show the doctors the exact location of the plaques as well as the amount of blockage these plaques are causing to the blood flow to the heart. However, there are risks to this procedure. These risks are rare, occuring in about 1 percent of patients. They include heart attack, injury to the arteries or veins, stroke, or kidney problems.

Cardiologists treat each person individually and recommend appropriate diagnostic tests depending on the extent of the person's symptoms and the results of previous tests. For example, if a person tells his doctor that he has noticed episodes of chest pain while walking long distances, the doctor will obtain an EKG to check the electrical tracings of the person's heart and see if there is a pattern of ischemia (diminished blood supply), or if there are tracings on the EKG that reveal a previous heart attack. He will order blood tests to check for cholesterol levels. Then, to further evaluate the heart, he may order a stress test. If someone comes into the emergency department after having severe, unremitting chest pain and the EKG tracings reveal that a significant amount of the heart is not getting an adequate supply of blood, then that person may be rushed to the cardiac catheterization lab where cardiologists perform angiograms, in an effort to locate the blockage causing the chest pain and lack of oxygen. Once the cardiologist locates the blockage and sees how extensive it is, he can better develop an immediate treatment plan for the person.

Reducing the Risk of Stroke from Coronary Artery Disease

Aspirin is commonly prescribed for preventing heart attacks in people with CAD. Since aspirin also reduces the risk of stroke, this medication may serve double duty for prevention of both heart attack and stroke. People who have had a heart attack in the past may be at risk of having a stroke. As we discussed previously, this is because when there is damage to the heart muscle, an area of the heart wall may not contract normally after a heart attack, leading to stagnation of the blood in this area. This can result in a blood clot forming within the heart. Stroke can result if a portion of this blood clot breaks off and travels to the brain. The usual treatment for this is Coumadin (warfarin), which prevents the formation of blood clots within the heart.

Problems with Rhythm: Atrial Fibrillation

Not all strokes due to heart disease are caused by coronary artery disease. Another common cause of stroke is an irregular heart rhythm known as *atrial fibrillation,* which is the most common type of heart rhythm abnormality. This irregular beating of the heart is caused by uncoordinated electrical activity and contraction of the *atria,* the upper chambers of the heart that receive blood from the veins and send it on to the ventricles (see Figure 8.2). Normally, the atria beat together and pump blood through the valves into the ventricles in a synchronized and rhythmic way. In atrial fibrillation, the atria generate many abnormal electrical stimuli, which cause the ventricles (the workhorse, pump portion of the heart) to beat too

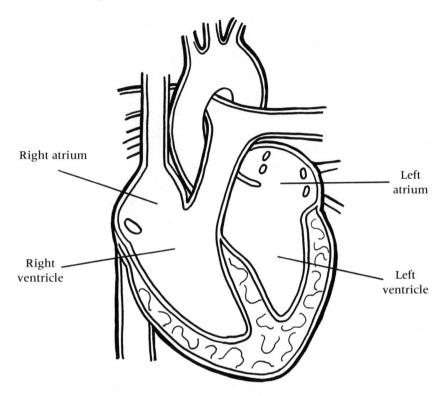

Figure 8.2. Cross-section of the heart showing all four chambers. Note that the figure shows the right side of the body to the viewer's left, as would be the case when examining someone from the front.

quickly. This uncoordinated heartbeat results in a less effective pumping of blood. The heart is an amazing organ, and this slight loss of efficiency is usually not a big problem for it, but the risk for stroke it can cause is a big problem.

The prevalence of atrial fibrillation increases with age. Approximately 2 percent of the general population has atrial fibrillation; this percentage rises to 5 percent in people over age 60. Atrial fibrillation is more common in men than in women.

Risk Factors for Atrial Fibrillation

Conditions that can lead to atrial fibrillation include heart problems and lung problems, as well as some lifestyle and other factors. These conditions are listed in Table 8.5. Less commonly, atrial fibrillation develops in an otherwise healthy young person for no apparent reason. Atrial fibrillation

Table 8.5. Risk Factors for Atrial Fibrillation

Heart and Heart-Related Problems
High blood pressure (hypertension)
Coronary artery disease
Heart attack
Heart valve disease
Weak or enlarged heart

Lung Problems
Pneumonia
Bronchitis/emphysema

Other Factors
Overactive thyroid gland
Alcohol abuse

---

in this situation appears to be less likely to cause a stroke than atrial fibrillation that is associated with one of the medical conditions listed.

How Atrial Fibrillation Can Lead to Stroke

The synchronized beating of the heart allows all the blood in the atria to flow into the ventricles and then out of the heart to the rest of the body. In atrial fibrillation, the desynchronized beating of the atria can allow some blood to collect or pool in the atrium, forming a clot. A piece of this clot can break off and travel through the arteries until it gets stuck in a small artery in the brain and causes a stroke.

Remember Don, the stroke survivor described earlier in this chapter? For fifteen years after his stroke, Don managed his coronary artery disease and high blood pressure. He restricted the fat in his diet, took his blood pressure medication, made exercise a regular part of his day, and lost weight. He suffered no further chest pain or medical problems until the day he collapsed in the bathroom while washing his hands. He could not move his right foot or put any weight on it. He had no warning signs before his collapse, which resulted from a second stroke.

In order to discover the underlying cause of Don's second stroke, his doctors performed an MRI to examine his brain and an EKG, a Holter monitor, an echocardiogram, and blood tests to examine his heart. (All of these tests are discussed in Chapter 3.)

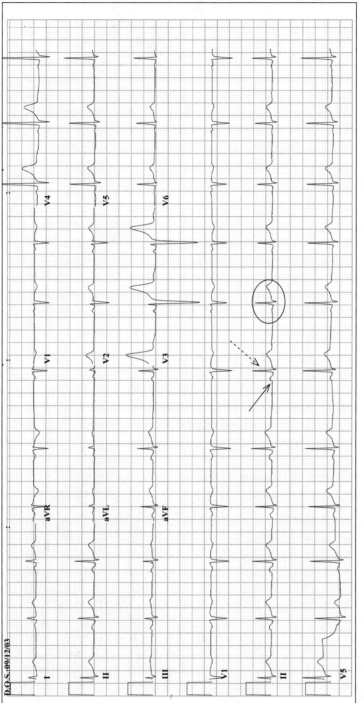

Figure 8.3. A normal electrocardiogram (EKG). The circled area represents one complete heartbeat. Note the regular rhythm of the heart's electrical activity and the small "P" wave (the solid arrow) preceding each of the larger "QRS" waves (the broken arrow).

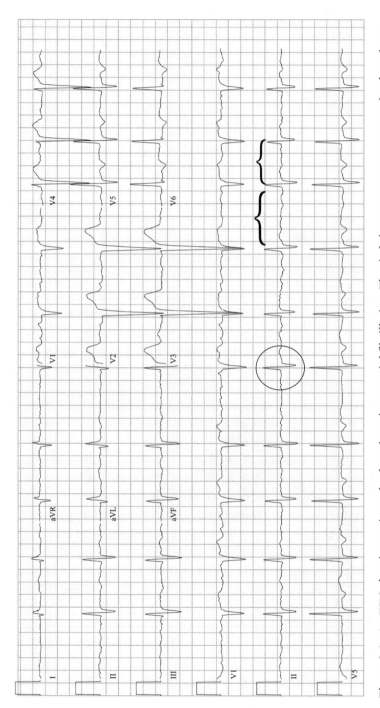

Figure 8.4. An EKG showing an irregular heartbeat due to atrial fibrillation. The circled area represents one complete heartbeat. Note the irregular rhythm of the heart's electrical activity, the irregularities in the time between heartbeats (shown with brackets), and the absence of a consistent "P" wave preceding each of the "QRS" waves.

The Holter monitor and the echocardiogram revealed Don's problem. The Holter monitor took recordings of his heart's rhythm and showed that he had frequent episodes of atrial fibrillation, which was most likely due to his high blood pressure and CAD. Compare the example of normal heart rhythm shown in Figure 8.3 to Don's EKG recordings in Figure 8.4. Don's echocardiogram showed that he had a blood clot in the left atrium of his heart. His brain MRI showed that a blood clot was blocking his left anterior cerebral artery. Don's case demonstrates how CAD and hypertension can damage the heart muscle as well as the electrical system of the heart, and how these problems can combine to lead to stroke.

Symptoms of Atrial Fibrillation

In some people atrial fibrillation causes no symptoms, but in others it can produce feelings of light-headedness, fainting, anxiety, fatigue, shortness of breath, or a noticeably increased and irregular heart rate. This type of heart rhythm disturbance can come and go in some people, while in others it is present continuously. Atrial fibrillation can cause a stroke even when it only occurs intermittently.

Diagnosing Atrial Fibrillation

Doctors must diagnose atrial fibrillation if it is present in patients who have had a stroke, because these people are at high risk of sustaining a second stroke. A physician can feel your pulse at your wrist and check to see if you have a normal rate and regular rhythm. If you have an "irregularly irregular" rhythm, then you may have atrial fibrillation. Normally, when you or a physician checks your pulse, he feels a steady regular beating at a relatively slow rate, about sixty to eighty times a minute. This may be depicted as:

• • • • • • • •

With atrial fibrillation, the pulse is entirely irregular and can be depicted as:

•• • • • •• •••• •• • • •• •

There are other causes of irregular pulse besides atrial fibrillation. An EKG and physician's evaluation are needed to determine if atrial fibrillation is responsible for the irregular pulse.

An EKG shows the electrical activity of the heart and is the gold standard in the diagnosis of atrial fibrillation. Again, Figure 8.3 shows a normal EKG, and Figure 8.4 shows an EKG of someone with atrial fibrillation. Atrial fibrillation may be *intermittent,* meaning that someone may have a regular pulse, then an irregular pulse for ten minutes, for example, and then a regular pulse again. For this reason, twenty-four-hour Holter monitors (essentially a twenty-four-hour EKG recording) are used to diagnose atrial fibrillation if it is suspected but is not seen on a routine EKG.

Controlling Atrial Fibrillation and Reducing the Risk of Stroke

In general, a person with untreated atrial fibrillation has a 5 percent to 6 percent chance of experiencing a stroke each year. In a young person with atrial fibrillation and an otherwise normal heart, the risk of stroke is relatively low. In an older person, even with an otherwise normal heart, the risk is higher. If you have atrial fibrillation plus a heart condition such as high blood pressure, rheumatic heart disease with associated mitral stenosis, or an artificial heart valve, your risk of stroke increases regardless of your age.

Atrial fibrillation can be treated in two major ways: restoring the heart rhythm to a normal rhythm and controlling the heart rate with medications. Recent studies have shown that these two approaches have similar long-term results in terms of lowering the risk of stroke.

For someone who has recently developed atrial fibrillation, many physicians will make an attempt to restore a normal heart rhythm. There are two ways to accomplish this goal: electrical cardioversion and chemical cardioversion. By *cardioversion,* we mean restoring a normal heart rhythm. With electrical cardioversion, there is a risk of stroke, so this method is only attempted in certain situations and after thorough investigation. For example, the procedure would not be performed if there were a thrombus (clot) located in the atrium, which could be seen on a *transesophageal echocardiogram* (a procedure in which an ultrasound probe is passed through the throat into the esophagus). Cardioversion generally requires pretreatment with anticoagulants (blood thinners) if the atrial fibrillation has been present longer than three days.

Electrical cardioversion delivers an electric shock to the heart through the chest wall. When this electrical shock reaches the heart, it momentarily stops the heart muscle cells from working. The heart then restarts itself, usually with a normal heart rhythm. This procedure is performed by a cardiologist and a nurse. The nurse places EKG leads on the patient's chest. The EKG tracing that shows the atrial fibrillation is constantly monitored, and so are the patient's blood pressure and heart rate. The patient is given intravenous (IV) sedation medicine to relax him and put him to sleep. While the patient is asleep, the cardiologist places two large hand-held electrode paddles on his chest. The electrical shock passes through these paddles. One shock lasts less than one second. Often it only takes one shock to reset the heart and bring it back to a normal rhythm. Sometimes, however, it takes multiple shocks. The procedure is quick (about five minutes) and usually the person receiving the electrical shock does not remember anything about it when it is done. After the procedure, the patient's chest may feel a little sore. The only evidence of the procedure may be ring-like marks on the patient's chest where the cardiologist had placed the electrode paddles. After several days, these marks fade and are not noticeable at all. Initially, the marks may be red, like a sunburn. In that case, an ointment can be applied to the marks to help them heal and reduce any discomfort they may cause.

Chemical cardioversion for atrial fibrillation involves administering medications to try to restore normal heart rhythm. These medications are called *anti-arrhythmia drugs* (*arrhythmia* means abnormal heart rhythm) and include quinidine, procainamide, disopyramide, propafenone, flecainide, amiodarone, and sotalol. These are powerful drugs with many side effects. If the medications are successful in restoring normal sinus rhythm, they will most likely need to be continued over the long term as maintenance therapy.

Deciding whether to use cardioversion is a difficult decision that needs to be made by a cardiologist. If cardioversion fails, doctors are increasingly likely to accept atrial fibrillation as a fact of life and to use medications to keep the overall heart rate in a desirable range (usually sixty to one hundred beats per minute). These rate-controlling medications include beta-blockers, calcium channel blockers, and digoxin. They are generally successful in slowing down the heart rate. However, they sometimes do not work for severe cases, and in that instance more invasive procedures are required. These procedures include destroying the heart's *A-V node* (the *atrioventricular node,* through which the heart's electrical impulses travel) and putting in a pacemaker. Another procedure for heart rates that are difficult to control involves a surgical technique called *the MAZE procedure,* in which a surgeon makes cuts in the atria; the cuts stop the abnormal electrical impulses. Most people with atrial fibrillation do not need these invasive procedures because they are able to control their heart rate with medications.

People with atrial fibrillation are at increased risk for stroke because they have an increased risk of blood clots in the heart. This is true whether the atrial fibrillation is chronic or intermittent. The use of Coumadin or other anticoagulant (blood-thinning) medications is usually recommended. Anticoagulants work on the clotting factors found normally in our blood. These clotting factors are present in a delicate balance that allows blood to flow easily through the blood vessels yet promotes clotting at a site of injury. If blood remains stagnant in the heart, as can happen with atrial fibrillation, it pools and gels together, forming a clot. Coumadin acts directly on the clotting factors in the blood, making it harder for them to form clots.

Aspirin may be used to thin the blood in people who are at lower than average risk for stroke (for example, someone who is young and has no medical conditions other than atrial fibrillation), or in people who are at high risk for complications from the use of Coumadin due to a history of intestinal bleeding or a history of falling frequently (which puts them at risk for trauma and subsequent internal bleeding). Aspirin works by a different mechanism than do drugs like Coumadin. It makes clotting more difficult by inhibiting *platelets,* the blood cells involved in forming clots in the body at the site of an injury.

Most people with atrial fibrillation take a medication to control their heart rate and a medication to prevent clotting. Many take anti-arrhythmia medicines as well. There are a great many treatment options to explore, and controlling atrial fibrillation can be challenging. Each person's condition must be considered on an individual basis. If you or someone you love has had atrial fibrillation, we suggest that you consult a cardiologist to help get this medical problem under control.

Problems with Pumping: Congestive Heart Failure

As we have seen, stroke can be caused by blockage and rhythm problems. Stroke can also result from a failure of the heart to pump blood effectively. *Congestive heart failure* (CHF), also known as *heart failure* or *fluid on the lungs,* is one such pumping problem. In CHF, the lungs and other areas of the body may become congested with fluid (primarily water) because the heart is not pumping blood out efficiently.

Congestive heart failure is caused by many different conditions. These are listed in Table 8.6.

Table 8.6. Risk Factors for Congestive Heart Failure

Coronary artery disease
Hypertension
Heart attacks
Unexplained weakening of the heart muscle (*idiopathic cardiomyopathy*)
Heart valve disease
Thyroid disease
Excessive alcohol use
Viral infection of the heart muscle (*viral myocarditis*)
Certain medication side effects

Risk Factors for Congestive Heart Failure

According to the American Heart Association, 4.9 million Americans live with CHF. Older people are most susceptible to this condition: although 10 percent of people older than 80 have this condition, less than 1 percent of people younger than 60 do.

How Congestive Heart Failure Can Lead to Stroke

In congestive heart failure, the blood does not pump through the heart and to the rest of the body efficiently. There is often a backup of blood in the heart. If the CHF is severe enough and the heart muscle is weak, blood can pool in the heart and clot. A piece of the clot can break off from the heart, travel to another location, and cause a stroke.

Symptoms of Congestive Heart Failure

People with congestive heart failure may experience any of the following symptoms:

Shortness of breath
Difficulty breathing when exercising (dyspnea on exertion)
Difficulty breathing when lying flat and sleeping (orthopnea)
Needing to urinate more frequently at night after lying down for a while (nocturia)
While sleeping lying flat, waking up short of breath and needing to sit upright or to stand by an open window (paroxysmal nocturnal dyspnea)

A chronic, nonproductive cough, worse when lying down

Swelling in the abdomen, ankles, and/or legs that makes an imprint when you push down on it with your fingertips (*pitting edema*)

Diagnosing Congestive Heart Failure

The treating physician often picks up clues regarding CHF from a person's history (including shortness of breath and waking at night unable to breathe), as well as from the physical exam (hearing fluid in the lungs with a stethoscope).

An echocardiogram is used to evaluate what kind of heart problem is causing the CHF. With an echocardiogram, the doctor can view the heart muscle to check for any areas that are thickened or thinned or appear weak, and examine the valves to see if they are able to open and close properly. An "echo" also allows important calculations to be made that can be followed over time to help in managing a person's congestive heart failure. These calculations include the size of the heart chambers and the *ejection fraction*.

The ejection fraction measures the efficiency with which the heart muscle pumps blood to the rest of the body. The heart does not normally completely empty of blood after each contraction; a normal ejection fraction is approximately 60 to 80 percent. If a person's heart has an ejection fraction of 30 percent or less, his heart is extremely weak, and blood may pool in his heart because it is not pumped out efficiently. Just as with a heart attack or atrial fibrillation, blood clots can form when the blood pools. Part of this clot can break off and travel to the brain, causing a stroke.

Reducing the Risk of Stroke from Congestive Heart Failure

Taking blood thinners can reduce the risk of a stroke when the risk is due to weak pumping action of the heart. If a person with a weak heart (an ejection fraction of less than 30 percent) also has one of the following conditions, she will typically need to take blood thinners to reduce the risk of stroke:

Atrial fibrillation

A significant heart attack in the past three to six months

A clot in the heart

A prior stroke or blood clot

Problems with the Heart's Anatomical Structure: Valve Problems

Four valves in the heart help regulate the flow of blood within this organ; how they function is a key factor in the efficiency of the heart's pumping action. The four heart valves are the *tricuspid, pulmonic, mitral,* and *aortic* valves. Maintaining the proper flow of blood through the heart is their main job. If a valve does not function properly, blood may leak from one chamber of the heart to another, which puts extra stress on the heart muscle. A valve may be diseased, damaged, or congenitally malformed. Abnormal valves can increase the risk of stroke.

Risk Factors for Valve Problems

Risk factors for valve problems include:

Rheumatic heart disease
Infection
Atherosclerosis
Congenital heart problems

In the past, the most common form of heart valve disease was due to rheumatic fever, which can damage any or all of the valves, most commonly creating a thickened mitral valve and also a hardened aortic valve that does not open and close properly. Rheumatic fever is caused by a streptococci infection that affects the throat ("strep throat") before affecting the heart. Though it still occurs, rheumatic fever is less common today, especially in more developed countries, thanks to the use of antibiotics to treat strep throat.

Other bacteria that infect the heart valve include enterococci and staphylococci aureus. An infection of the heart valve is called *endocarditis.* The infection can cause damage to the valves, especially the aortic or mitral valve, and the damage causes malfunction. Antibiotics are usually sufficient for treatment, but in severe cases surgery may be required to replace the heart valve.

Infection is not the only condition affecting heart valves. In older individuals, cholesterol plaque can damage the heart valves as well as the arteries. Atherosclerosis is associated with calcification (hardening) of the aortic valve, which directly leads to its inability to open and close properly, and a narrowing of the heart valve opening (*aortic stenosis*). Large heart attacks can sometimes cause valve problems, as well, most commonly affecting the mitral valve.

Some people are born with defects in their heart valves. *Mitral valve prolapse,* one of the milder forms of heart valve disease, is found in 4 percent of the population. Whether a mitral valve prolapse increases the risk of stroke remains controversial. If you have mitral valve prolapse you are more likely to develop a condition where blood leaks back into the right atrium instead of being propelled forward in the heart (*mitral regurgitation*). Another congenital defect is an aortic valve made of only two leaflets (parts that look like small leaves), rather than the usual three. A valve with two leaflets is called an *aortic bicuspid valve.* If you have this type of defect, you are more likely to develop calcifications on your aortic valve at an early age, which means you are more likely to have valve problems and then suffer endocarditis (infection of the valve). Endocarditis puts a person at increased risk for stroke.

How Heart Valve Problems Can Lead to Stroke

Abnormal heart valves (whether they be congenitally malformed, damaged, or leaking) can serve as a resting ground for bacteria that have made their way into the circulation. Bacteria can enter the bloodstream through routine events such as a dental cleaning or through less common means such as injecting illicit drugs into a vein. Once in the bloodstream, the bacteria find a protected environment on diseased or malformed heart valves, where they may grow and multiply. Ultimately, fragile growths known as vegetations may occur on the valves. Portions of these vegetations can break off and travel through the bloodstream to the brain, where they can block blood flow and cause a stroke. Prompt recognition of an infected heart valve is essential to prevent stroke and other complications. Antibiotics are often sufficient treatment, though in some cases valve destruction is so extensive that surgery is required to replace the heart valve. What happened to Mary demonstrates the connection between heart valve disease and stroke.

Mary, a 40-year-old mother of two young children, fell to the ground when her right leg suddenly became weak. While she was being evaluated at the hospital, she had difficulty speaking and trouble using her right arm. Her hospital evaluation revealed severe mitral valve prolapse and evidence of a valve infection. Her doctors also learned that Mary had had extensive dental work ten days before her stroke, and that she did not receive antibiotics before getting the work done. Mary was treated with antibiotics and her infected mitral valve healed well. She recovered from her stroke, too, and was instructed to take prescribed antibiotics before any dental or surgical procedures in the future.

Symptoms of Heart Valve Problems

Heart valve problems often lead to symptoms of congestive heart failure. Because the heart is not able to pump blood properly through the malformed valve, blood may "back up" in the heart, causing congestion. The symptoms vary depending upon which of the four heart valves is affected and the type of damage. For example, someone with an aortic valve narrowing (*aortic stenosis*) due to atherosclerosis could be asymptomatic until he reached 60, at which time he might develop congestive heart failure and chest pain and might start fainting because of the lack of blood reaching the brain. Someone with a history of rheumatic fever, on the other hand, may develop a mitral valve problem called *mitral stenosis* and start feeling shortness of breath (*dyspnea*), difficulty sleeping flat (*orthopnea*), and sudden awakening at night feeling unable to catch a breath (*paroxysmal nocturnal dyspnea*).

Diagnosing Heart Valve Problems

A standard echocardiogram of the heart allows diagnosis of most heart valve problems. In some cases more detailed images are obtained via a special test called a *transesophageal echocardiogram,* in which an ultrasound probe is passed through the throat into the esophagus. This type of echocardiogram often allows the best view of the valves.

Decreasing the Risk of Stroke from Heart Valve Problems

Whatever the cause of the valve abnormalities, an abnormal heart valve remains a potential site of infection. Antibiotics are recommended before many surgical procedures and dental procedures, to prevent bacteria from gaining a foothold on an abnormal valve.

The risk of stroke associated with damaged heart valves varies depending on which valve is affected and how it is damaged. Treatment is individualized, and may consist of anything from observation with annual exams without any formal intervention (in minor valve abnormalities) to aspirin to Coumadin in some cases. When severe valve problems are present, the natural heart valve may need to be replaced by an artificial heart valve. There are two major types of artificial heart valves: mechanical and tissue (*bioprosthetic*) valves. The former are constructed of metal, plastic, carbon-fiber, and composite materials. The tissue or bioprosthetic valves come from animal tissues—most commonly from cows or pigs. Mechanical valves are particularly prone to blood clot formation. For this reason, people with mechanical valves must take blood thinners (typically Coumadin) daily and monitor their blood levels carefully. Bioprosthetic valves are less likely to cause abnormal blood clot formation, but people who have them typically require anticoagulation medications for at least the first three months after surgical placement.

Holes in the Heart: Patent Foramen Ovale

A *patent foramen ovale* (PFO) is a small opening between the two atria (see Figure 8.5). This congenital condition results when the wall separating the two atria fails to close normally at the time of birth. PFOs are usually diagnosed via echocardiogram, and a special "bubble test" is also used to check for this hole. Echocardiography has revealed that small PFOs are quite common; as many as one-third of adults have this problem. Typically, PFOs are very small, less than one-quarter inch in diameter, and they cause no symptoms. The challenge is to figure out whether an individual's PFO is causing or has caused her trouble.

The Association between Patent Foramen Ovale and Stroke

Normally, blood flows from the right atrium to the right ventricle to the lungs, where it is oxygenated, then to the left atrium, the left ventricle, the aorta, and finally to the rest of the body. PFOs allow blood to flow from the right atrium directly into the left, rather than in the normal direction. The larger the PFO, the greater chance for a stroke, because more blood is allowed to flow abnormally. With the normal flow, any small bubble or piece of clot coming from the veins into the heart would get lodged or stuck in the lungs, where there are tiny capillaries to trap it. Infarcting (cutting off the blood supply to) a tiny area of the *lung* may produce no symptoms at all and cause very little problem, as the rest of the lung takes over. This is not the case with the *brain*. A tiny infarct in an important area such as the midbrain could cause big problems. In other words, abnormal flow from the right atrium directly to the left atrium bypasses the "filtering" function of the lungs, which traps any blood clots or other material that may be in the blood entering the heart. Thus, instead of being filtered out in the lungs, a blood clot can enter the aorta, travel to the brain, and cause a stroke. A

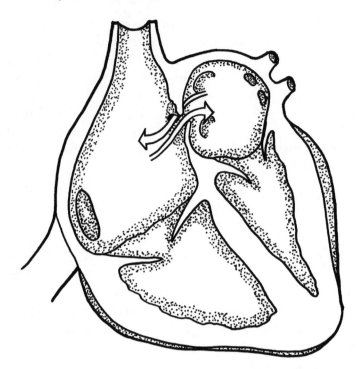

Figure 8.5. *Patent foramen ovale, a hole between the two sides of the heart. Blood can flow between the two sides and allow a blood clot to pass through this hole.*

PFO often causes stroke in combination with a blood clot in the legs known as a *deep venous thrombosis,* or *DVT.* Deep vein thrombosis often occurs after prolonged immobility, such as a lengthy car trip or airplane flight. Certain conditions—such as pregnancy, the use of estrogen-containing oral contraceptives, cancer, and blood disorders that cause increased clotting tendency—are known to increase the risk of deep vein thrombosis.

Reducing the Risk of Stroke from a Patent Foramen Ovale

A patent foramen ovale is a potentially treatable cause of stroke. Treatment may include medications such as aspirin or Coumadin to prevent blood clots from forming. There is also an invasive technique to close the PFO, which is performed by specialized cardiologists in a cardiac catheterization lab. It involves threading a catheter from the groin to the heart through the blood vessels, as is done in an angiogram. For a PFO, an umbrella-like device is implanted in the heart to close the hole. (This is discussed in Chapter 14.)

Tom, a 52-year-old lawyer, was working on a big case, and sat at his desk for hours at a time. At one point, he got hungry for dinner, got up from his desk, and collapsed. He was brought to the hospital emergency department, where a stroke was diagnosed. An echocardiogram revealed a PFO, and ultrasound of his legs revealed a blood clot in the leg (deep venous thrombosis, or DVT). The physician informed Tom that a small piece of the clot in his leg broke off and traveled through his veins to his right atrium, where it traveled through his PFO to the left atrium, and then to the left ventricle, the aorta, and eventually an artery in his brain. As his doctors further explored the cause of the blood clot formation, they found that Tom had a previously undiagnosed lung cancer, which appeared to have increased his risk of developing a blood clot in his leg.

Your heart and blood vessels are critical to your brain. Heart conditions such as coronary artery disease, myocardial infarctions (heart attacks), atrial fibrillation, congestive heart failure, valve problems, and PFOs can cause stroke. Knowing the cause of a stroke is essential to preventing a second one. Maintaining a healthy heart is important for its own sake *and* for stroke prevention.

Chapter 9

• •

High Blood Pressure and Stroke

Robert grew up in a small town in the rural Midwest. Until he had a stroke, he rarely went to see a doctor. He believed in being self-reliant, and as long as he was fairly healthy, he didn't think regular checkups were all that important. When Robert ended up in the hospital with blurred vision and numbness on his left side, things changed. Clearly this was not something he could manage on his own.

The doctors at the hospital did several tests to find out what caused Robert to have a stroke. They discovered that Robert had high blood pressure and told him that because of this problem, he would continue to be at risk for developing another stroke unless he made some changes to his diet, took medicine, and made regular visits to the doctor to monitor his blood pressure. Robert willingly accepted this plan—he was, after all, a take-charge kind of person. Eventually his blood pressure was controlled, and he lived comfortably for many more years.

If you or someone you love have had a stroke and have learned that you have high blood pressure like Robert, it will be important for you to control this problem to prevent another stroke. If you have hypertension, you are seven times more likely to have a stroke than if you have normal blood pressure. If you have hypertension and you have already had a stroke, your risk of having another stroke because of hypertension is high, and your high blood pressure must be aggressively treated and regularly monitored. The best way to reduce the risk of a second stroke is to reduce the risk factors that you can control, take your medication faithfully, and monitor your blood pressure regularly. In this chapter, we will define hypertension, discuss risk factors, medications, and blood pressure levels, and describe how hypertension can lead to stroke as well as the damage it does to blood vessels and the damage it can do to the brain. With this information you will be better equipped to manage and tackle this disease.

What Is Blood Pressure?

Dorland's Illustrated Medical Dictionary, 27th edition, defines *blood pressure* as "the pressure of the blood on the walls of the arteries, dependent on the energy of the heart action, the elasticity of the walls of the arteries, and the volume and viscosity of the blood." Blood pressure, or the pressure on the walls of the arteries, is directly related to the amount of blood pumped out of the heart each minute (*cardiac output*) and the oppositional force encountered by the blood as it enters the blood vessels (*peripheral vascular resistance*).

Scientists have created a mathematical formula that relates blood pressure, cardiac output, and peripheral vascular resistance. The formula is:

Blood Pressure = Cardiac Output × Peripheral Vascular Resistance

We can use the garden hose analogy to explain the regulation of blood pressure, which is a complex process. Think of the faucet as the aorta (the place where the blood exits the heart and enters the circulation) and the garden hose as an artery. As water comes out of the faucet and enters the hose, the force of the water puts pressure on the walls of the garden hose. If more water comes out of the faucet at a faster speed, then more pressure will be put on the walls. Another way to increase the pressure on the walls of the garden hose is to squeeze the hose with your hand. By squeezing the hose, you decrease the size of the hole through which the water flows. It is much harder for the water to flow through a small hole. By narrowing the size of the hole, you increase the force the water needs to travel through the hose (this is similar to the peripheral vascular resistance in blood vessels).

The pressure on the walls of the garden hose can be increased by increasing the amount of water entering the hose or by decreasing the inner open space of the hose. Similarly, the pressure on the walls of the artery can be increased by (1) increasing the amount of blood being pumped out of the heart each minute or (2) decreasing the inner space (the *lumen*) of the artery (*vasoconstriction*). The amount of blood being pumped out of the heart each minute can be increased in many ways, including speeding up the heart rate, intensifying the force of the heart's contractions, and expanding the volume of blood by increasing the amount of water in the blood (this happens if you eat more salt or drink more water). Many different hormones and other biologically active compounds made by the body work to decrease the lumen of the arteries. Epinephrine, norepinephrine, leukotrienes, enodothelin, and thromboxane are examples of these substances.

Normally, the blood moving through arteries puts some pressure on the walls. If there is not enough blood traveling through someone's arteries because he is dehydrated or has suffered massive blood loss, then there will not be enough pressure on the arterial walls. In this case, he may faint because the blood is not able to travel to his brain. To function normally, people need some blood pressure inside the arterial walls. However, when the pressure gets too high in the arterial walls because a narrowed lumen in the artery makes it difficult for the blood to pass through, high blood pressure can cause damage to the body. This situation will be discussed in detail in this chapter.

When a physician or nurse measures your blood pressure, they usually report two numbers to you. For example, they may say, "140 over 90." The first number mentioned is the systolic pressure and the second number is the diastolic pressure. What do *systolic* and *diastolic* mean? The heart is an amazingly strong muscle whose job is to pump blood to the rest of the body. It accomplishes this job by contracting and relaxing. The time during which the heart muscle is contracting is called *systole,* and the time during which the heart muscle is relaxing is called *diastole.* Blood pressure measures the pressure on the walls of the arteries during these two different periods. Generally, the pressure on the walls of the arteries is higher during the period when the heart is contracting (systole). At this time, the heart is forcing blood out into the aorta and to the rest of the arteries in the body. The pressure in the walls of the artery drops as the heart relaxes and fills up again with more blood (diastole). Both numbers are important, and that is why both numbers are measured and recorded when blood pressure is taken. Blood pressure is measured in millimeters of mercury, which are recorded as mmHg.

What Is High Blood Pressure?

High blood pressure, also called *hypertension,* occurs when the blood flowing through the veins and arteries meets resistance. This elevates pressure, which can damage the blood vessels, and this damage contributes to blockages within the arteries. In addition, the heart must work harder to pump the blood, and this extra effort can lead to heart disease and, as a result, stroke.

High blood pressure is generally defined as blood pressure above 140/90 millimeters of mercury (mmHg) in an adult. In this reading, the systolic

Table 9.1. Interpreting Blood Pressure Results

Blood pressure	Systolic	Diastolic
Normal	<130	<80
Pre-hypertension	130–139	80–89
Mild hypertension	140–159	90–99
Moderate hypertension	160–179	100–109
Severe hypertension	180–209	110–119
Very severe hypertension	>210	>120

pressure (the number on top) is above 140 and the diastolic pressure (the number on the bottom) is above 90. High blood pressure elevations between 130/80 and 140/90 are known as pre-hypertension. The severity of hypertension is graded depending on the systolic and diastolic numbers obtained (see Table 9.1).

Hypertension is known as the "silent killer" because it damages blood vessels in the body while a person has no symptoms and therefore no idea what is happening. In fact, although an astounding 65 million people in the United States have hypertension, 1 in 3 of these people do not even know that they have high blood pressure. High blood pressure doesn't directly cause symptoms; rather, the symptoms that occur are due to organs being damaged by hypertension. In most cases, high blood pressure does not cause symptoms for fifteen to twenty years. During these fifteen to twenty damaging years, hypertension targets the heart, brain, kidneys, and eyes. People with long-standing (chronic) hypertension may eventually experience coronary artery disease, congestive heart failure, heart attacks, strokes, renal failure, and blindness.

Causes of High Blood Pressure

In 90 to 95 percent of people with hypertension, no specific medical cause of the hypertension can be identified. These people are diagnosed with *essential hypertension*. The exact mechanism of essential hypertension is not well understood, and researchers continue to investigate its causes. We do know that there are several potential contributing factors to the development of essential hypertension (see Table 9.2). Five to ten percent of people with hypertension have *secondary hypertension*. Secondary hypertension can be caused by specific medical and other conditions, including:

Table 9.2. Factors Contributing to High Blood Pressure

Genetics
Salt consumption
Obesity
Alcohol consumption
Poor nutrition in utero (poor fetal nutrition)
Overgrowth of cells in the blood vessels, making the lumens smaller
Endothelial cell damage resulting in failure to produce a substance called
    nitric oxide, which relaxes the blood vessels and opens the lumen
The effect of certain hormones, including catecholamines, renin, and
    insulin, on the blood vessels

Kidney disease (the most common identifiable cause of hypertension)
Endocrine disorders (hormonal problems, such as hyperthyroidism or
    hypothyroidism, parathyroidism, or Cushing's syndrome)
Drug use, including alcohol withdrawal and amphetamine intoxication
Medication use, including corticosteroids

If your doctor has been able to determine the cause of your high blood pressure, most likely controlling the cause (for instance, treating a thyroid problem) will also help to keep your blood pressure under control. Even if you don't know the exact cause of your hypertension, you can take steps to minimize the factors that may be contributing to it. We'll look at these risk factors next.

Risk Factors for High Blood Pressure

Of the many risk factors for hypertension, some can be controlled and others cannot (see Table 9.3). Black Americans are twice as likely to develop hypertension as white Americans. People whose parents or close relatives had hypertension are also more likely to develop this health problem. If you are older than 35, your risk is higher than it was when you were younger. Finally, men are more likely to develop hypertension during mid-life than women are, but after menopause women catch up.

Even if you are a 65-year-old black man and both of your parents had hypertension, there are things you can do to keep your blood pressure under control and reduce your risk of stroke. Working on controlling these "controllable" risk factors can decrease your blood pressure and save your life! Limit-

Table 9.3. **Risk Factors for High Blood Pressure**

Risk Factors You Can Change or Influence
Too much salt (sodium) in your diet
Being overweight
Poor exercise habits
Excessive alcohol use

Risk Factors You Cannot Change or Influence
Race
Family history
Age
Sex

ing salt (sodium) intake to less than 2,400 mg a day lowers blood pressure in most people. The best way to reduce salt in your diet is to take table salt away from your dinner table and refrain from adding it to any foods you eat. Prepared foods are often particularly high in salt. For example, half a cup of prepared spaghetti sauce contains about 700 mg of sodium, a piece of wheat bread has about 200 mg of sodium, a can of soup has about 2,400 mg of sodium, and a can of reduced-sodium soup has 1,700 mg of sodium. The sodium content varies depending on the brand. It is best to avoid canned foods, but if you must have canned soup, select the reduced-sodium type. Checking the labels of foods you eat will help you to cut down on salt intake.

Losing weight lowers blood pressure in most people, especially those carrying their fat in the middle of their bodies, carrying fat around their waist as opposed to around their hips. Increasing exercise not only helps with weight loss but also has been shown to lower blood pressure on its own. (Diet, weight loss, and exercise will be covered in more detail in Chapters 15 and 16.)

Another way to modify your risk factors for hypertension is to monitor your alcohol use. Limiting alcohol intake to one drink a day lowers blood pressure in individuals who had formerly consumed larger amounts of alcohol on a daily basis. If you are not convinced that reducing the salt in your diet or drinking less alcohol will help lower your blood pressure, try it for a period of six months and see what happens.

Although these modifications are helpful, they are often not the only form of treatment needed. Most people with hypertension require medication to control their blood pressure adequately. However, the more people reduce their risk factors, the less medication they need. We will describe the medical management of high blood pressure later in this chapter.

How High Blood Pressure Leads to Stroke

Hypertension causes strokes by damaging blood vessels all over the body, including in the brain. There is a close association between atherosclerosis and high blood pressure. In fact, high blood pressure accelerates the development of atherosclerosis, so people with hypertension are more likely to develop a cholesterol plaque in the arteries in their brains and suffer a stroke. Hypertension is also known to weaken the arteries in the brain, making them more likely to rupture and create a bleed in the brain (a hemorrhagic stroke).

The arteries are not the only blood vessels harmed by high blood pressure. This disease also targets smaller vessels, called *arterioles,* which are damaged by atherosclerosis as well as by two other processes: hyaline *arteriolosclerosis* and *hyperplastic arteriolosclerosis.* All of these narrow the lumen (the inner open space) of the arteriole, making a blockage more likely. They also ruin the nice neat layers of the arteriolar walls, disturbing their structure and possibly weakening them. High blood pressure is associated with tiny outpouchings (areas where the linear artery balloons out to form a pouch), called *Charcot-Bouchard microaneurysms,* in very small blood vessels that have weak walls and are prone to bleeding.

High blood pressure causes both *infarcts* (blockages) and hemorrhages in large and small blood vessels in the brain by several different mechanisms. We will discuss a few of these mechanisms in more detail.

Atherosclerosis

As we explained in Chapter 8, our arteries are lined with important cells called *endothelial cells.* These E cells serve as the "bouncers" that let cells into and keep cells out of the blood vessels. When the endothelial cells are damaged by high blood pressure, the monocytes (a type of inflammatory cells that usually fight infection) enter the blood vessel and engulf LDL cholesterol. They also call in smooth muscle cells to join the party and ultimately create a cholesterol plaque. This process is called *atherosclerosis,* also known as hardening of the arteries.

If you have hypertension, you may develop atherosclerosis much faster than people with normal blood pressure because of the damage high blood pressure does to the endothelial cells in your arteries. If you are susceptible to coronary artery disease because of diabetes, high cholesterol, or a family history of coronary artery disease, you need to be *especially* vigilant about controlling your blood pressure.

Hyaline Arteriolosclerosis

The small blood vessels called *arterioles* have a similar structure to the arteries discussed in Chapter 8. High blood pressure allows an extra substance, known as *hyaline*, to be more readily deposited in the walls of these small blood vessels, through a process called hardening of the arterioles, or *hyaline arteriolosclerosis*. If we look under the microscope at the arterioles of elderly people who do not have high blood pressure, we may see a few deposits of hyaline, because this can accumulate during the normal aging process. However, if we look under the microscope at the arterioles of people with long-standing hypertension, we see many more deposits of hyaline in a larger number of the arterioles compared with people of the same age who have normal blood pressure. The high pressures in the arterioles of people with hypertension encourage the deposit of hyaline in the arterioles.

What do the hyaline deposits do to the arteries? This extra substance makes the walls of the arterioles thicker and disrupts their normal structure. Adding material to their walls makes the arterioles narrower, and narrower lumens make it easier for a piece of clot or plaque (embolus) traveling in the bloodstream to get lodged in the arteriole and cause a stroke. Also, if the lumen's area is severely decreased, not enough blood may be allowed through the arteriole to feed that part of the brain, which could lead to a stroke. Many scientists and doctors believe that disrupting the normal structure of the arteriole weakens it, and with weaker walls, the arteriole is more likely to rupture and bleed. *Hyaline arteriolosclerosis* (hardening of the arterioles) creates an environment ripe for a stroke, either by entirely blocking the very small lumen in an arteriole or by causing the thick, weak walls of the arterioles to burst and bleed.

Hyperplastic Arteriolosclerosis

A process called *hyperplastic arteriolosclerosis* is another type of hardening of the arterioles in which the openings of the arterioles are narrowed. In cases of severe hypertension with diastolic pressures higher than 110 mmHg, the extremely high pressures in the arterioles may foster extra growth of the cells already present in the arteriolar wall, such as the smooth muscle cells and the lining of the arterioles, called the *basement membrane*, that separates them from the rest of the tissues. These changes might even cause the death of some of the cells in the arterioles and the deposit of extra proteins, including *fibrin*. All these changes can decrease the size of the opening in the arteriole, and this decrease can in turn lead to a blockage of blood flow and a stroke.

Charcot-Bouchard Microaneurysms

High blood pressure can also cause very small pouch-like areas to protrude from the blood vessels. These outpouchings, called *Charcot-Bouchard micro-aneurysms,* usually develop in an area of the brain called the *basal ganglia,* which controls movement. The tiny aneurysms have thin, weak walls that are likely to rupture under high pressures, causing a bleed in the brain that can lead to stroke.

Damage to the Brain Caused by High Blood Pressure

Lacunar Infarcts

Susan, a 66-year-old attorney with a long history of high blood pressure, was having tea with a friend when she suddenly felt a numbness in her left hand. When she touched her left hand and arm, she could not feel anything. However, when she touched her right hand and arm, she could feel everything. Then Susan noticed that her left leg was also affected. She called 9-1-1 and was rushed to the hospital.

At the hospital, Susan's blood pressure measured 180/100. An MRI revealed that Susan had a lacunar infarct in her right thalamus. Her blood pressure was carefully controlled and she was started on aspirin. After being discharged from the hospital, Susan went home. She gradually regained the sensation on her left side. Her blood pressure medication was changed and increased. She continued taking aspirin.

Each artery deep in the brain and each smaller arteriole supplies a specific area of the brain. Lacunar (meaning "lake-like") infarcts are small areas of damaged or destroyed brain tissue that occur as a result of blockages in these small "garden hoses" that supply the brain. Most commonly the arteries that cause lacunar infarcts are the *penetrating arteries.* As their name suggests, these penetrate deep within the brain. Blockages in these arteries can be caused by any of the three processes described earlier: atherosclerosis, hyaline arteriolosclerosis, and hyperplastic arteriolosclerosis.

The symptoms of lacunar infarcts vary widely based on their location and their severity. Many of these strokes are so small they are silent, meaning there are no symptoms or deficits associated with them. When a lacunar infarct occurs in a very important brain structure, however, it can cause major symptoms. There are a few lacunar syndromes that are easily identified by the symptoms they create. For example, a lacunar infarct in the posterior limb of the internal capsule will create weakness without any sensory changes. A lacunar infarct in the thalamus can create sensory changes without any weakness. Another common lacunar syndrome occurs with a stroke in the *pons* (part of the brainstem) and causes difficulty speaking (due to weak facial muscles) as well as a clumsy hand.

Treating Lacunar Infarcts. Lacunar infarcts are treated by controlling the underlying cause—the high blood pressure—and by using medications to prevent the narrowed arterioles from becoming completely blocked with a blood clot. The treatment of the high blood pressure involves the same strategies for risk factor reduction (weight loss and exercise) and medications as treatment of hypertension does. Medications used to prevent clotting of the narrowed arterioles include aspirin, clopidogrel (Plavix), and an aspirin and dipyridamole combination (Aggrenox).

Multi-Infarct Dementia

If many small strokes occur in the brain, a person can develop a condition called *multi-infarct dementia.* The infarcts are usually not caused by any one process alone, but instead they may be the result of several different processes discussed in this chapter and in Chapter 8. These processes include

cholesterol plaques blocking blood flow in the arteries in the brain;
hardening of arterioles in the brain caused by high blood pressure; and
blood clots or cholesterol plaques traveling to the brain from the carotid artery or heart and blocking blood flow.

In multi-infarct dementia, there are many strokes on both sides of the brain in several different locations. People with multi-infarct dementia may have a wide variety of symptoms because so many parts of the brain could be affected. They may experience

mental deterioration with memory loss and difficulty naming objects (dementia);
walking problems (gait abnormalities);
facial muscle problems such as difficulty talking and difficulty opening the eyelids; and
weakness or numbness in one or more body areas.

The best way to avoid future strokes and further deterioration is to address the causes of the infarcts, which vary from person to person but generally include high blood pressure and atherosclerosis.

Hypertensive Hemorrhages

High blood pressure may lead to rupture of arteries and bleeding or hemorrhaging into the brain. How much damage the bleeding causes and what symptoms it causes depends on the location and size of the bleed. The penetrating arteries that feed the brain are most commonly associated with hypertensive hemorrhages. These arteries feed regions deep within the brain, including

> the basal ganglia (a major center for the control of movement, made up of the caudate nucleus, putamen, and globus pallidus);
> the thalamus (an important relay station for sensory signals traveling in the brain);
> the pons (an area in the brainstem close to the respiratory, cardiac, and gastrointestinal centers; messages from the spinal cord, cerebral cortex, and cerebellum travel through the pons); and
> the cerebellum (a major center for balance and coordination).

Most hypertensive hemorrhages (50 to 60 percent) occur in an area of the brain called the *putamen,* which is part of the basal ganglia and plays an important role in the control of movement. The putamen is near a critical structure known as the *internal capsule,* through which all the motor signals from the brain travel to get to the rest of the body. Bleeding into the putamen on one side of the brain may damage the internal capsule and stop motor messages from being transmitted on the opposite side of the body. This interruption of signals results in weakness or paralysis on the side of the body opposite the affected putamen. A similar process and resulting weakness may happen when the hemorrhage occurs in the *thalamus,* which is also adjacent to the internal capsule. Thalamic hemorrhages usually create a significant sensory impairment, as well. Remember the case of Susan, who had a lacunar infarct in her thalamus small enough that it affected only one specific part of the thalamus and caused only sensory loss. In the case of a thalamic hypertensive hemorrhage, the amount of brain tissue affected is much greater, causing problems in both motor and sensory parts of the brain.

When a hemorrhage occurs in the part of the brain called the pons, it often causes more than just weakness. The pons is in the brainstem, where all the vital centers (including the respiratory center) are housed. With a bleed in the pons, a person may suddenly fall into a deep coma and be unable to move her arms or legs. This type of hemorrhage can be devastating and can result in death. A hemorrhage in the cerebellum, a key center for balance, coordination, and walking, may also be devastating. The person may first experience the sudden onset of vertigo (dizziness) and difficulty walking. As blood accumulates in the small space in the back of the head where the cerebellum is located, the person may start vomiting. The swelling of the cerebellum can then block the normal flow of the fluid within and around the brain (known as cerebrospinal fluid), causing increased pressure to develop within the brain. This increased pressure in a confined space may cause part of the brain to be pushed down through the hole at the base of the skull toward the spinal cord. This condition is called a *cerebral herniation* and is life-threatening because the brain's critical center for basic functions such as breathing may be damaged or destroyed. Hemorrhages in the cerebellum must be monitored carefully and may require surgery to remove the accumulating blood and ease the pressure on the adjacent brain tissue.

With hypertensive hemorrhages, most people experience a severe headache with the onset of the bleeding in the brain. The blood in the brain also creates increased pressure inside the skull, which can cause vomiting and drowsiness or coma. *It is imperative that people go to the doctor or to the emergency room if they have a sudden, severe headache.* A severe headache may mean that blood is building up in the brain and may require emergency treatment. Most "regular" (that is, tension or migraine) headaches develop more gradually, over the course of the day. Tension headaches rarely cause severe pain; migraine headaches can be more severe, but most people with migraines are familiar with their own pattern of headache. If in doubt, seek immediate medical attention, since time is of the essence when treating a cerebral hemorrhage. Some hemorrhages rapidly progress to coma, so getting to the hospital as quickly as possible is essential. Surgery may be required depending on the size and location of the bleeding.

Treating Hypertensive Hemorrhages. Treatment for most hypertensive hemorrhages is "supportive," involving close monitoring by physicians of the progress of the hemorrhage, controlling elevated blood pressure, and preventing complications. If the hemorrhage is due to a blood-thinning medication such as Coumadin, medications may be given to reverse the effects of the blood thinner. In people with very large hemorrhages, or with hemorrhages causing pressure on a vital structure within the brain, surgery may be needed to remove the accumulating blood and relieve the pressure.

Often a section of the skull is temporarily removed to alleviate pressure within the head.

> Ralph, a 50-year-old accountant with a history of high blood pressure since his twenties, was playing golf when he started to complain of a headache. The pain was located in the back of his head. He had suffered from migraine headaches ever since he was a teenager, but this was nothing like his migraines. Despite his headache, Ralph continued playing the golf match. After two more holes, Ralph started having trouble walking straight. He felt off balance. Then he started vomiting. His golf partners called 9-1-1. Ralph lost consciousness before the ambulance arrived.
>
> At the hospital a CT scan revealed a large bleed in Ralph's cerebellum. He was rushed to the operating room, where neurosurgeons removed the blood. After a long stay at a rehabilitation facility, Ralph was discharged home. He had some residual balance problems, but with the guidance of a recreational therapist, he was eventually able to return to playing golf. His blood pressure regimen was adjusted to prevent another brain hemorrhage.

Diagnosing High Blood Pressure

Your doctor can diagnose hypertension after he has measured your blood pressure several times on different office visits. Because blood pressure normally fluctuates, a single elevated blood pressure reading does not mean a diagnosis of hypertension. Blood pressure must be high for several readings on different days for a doctor to make this diagnosis.

In the doctor's office, some people experience "white coat" hypertension, meaning that when they see the doctor, their blood pressure rises. The most likely explanation for this phenomenon is that the patients are nervous in the doctor's office, which increases *catecholamines*—hormones such as adrenaline that are associated with the "fight or flight" response. These hormones increase the heart rate and cause the heart to pump more forcibly. They also cause the blood vessels to tighten (*vasoconstriction*). All of these factors can lead to increased blood pressure, so to confirm a diagnosis of hypertension many doctors recommend that patients take their blood pressure at home or have a qualified health care professional take it in the comfort of the patient's home.

Controlling High Blood Pressure

As noted earlier, the first step in the treatment of high blood pressure is modifying your lifestyle. Some of the same lifestyle modifications that can help reduce your risk of stroke, such as exercising and losing weight, also lower blood pressure. In a sense, these lifestyle changes give you a double benefit—they reduce stroke risk by themselves and they also reduce your blood pressure, which is another risk factor for stroke. (Weight loss is only recommended for people who are overweight.) Although we provide some general recommendations in Chapter 15 (on diet) and Chapter 16 (on exercise), we recommend that you check with your doctor about the best ways to exercise and lose weight.

Exercise can be a key ingredient in controlling high blood pressure, but only a commitment will make it work. The right type of exercise performed regularly and for a long enough time is critical in using exercise as a means of blood pressure control. *Aerobic exercise, such as walking, swimming, or bicycling, is the only type of exercise that has been found to be beneficial for blood pressure control.* Performing aerobic exercise, also called cardiovascular conditioning, does not mean that you cannot also perform strength training, flexibility, or other exercises, but these exercises should be added to an aerobic exercise regimen rather than taking the place of it.

Diet has also been shown to be useful in controlling blood pressure. The Dietary Approaches to Stop Hypertension (DASH) study found that a diet high in fruits, vegetables, and low-fat dairy foods, combined with a reduction in consumption of total fat and saturated fat, was helpful in lowering blood pressure. The DASH study concluded that people can lower their blood pressure even more effectively by combining these dietary changes with a reduction in salt intake. Some people are more sensitive to dietary salt than others, but reducing the salt in your diet, with or without making other dietary changes, cannot hurt and may help reduce your blood pressure.

Alcohol can temporarily elevate blood pressure, so alcohol intake should be minimized or avoided by people seeking to lower their blood pressure through lifestyle changes.

Reducing stress is sometimes helpful in lowering blood pressure, though this may be very difficult to accomplish. Many types of stress, such as financial, work, or family stresses, may be beyond your control to some extent. Nonetheless, evaluating the sources of stress in your life and working to minimize them may help control your blood pressure. Adopting techniques such as meditation to reduce the impact of stressful circumstances on your feelings of stress may be useful, and you may wish to consult with a psychologist for more information about stress reduction.

Many people with high blood pressure find that even with these lifestyle changes their blood pressure remains elevated and requires treatment with prescription medications. Choosing among the many different blood pressure lowering medications is a topic of ongoing discussion in medicine. The situation is complicated further by the fact that many people do not achieve adequate control of their blood pressure with one medication alone—they must take two or more medications.

Though there is ongoing debate about the best medications for the initial treatment of high blood pressure, most doctors would agree that some of the best choices are *diuretics* ("water pills") such as hydrochlorothiazide (Hydrodiuril), beta-blockers such as atenolol (Tenormin) and metoprolol (Toprol), ACE inhibitors such as lisinopril (Zestril) and enalapril (Vasotec), and angiotensin receptor blockers such as valsartan (Diovan) and candesartan (Atacand). Medications usually reserved for more resistant cases include calcium channel blockers such as amlodipine (Norvasc), alpha-blockers such as doxazosin (Cardura), and anti-hypertensives that work on the central nervous system such as clonidine (Catapres).

In the past, doctors' general practice was to keep increasing the dose of a single medication until blood pressure was controlled, the maximum dose was reached, or side effects developed. Many physicians have altered their approach, however, and now prefer to use lower doses of medications to avoid side effects, adding a low dose of a second or third medication if needed to achieve blood pressure control.

Table 9.4 lists common blood pressure medications and their classes; Table 9.5 describes how they work and their common side effects. More information about specific medications is available on the Internet and from most pharmacies.

Some blood pressure medications are available in combination form, with two or more medications combined into one pill to reduce the number of pills a person with high blood pressure needs to take. There is often a trade-off between convenience and cost, however, as these medications may be less expensive individually than in combination form.

A review of the package inserts from these blood pressure medications reveals that many different side effects can occur. Most people don't experience any of these side effects, but any side effect you notice should be taken

Table 9.4. Blood Pressure Medications

Brand Name	Generic Name	Class of Medication
Aceon	Perindopril	ACE inhibitor
Adalat	Nifedipine	Calcium channel blocker
Altace	Ramipril	ACE inhibitor
Atacand	Candesartan	Angiotensin receptor blocker
Avapro	Irbesartan	Angiotensin receptor blocker
Benicar	Olmesartan	Angiotensin receptor blocker
Calan	Verapamil	Calcium channel blocker
Capoten	Captopril	ACE inhibitor
Cardene	Nicardipine	Calcium channel blocker
Cardura	Doxasozin	Alpha-blocker
Catapres	Clonidine	Centrally acting medication
Corgard	Nadolol	Beta-blocker
Cozaar	Losartan	Angiotensin receptor blocker
Diovan	Valsartan	Angiotensin receptor blocker
Hydrodiuril	Hydrochlorothiazide	Diuretic
Hytrin	Terazosin	Alpha-blocker
Inderal	Propanolol	Beta-blocker
Isoptin	Verapamil	Calcium channel blocker
Lopressor	Metoprolol	Beta-blocker
Micardis	Telmisartan	Angiotensin receptor blocker
Minipress	Prazosin	Alpha-blocker
Normodyne	Labetalol	Alpha-/beta-blocker
Norvasc	Amlodipine	Calcium channel blocker
Prinivil	Lisinopril	ACE inhibitor
Procardia	Nifedipine	Calcium channel blocker
Tenormin	Atenolol	Beta-blocker
Teveten	Eprosartan	Angiotensin receptor blocker
Toprol	Metoprolol	Beta-blocker
Trandate	Labetalol	Alpha-/beta-blocker
Vasotec	Enalapril	ACE inhibitor
Zestril	Lisinopril	ACE inhibitor

Table 9.5. **Blood Pressure Medication Effects by Class**

Medication Class	How They Work	Possible Side Effects
Alpha-blockers	Dilate blood vessels	Can cause low blood pressure when a person rises suddenly from a seated position
Alpha-/beta-blockers	Combine blood vessel dilation of alpha-blockers with heart rate slowing effects of beta-blockers	Low blood pressure
Angiotensin converting enzyme (ACE) inhibitors	Block the creation of angiotensin, a chemical that causes blood vessels to constrict	Chronic cough, allergic reactions
Angiotensin receptor blockers (ARBs)	Blocks the action of angiotensin, a chemical that causes blood vessels to constrict	Allergic reactions
Beta-blockers	Slow the heart and reduces the force of heart contraction	Fatigue, reduced exercise ability, sexual dysfunction
Calcium channel blockers	Dilate blood vessels	Ankle swelling, constipation
Centrally acting medications	Affect neurotransmitters in the brain that regulate blood pressure	Depression
Diuretics ("water pills")	Cause fluid and salt to be excreted by the kidneys	Frequent urination, low potassium levels

seriously, even if it does not appear on the "official" list. We advise people to let their doctors know about any adverse effects of a drug they are taking, so their doctors can advise them whether it should be discontinued and, if so, whether to stop taking the medication abruptly or taper it down. The doctor may also want to discuss an alternative treatment.

How low should you go? The Joint National Committee (JNC) on hypertension officially recommends that individuals diagnosed with hypertension reduce their blood pressure to below 130/85 through a combination of lifestyle changes and medication. People with diabetes are at higher risk of complications from hypertension, and some experts advocate lower blood pressure goals for these people. Even for individuals with "pre-hypertension," defined as a systolic blood pressure between 130 and 139 or a diastolic blood pressure between 80 and 89, lifestyle changes are appropriate, and medications may be needed for people at higher risk. There is no clear dividing line—or target blood pressure goal—for stroke risk. The risk seems to go down with the blood pressure, though side effects (such as dizziness and fainting) are a risk of lowering blood pressure too much. Your physician should determine the blood pressure goal that is appropriate for you. The JNC's guidelines are intended only as a general rule, not as advice for any specific individual.

Again, people with both high blood pressure and diabetes have been found to have a higher risk of stroke and other cardiovascular complications than people with either condition alone. Good control of high blood pressure is particularly critical for people with both diabetes and hypertension.

Because hypertension is a silent killer, everyone should have their blood pressure checked regularly. Regular monitoring of high blood pressure is critical for stroke survivors. If you have had a stroke and you have high blood pressure, lowering your blood pressure is one of the most important ways to lower your risk of a second stroke. Being aware of all the risk factors for hypertension and doing everything you possibly can to modify the risk factors you can control will help lower your blood pressure. Taking blood pressure medication routinely and closely monitoring blood pressure are essential components of a program to avoid the complications of chronic hypertension.

Chapter 10

• •

Diabetes and Stroke

Diabetes, like high blood pressure, is sometimes a "silent" health problem that is not discovered until after a person has had a complication like a stroke or a heart attack. Diabetes often goes undetected for several years before its damage to the body becomes apparent. Diabetes can harm the eyes, the kidneys, the nervous system, and the blood vessels. Half of all people who discover that they have diabetes already have cardiac complications from it.

Diabetes is a risk factor for many serious medical conditions. For example, compared to people who do not have diabetes, people with diabetes have

two to four times the risk of having a stroke and, after their first stroke, two to four times the risk of having a second stroke;

twice the risk of having a heart attack;

a hundred-fold increase in the risk of developing gangrene of the leg caused by atherosclerosis; and

four to five times the risk of developing congestive heart failure.

If you or someone you love has diabetes, these statistics may frighten you. But there are steps you can take to improve your health and reduce the chance of serious complications from diabetes. Research studies have shown that improving the control of diabetes can significantly reduce the risk of developing complications such as stroke. This chapter provides a guide to understanding your diabetes and taking action to help prevent complications.

Even if you have had diabetes for a long time, or if you already have complications such as heart disease from diabetes, there are many ways you can get your diabetes under control and reduce your risk of having a stroke or other problem in the future. In this chapter, we'll explain how diabetes affects the body and how the disease can lead to stroke. We'll also tell you about the risk factors for and complications of this disease. By being aware that you have diabetes, controlling your blood glucose levels, and working to reduce other risk factors for stroke and cardiovascular disease, you can substantially reduce the risk of these complications.

Types of Diabetes

According to the American Diabetes Association, 18.2 million people in the United States have *diabetes mellitus.* This term literally translates to "honey sweet diabetes," because people with diabetes have too much glucose (a type of sugar that serves as fuel for the body) in their bloodstreams. It is estimated that only 13 million people have been diagnosed with diabetes and are aware of their disease, meaning that 5.2 million people have diabetes but do not know it. Of these 13 million people with diagnosed diabetes mellitus, approximately 5 to 10 percent have Type I diabetes, and 90 to 95 percent have Type II. Two other conditions—insulin resistance and insulin resistance syndrome—carry risks similar to the risks of diabetes.

Type I Diabetes

Type I diabetes is most commonly diagnosed in adolescents between the ages of 10 and 14; for this reason it is often called *juvenile* diabetes. However, this disorder can strike at any age and is a life-long condition once it occurs. Some people have a genetic susceptibility to this disease.

In 10 percent of people with Type I diabetes, the cause is unknown. For everyone else, the cause is thought to be an autoimmune disease in which the body attacks its own pancreatic *islet beta cells*—the cells responsible for producing a hormone called *insulin.* Normally, insulin helps to move glucose out of the bloodstream and into the cells for use as energy. Without insulin, glucose levels remain high in the bloodstream. The cells are starved for fuel, since they are unable to use the glucose in the bloodstream without insulin to help bring it inside the cells. As a result, the body breaks down fat (*adipose tissue*) for energy. Fat breakdown creates a high level of free fatty acids in the bloodstream. When oxygen combines with these free fatty acids, *ketone bodies* (acetoacetic acid and beta hydroxybutyric acid) are formed. High levels of ketones produce a condition called *ketoacidosis,* which can cause disorientation or even loss of consciousness (known as *diabetic ketotic coma*). Diabetic ketoacidosis is a medical emergency and should be treated in a hospital.

Because Type I diabetes is caused by insufficient levels of insulin produced by the pancreas, the only effective treatment is to receive insulin by injection or other technique (such as an insulin pump), or to restore insulin production through a transplantation of pancreas tissue (still a relatively uncommon procedure).

Type II Diabetes

Ninety to ninety-five percent of people with diabetes have Type II diabetes. Type II diabetes is most commonly diagnosed in people older than 45. Risk factors for Type II diabetes include obesity with fat carried around the waist, low levels of physical activity, and a family history of the disease. Ethnic groups that appear to have a greater propensity for developing Type II diabetes include African Americans, Hispanics, Native Americans, Asian Americans, and Pacific Islanders.

In Type II diabetes, the initial problem is insulin resistance, which leads to pancreatic beta cell failure. The term *insulin resistance* means that cells throughout the body do not respond normally to insulin, and glucose levels in the bloodstream remain high. The pancreas responds to the rising blood glucose levels by making more and more insulin, yet the body still is unable to use the glucose efficiently. At first, the body is able to compensate for insulin resistance by raising the insulin level, but eventually the blood sugar level starts to rise in spite of the increased insulin production. The cells in the pancreas that make insulin (*beta cells*) cannot keep up with the demand, and there is a relative shortage in the supply of insulin in the body. In other words, the pancreatic beta cells become exhausted and fail. Some people with Type II diabetes may require shots of insulin to control their blood sugars. The problem of ketoacidosis is uncommon among people with Type II diabetes, but very high blood sugar levels in Type II diabetes can also lead to confusion and even coma.

Insulin Resistance

According to the American Diabetes Association, in addition to the millions of people with Type II diabetes, an astonishing 41 million Americans have insulin resistance—a sort of "pre-diabetes." These people do not have pancreatic islet beta cell dysfunction and failure, and they have not been diagnosed with diabetes; however, they already have mildly elevated levels of blood glucose. These levels are not high enough to be labeled diabetes, but they are not normal, and 25 percent of these individuals will eventually develop Type II diabetes.

Some people who have insulin resistance pre-diabetes can modify their risk factors for Type II diabetes and prevent the progression of their condition to diabetes, or at least slow it down. If you have insulin resistance, there are two keys to fighting back against developing diabetes: first, lose weight (if you are overweight); and second, exercise regularly. Weight loss increases the body's sensitivity to insulin. Regular exercise also has this effect on the body, and can help with weight control, providing a "two-for-one" benefit. Increased physical activity decreases blood glucose levels because when you expend energy, your cells use up glucose—the number one fuel source for the body. People with diabetes need to monitor their blood sugars and carbohydrate intake prior to exercise. (Chapter 16 discusses this situation in more detail.)

Insulin Resistance Syndrome

Insulin resistance syndrome is not a type of diabetes but is very common among people with insulin resistance and Type II diabetes. It is also known as metabolic syndrome, syndrome X, and Raeven's syndrome. Not only does this syndrome have many different names, it is associated with many different medical problems and blood test abnormalities. These medical problems and blood test abnormalities are listed in Table 10.1. As you can see from the list, this syndrome includes several risk factors for stroke. It is called a syndrome because it is a collection of medical problems (such as obesity, Type II diabetes, and hypertension) and blood test abnormalities (such as high LDL level, low HDL level, increased clotting factors, and increased uric acid) found in the same patient. No single disease process accounts for all of the medical problems and blood test abnormalities in this syndrome. In fact, there are multiple disease processes involved. Just because someone has hypertension and Type II diabetes does not mean that he has insulin resistance syndrome. However, if a person has several components of the syndrome, such as insulin resistance, hypertension, Type II diabetes, high LDL levels, low HDL levels, and a high uric acid level, then it makes sense to check for some of the other medical problems associated with the syndrome. Approximately 50 million people in the United States have insulin resistance syndrome. They are at markedly increased risk for atherosclerosis, heart attack, and stroke. If you have insulin resistance or diabetes, it is important to check for this syndrome and monitor blood tests to reduce your risk of a second stroke.

Complications of Diabetes

For someone with diabetes, tight control of the blood sugar is critical to slow down the progression of the disease and possibly prevent the compli-

Table 10.1. Medical Conditions Associated with Insulin Resistance Syndrome

---

Insulin resistance
Impaired glucose tolerance
Type II diabetes
Central obesity (obesity of the abdominal area)
High blood pressure
High LDL cholesterol
Low HDL cholesterol
High uric acid levels (which is associated with gout)
Decreased levels of factors in the blood that help to prevent clotting

---

cations associated with the disease. Diabetes can affect almost any organ in the body but most commonly damages the eyes, kidneys, nervous system, and vascular system.

Eyes

In the short term, very high blood sugar (glucose) levels can cause blurry vision because they may alter the ability of the lens of the eye to adjust its shape and to focus. There is a delicate balance in the glucose concentration of the fluid around the eye, called the *aqueous humor,* and the lens of the eye. If there is too much glucose in the fluid around the eye, it will absorb fluid from the lens and change the shape of the lens. When the blood glucose levels go back down, the fluid returns to the lens and vision returns to normal. Other changes in the eye, such as cataracts, glaucoma, and, in severe cases, blindness, may develop after years of exposure to high glucose and are not so easily reversible. According to the American Diabetes Association, diabetes is the number one cause of new onset blindness, with about 12,000 to 24,000 people a year becoming blind because of this disease.

A detailed eye examination tells a physician a great deal about the effects of diabetes on the eyes. With an ophthalmoscope, the physician can peer into the back of the eye (the *retina*) and may find tiny outpouchings of blood vessels called *microaneurysms.* These microaneurysms are the early signs of diabetes affecting the eyes. As the disease advances, more and more changes take place in the eye, and may include fluid leaking out of the blood vessels and creating tiny spots known as *exudates,* visible only through an ophthalmoscope. When these spots occur in the area of the retina responsible for vision (*macula*), vision can be affected.

Other findings on an ophthalmologic exam may include hemorrhages in the blood vessels in the retina or the development of new blood vessels within the retina. If new blood vessels form in the area of the eye that drains the fluid (*the anterior chamber*), a real problem develops because the fluid in the eye cannot drain properly with the new blood vessels in the way. If it is not treated promptly, the buildup of fluid in the eye can cause increased pressure in the eye (*glaucoma*), pain, and loss of vision. After the formation of new blood vessels in the retina and the vitreous cavity, which lies next to the retina, fibrosis develops. A fibrous membrane can develop in the vitreous cavity and pull on the retina, causing a retinal detachment and loss of vision.

Kidneys

Diabetes targets the kidneys. People who have had Type I diabetes for twenty years have a 30 to 40 percent chance of developing kidney disease (*nephropathy*). In contrast, people with Type II diabetes have a 15 to 20 percent chance of developing nephropathy after twenty years. Like the eyes, the kidneys are important organs. However, most people do not appreciate the complexity and the significance of normal kidney function. There are two kidneys in the body that function to filter the blood, and they have three main filtering functions:

1. To rid the blood of waste and toxins
2. To hold on to the important nutrients in the blood, such as proteins and glucose
3. To maintain a healthy balance of sodium, potassium, calcium, hydrogen, bicarbonate, and water in the blood

You may be wondering how two small organs accomplish all of this. Each kidney is made up of a million tiny *nephrons,* and each nephron is its own functional filtration unit. This means that the body uses two million little filters to clean and maintain the blood. Diabetes attacks these tiny filtration units. In the nephrons, there are specialized blood vessels for filtering the blood called *glomeruli.* The glomeruli are made up of arterioles that bring the blood into the kidney. These arterioles lead into capillaries, which are even smaller blood vessels than the arterioles. Capillaries have very thin walls that allow for the transfer of substances from the bloodstream to the body's tissues.

Scientists believe that the high levels of glucose seen in people with diabetes damages the glomeruli in their kidneys. The damage causes one of the membranes in the capillaries (the *basement membrane*) to become thickened. The thickened membrane becomes leakier and less able to properly perform its filtering functions. The end result is that protein leaks out. Initially, only the building blocks of proteins, the small amino acids, leak out of the bloodstream and end up in the urine. Remember that it is the nephrons' job to keep protein in the bloodstream. This function is disrupted by the damage caused by diabetes.

Damage to the filtering system of the kidney can be detected by a simple urine test. If the proteins are not kept in the bloodstream by the nephrons, they end up in the urine. Within a few years after the onset of diabetes, *microalbuminemia* (tiny particles of the protein *albumin*) can be detected in the urine. At this point, a person with diabetes may not have any symptoms at all from this microalbuminemia. After ten or fifteen more years of damage, the filtration units of the kidneys allow larger proteins to escape into the urine. This is called *proteinuria.* After five or ten additional years of high blood sugar, the damage becomes devastating to the millions of nephrons in the kidney, and the kidney is unable to perform its filtering functions. When this happens, it is called *end-stage renal disease (ESRD)*, or kidney failure. There is so much damage that the kidneys can no longer get rid of all the waste and toxins in the blood, hold on to all the important nutrients in the blood such as proteins and glucose, or maintain a healthy balance of sodium, potassium, calcium, hydrogen, bicarbonate, and water in the blood.

Unlike people with microalbuminemia, people with end-stage renal disease have many symptoms. They experience swelling from excess fluid escaping from the bloodstream and entering the tissues. The swelling can be in the ankles and legs, and even around the eyes in the morning after lying flat all night. The retention of fluid causes weight gain. Other symptoms of end-stage renal disease include poor appetite, nausea, vomiting, fatigue, itching, and headache.

A person with end-stage renal disease needs *dialysis (hemodialysis* or *peritoneal dialysis)* to relieve them of symptoms, rid their bodies of toxins and waste products, and correct the imbalances created by the kidneys' failure to filter. Hemodialysis is a medical procedure in which an artificial kidney machine does the job of the two million nephrons in the failed kidneys. Hemodialysis needs to be completed three times a week, usually at a specialized dialysis center or a hospital, and each time the hemodialysis takes about three to five hours.

Peritoneal dialysis does not require any machines. It uses the *peritoneal membrane* (the lining of the abdomen) and a special dialysis solution to rid the body of wastes and to remove excess fluid. This solution, which includes sugar and minerals mixed with water, is introduced into the peritoneum through a little tube in the abdominal wall. After a few hours, the sugar has attracted the waste, toxins, and extra fluid out of the peritoneal membrane blood vessels and pulled these products into the solution. The "used" solution is removed from the peritoneum via the tube in the abdominal wall. This procedure is repeated again with a fresh dialysis solution, and the blood is cleaned. Peritoneal dialysis is done several times a day.

Dialysis is not painful but it is a complicated, time consuming, exhausting process. The best way to avoid it is to watch your blood sugars and keep them under control. If you have diabetes, you can protect your kidneys by not exposing them to high glucose levels.

Nervous System

Nervous system complications of diabetes can be annoying and sometimes painful. People with diabetes often experience injury to the nerves in their body; this damage is known as *neuropathy*. The damage to the nerves generally affects the longest nerves first, so the first symptom of diabetic neuropathy is typically a decrease in sensation in the feet, including a decrease in the ability to sense pain, temperature, and vibration. Some patients describe "burning sensations" in their legs at night. By the time the sensory changes progress to involve the area up to the knee, the fingertips and hands are usually affected as well. While changes in sensation are the most common symptoms of diabetic neuropathy, more severe neuropathy can cause weakness in the feet and hands due to involvement of the motor nerves in those areas.

In addition to controlling movement and supplying sensation, nerves control many of the more automatic functions of the body. This portion of the nervous system, known as the *autonomic nervous system*, may also be affected by diabetes. The autonomic nervous system regulates blood pressure, so people with diabetes who have problems with this system sometimes experience lightheadedness upon standing, due to pooling of blood in their lower extremities (this is called *postural hypotension*). They can also experience alternating episodes of diarrhea and constipation as well as difficulty urinating, with a weak stream. Many men with long-standing diabetes experience erectile dysfunction as a result of autonomic nerve damage.

People with diabetes are prone to infections in their feet because of their impaired sensory system. Pain is an important warning system for the body, letting a person know that a body part may be at risk for damage. Because people with diabetic neuropathy cannot reliably sense pain in their feet, they are more likely to stub their toe, for example, and not even feel it. They may not notice that they have a cut on a foot, and then may not notice it progressing to an ulcer. Diabetes impairs the circulation in the feet, and in severe cases may lead to the inability to fight skin infections or even to gangrene. People with diabetes should never walk around barefoot. They should take meticulous care of their feet by cleaning them regularly and having a podiatrist trim their toenails. Extra-depth and extra-width shoes are often a good choice for someone who has diabetes. Proper shoes are wide enough and deep enough to allow a comfortable fit without causing pressure anywhere on the foot. Shoes are so important, in fact, that many health insurers (including Medicare) will pay for shoes for their clients with diabetes.

Vascular System

Most of the complications of diabetes are caused by poor circulation, which is caused by damage to blood vessels ranging from the largest vessel (the aorta) to the smallest (the capillaries). In the larger blood vessels, including the aorta and the large and medium-sized arteries, the damage is caused by atherosclerosis. People with diabetes tend to have extensive atherosclerosis and tend to get it at an earlier age than people without diabetes. The excess glucose, and in Type II diabetes the excess insulin, in the bloodstream of people with diabetes damages the endothelial cells in the arteries and creates an environment conducive to the progression of atherosclerosis. Also, vital clot-forming particles in the blood known as *platelets* become "stickier" and more likely to adhere to the blood vessel walls in people with diabetes. When these platelets stick to an atherosclerotic plaque, the plaque becomes larger. The tendency toward accelerated atherosclerosis makes stroke, coronary artery disease, and peripheral vascular disease common problems for people with diabetes.

Despite the problems it creates, atherosclerosis is not the primary culprit for damage in the smaller blood vessels (the arterioles and capillaries). As in high blood pressure, in diabetes the arterioles are damaged by the deposit of an extra protein called hyaline, which is mostly made up of the fibrous protein *collagen*. This condition is called *hyaline arteriolosclerosis*. The capillaries can also be damaged by the deposit of hyaline, in a process called *microangiopathy*. In people with diabetes, capillaries all over the body, including those in the skin, skeletal muscle, nervous system, retina, and kidneys, are affected by microangiopathy. Microangiopathy in the capillaries of the skin makes the healing of a small cut on the foot difficult because oxygen and nutrients cannot reach the site of injury.

The Association between Diabetes and Stroke

Why do people with diabetes have two to four times the risk of a stroke compared to those who do not have diabetes? As we have seen in this chapter, the vascular system is one of the major targets for this disease. The combination of high glucose levels and high insulin levels damaging the endothelial cells of the arteries make atherosclerosis a prominent feature of Type II diabetes. (Chapter 8 discusses atherosclerosis in detail.) Diabetes leads to stroke primarily, but not solely, through atherosclerosis. People with diabetes are also more prone to form blood clots (they are more *hypercoagulable*). We all have factors in our blood that help us to form clots, break up clots, and stop clots from forming. Usually these different factors are present in our blood in a balance that allows proper functioning: clotting when we need to clot and preventing blood clots when we need to allow blood flow. People with diabetes tend to have increased levels of blood factors that form clots. On top of this, they also tend to have "stickier" platelets. Platelets normally function in the blood to allow clot formation when needed. However, when they are extra sticky, they may stick to atherosclerotic plaques, increasing their size, or stick to each other, forming a clot. Because people with diabetes have an increased tendency to form blood clots, they are more susceptible to stroke.

High blood pressure is common among people with diabetes. In fact, one in three individuals with diabetes also has high blood pressure. The damage high blood pressure does to the arteries plus the damage diabetes itself does makes people who have both high blood pressure and diabetes more likely to have a stroke. (Chapter 9 discusses high blood pressure in detail.)

Diagnosing Diabetes

Symptoms of Diabetes

It is a good idea for everyone to be aware of the symptoms of diabetes (see Table 10.2). If you develop these symptoms—even just a few of them—you should see your doctor for a diagnostic test. These symptoms may occur

Table 10.2. **Symptoms of Diabetes**

Frequent urination

Persistent thirst

Weakness or fatigue

Blurred vision

Increased appetite and intake of food with weight loss

Night-time bed wetting (*enuresis*)

Infections in the vaginal area (*vulvovaginitis*)

Itching (*pruritus*)

Sensory changes or weakness in the arms or legs (*peripheral neuropathy*)

---

with other conditions, and someone with these symptoms does not necessarily have diabetes. On the other hand, many people with diabetes have no symptoms at all. For this reason, everyone over the age of 45 should take a fasting glucose test. If the test is normal, it should be repeated again in three years.

The Fasting Blood Glucose Test

Diabetes can be diagnosed by a simple blood test called the *fasting blood glucose test*. After twelve hours of fasting, about one tablespoon of blood is drawn from a vein and sent to a laboratory to measure the concentration of glucose in the blood. A level of 126 milligrams per deciliter (mg/dL) or higher is abnormal and may signal diabetes. Having one high reading, however, does not necessarily mean that you have diabetes. In fact, two or three high readings on different days are required to make a definite diagnosis.

The Oral Glucose Tolerance Test

Another test for diabetes is the *oral glucose tolerance test.* If someone has had one or two inconclusive fasting blood glucose tests, they may be given the oral glucose tolerance test to confirm the diagnosis of diabetes. The oral glucose tolerance test is more time consuming, but it also provides more information. This test involves two tests of blood sugar levels. The first level is checked after at least twelve hours of fasting. The person is then given a very sweet drink containing a substantial amount of glucose. Two hours after receiving the glucose drink, the person's blood glucose is measured again. Normally, the body's concentration of glucose will increase slightly after ingesting a large amount of sugar. If it increases by a large amount,

Table 10.3. Oral Glucose Tolerance Test

	Normal	*Impaired Glucose Tolerance*	*Diabetes*
Fasting blood glucose	<110 mg/dL	110–125 mg/dL	>125 mg/dL
2 hours after glucose load	<140 mg/dL	140–199 mg/dL	>199 mg/dL

however, there is a problem with the body's ability to use the glucose in the bloodstream and move it into the cells, where it belongs. Table 10.3 shows how the test results are interpreted.

Treating Diabetes

Control of blood sugar can help reduce the risk of stroke and other complications of diabetes. If you have diabetes, the first step in controlling your condition is to improve your diet and increase your level of exercise. Diet is discussed in Chapter 15, and exercise is discussed in Chapter 16. Both of these chapters include sections for people with diabetes. In brief, foods with simple carbohydrates and sugars (for example, chocolate cake, ice cream, and refined breads and snacks such as donuts and pastries) all cause a rapid rise in the blood sugar level and worsen control of diabetes. Conversely, exercise reduces blood sugar, and with it, the dose of diabetes medications or insulin needed. As a bonus, controlling diet and increasing exercise will also help with weight reduction, an important goal for anyone with Type II diabetes who is above their ideal body weight.

Controlling blood sugar, exercising regularly, and maintaining a healthy diet have been shown to be helpful in reducing the risk of stroke in people with Type I and Type II diabetes. Many people with diabetes (including all individuals with Type I diabetes) find that exercise and diet alone are not enough to control their blood sugar levels, however. They also need medical treatment. As discussed earlier in this chapter, people with Type I diabetes require insulin, but many people with Type II diabetes do not, although they may require other medications for blood sugar control.

For individuals using insulin to control their diabetes, new types of insulin and new regimens are now available to help achieve control. Some people benefit from a new form of very long-lasting insulin called insulin glargine (Lantus), which provides a long-lasting base level of insulin. In some cases, this may be combined with a new very short-acting insulin known as insulin lispro (Humalog), which can be taken immediately before a meal, when insulin is most needed. Many people with Type II diabetes can achieve good control with more conventional insulins (such as NPH insulin and regular insulin). Insulin regimens need to be customized to an individual's metabolism. Some people with Type II diabetes take combinations of insulin and oral medications for blood sugar control.

Insulin pumps are used by some people with Type I diabetes to provide both a baseline level of insulin and increased doses at mealtimes. Pumps are commercially available in a number of different options. Currently available pumps are external, and require the user to insert a small tube (known as a *cannula*) under the skin to deliver the insulin. The pumps require the user to determine how much insulin is needed. Fully implantable pumps (pumps that are surgically placed beneath the skin) are being tested but are not yet widely available.

The number and types of oral medicines available for the treatment of Type II diabetes have expanded substantially in recent years. The older oral medicines, known as *sulfonylureas,* remain important in controlling diabetes. These medications work by increasing the body's release of insulin from the pancreas. They include glyburide (Micronase, Diabeta), glipizide (Glucotrol), glimepiride (Amaryl), and others. The meglitinide medications, which include repaglinide (Prandin) and nateglinide (Starlix), also stimulate the pancreas to release more insulin, though these medications are not chemically related to the sulfonylureas and may work in a slightly different fashion. Both sulfonylurea and meglitinide medications can cause excessively low blood sugar as a complication, so anyone taking these medications should monitor their blood sugar closely.

Metformin (Glucophage) is the only medication currently available in the biguanide class of medications. It reduces blood sugar levels by reducing sugar production in the liver and increasing sensitivity to insulin in several organ systems, including the liver and muscles. It also appears to affect sugar metabolism in the intestines, further contributing to its effect on blood sugar. Metformin is less likely to cause excessively low blood sugar than sulfonylurea medications. Sulfonylurea medications (or meglitinide medications) are often used in combination with metformin to achieve more effective reductions in blood sugar than with either medication alone. Certain conditions can affect the metabolism of metformin and cause a dangerous buildup of a chemical known as *lactic acid* in the blood. These conditions include reduced kidney function, liver disease, alcohol overuse, congestive heart failure, and acute illness (such as a severe infection). Individuals with diabetes who have one or more of these conditions need to alert their physician, who may decide not to prescribe metformin for them.

Another class of oral medications used for control of diabetes is the thiazolidinediones (often known as "glitazone" medications), which include pioglitazone (Actos) and rosiglitazone (Avandia). These medications increase insulin sensitivity in the liver and muscles by increasing the utilization of sugar and decreasing sugar production. Medications in this class have caused liver inflammation in some people.

Acarbose (Precose) and miglitol (Glyset) help smooth out the peaks in blood sugar by delaying the absorption of sugar from the intestines, though they work in somewhat different ways to accomplish this goal. These medications are often used in combination with other oral medications described earlier.

How effective is your diabetes control? There are two ways to check this, both of which are important. The finger-stick test, in which a small drop of blood is tested, is a key technique for monitoring your blood sugar. The results provide important information about your personal blood sugar patterns. This is the only way to know what times of day your blood sugar may be too high or too low. For example, you might find that your blood sugar is very high around breakfast time but falls to a dangerous level in the midafternoon. Regularly checking your finger-stick blood glucose level and reviewing a log of your blood sugar levels with your physician is an essential step toward achieving good blood sugar control and reducing your risk of having a stroke.

Another test that can check the overall level of blood glucose over time is known as a *hemoglobin A1C.* In contrast to checking your blood sugar at a single moment in time, the hemoglobin A1C test lets you and your physician know your average blood sugar levels over the past six to eight weeks. Make certain that your doctor not only checks this level but discusses the results with you. The American Diabetes Association recommends keeping this level below 7 percent, though a different goal may be appropriate based on individual circumstances. Both finger-stick glucose testing and hemoglobin A1C levels should be monitored to achieve the best overall diabetic control.

If you have diabetes and you have had a stroke, the best way to reduce your chance of a second stroke is to work on controlling your blood glucose levels. If you are overweight, lose weight. If you do not currently exercise, make exercise a routine you enjoy regularly. If you already exercise, ask your doctor whether what you are doing is sufficient or whether you can improve your exercise regimen. If your doctor prescribes medication to lower your blood glucose level, take it faithfully. Finally, monitor your blood glucose carefully and keep an accurate log and review it with your doctor. All of these steps can help to prevent another stroke.

• •

Chapter 11

Other Causes of Stroke

In the last three chapters, we discussed the most prevalent causes of stroke: common heart and blood vessel problems, high blood pressure, and diabetes. The vast majority of people who have a stroke have one or more of these three medical conditions. There are many other reasons why someone might have a stroke, however. In this chapter, we will focus on rarer categories of medical conditions and factors that can cause stroke:

1. Diseases of the blood
2. Rare problems with the blood vessels
3. Rare heart conditions
4. Infectious or inflammatory conditions
5. Side effects of medications

Each of the following five sections includes a table that lists some of the unusual causes of stroke in each particular category. In this book we cannot review every diagnosis in detail, though we do describe a few of the more common diagnoses in each section. We primarily want to provide an overview of why strokes happen to people who may not have the more common risk factors of stroke.

Diseases of the Blood

We have long known that blood is essential to survival, but we didn't always understand why. In 1875 the French scientist Paul Bert sent a hot-air balloon called *The Zenith* 7,900 meters into the air, which was the highest altitude that had then been reached by humans. When the balloon came down, two of the three men on board were dead. Bert concluded that at low atmospheric pressures, people need supplemental oxygen to make sure that the blood carries enough oxygen for survival. Certainly this was

Table 11.1. Diseases of the Blood That May Lead to Stroke

Protein S deficiency
Protein C deficiency
Antithrombin III deficiency
Sickle cell anemia
Polycythemia vera
Antiphospholipid antibody syndrome
Factor V leiden mutation
Prothrombin G20210 mutation
Beta thalassemia
Homocysteinemia
Thrombotic thrombocytopenic purpura
Disseminated intravascular coagulation
Idiopathic thrombocytopenic purpura
Hypercoagulable states resulting from:
    Cancer
    Nephrotic syndrome
    Inflammatory bowel disease

Sources: Wade S. Smith, Stephen L. Hauser, and J. Donald Easton, "Cerebrovascular Diseases," in *Harrison's Principles of Internal Medicine,* 15th edition, ed. Eugene Braunwald et al. (New York: McGraw-Hill, 2001); Timothy J. Counihan, "Cerebrovascular Disease," in *Cecil Essentials of Medicine,* 6th edition, ed. Thomas E. Andreoli et al. (Philadelphia: W. B. Saunders, 2004); H. A. Klausner and C. Lewandowski, "Infrequent Causes of Stroke," *Emergency Medicine Clinics of North America* 2, no. 3 (August 2002).

a tragic way to discover this concept; however, over time this and many other experiments helped us understand how the blood works and why it is so important.

Problems with our blood can lead to many different kinds of medical conditions, including stroke (see Table 11.1). This section is not a comprehensive discussion of how blood functions. Rather, the overview provided here will help you understand how a problem with your blood might be a factor in your risk of stroke. Many problems with the blood are easily diagnosed with simple lab tests. If you have a blood disorder, your doctor will provide you with details about your particular condition. You might want to consider seeing a *hematologist* (a physician who specializes in treating blood problems), if you have a blood disorder. Note that a number of these conditions are inherited and are passed down from generation to generation.

A number of medical conditions cause the blood to form clots, and clots can lead to a stroke. Our bodies normally produce natural anticoagulants, proteins that circulate and help to prevent our blood from clotting inappropriately. When the level of these proteins is abnormally low, clotting is more likely. People with this problem may be more likely to have a stroke. A stroke may also be caused by abnormalities in the size and shape of red blood cells, as occurs in people with *sickle cell anemia.* Too many red blood cells circulating in the bloodstream, which occurs in *polycythemia vera,* may also result in stroke.

Protein S, Protein C, and Antithrombin III Deficiencies

Protein S, protein C, and antithrombin III all work to help prevent clotting in the blood. When there is a deficiency of any of these naturally occurring anticoagulants, clotting is more likely. The clots may form in the deep veins of the leg or in the blood vessels in the lungs or in the heart. If there is a hole in the heart such as a patent foramen ovale (PFO), a piece of the clot can break off, travel through the hole, and enter the blood vessels supplying the brain, where it can cause a stroke.

Although these conditions are not common, it is important to recognize that they cause strokes in some people. Blood tests to check for the levels of these proteins are commonly performed when a person has a stroke without a clear cause. Treatment involves long-term use of the medication Coumadin in order to prevent blood clots from forming. Smoking should also be absolutely avoided, since smoking increases the risk of stroke in individuals who have a tendency to form blood clots. Smoking increases the risk of stroke in many ways:

1. By decreasing HDL (good cholesterol), which increases the chances of atherosclerosis
2. By damaging the endothelial cells with toxins such as carbon monoxide, increasing the chance of atherosclerosis
3. By making platelets more likely to clump together and clot
4. By affecting *fibrinogen* (a blood protein involved in forming clots), making clotting more likely

Sickle Cell Anemia

Sickle cell anemia is another blood disorder that can lead to blood clots. Stroke is not a common effect of sickle cell anemia, but it certainly can happen. Although this disease is most commonly found in African Americans, people of many ethnic origins have it, including people from the Middle East, the Mediterranean, and India.

Sickle cell anemia is an inherited condition in which the bone marrow makes some normal red blood cells and some malformed ones with abnormal hemoglobin (*hemoglobin S* or *HbS*). Hemoglobin is the component of a red blood cell that carries oxygen, a critical function for the survival of all cells and tissues in the body. This abnormal hemoglobin is extremely sensitive to the amount of oxygen, water, and acids in the blood. If the blood is high in acids or low in oxygen or water, then the hemoglobin S will go through an intricate molecular transformation which alters the red blood cell's membrane, making it less flexible. It also changes the shape of the red blood cells. Instead of being round, they are shaped like a sickle (crescent or C-shaped). Sickling of the red blood cells is reversible. If oxygen and water are restored to the red blood cells or the acid level in the blood is reduced to normal, the sickle cells can revert back to a round shape. However, after several transformations into sickle cells and back to round cells, the red blood cells with the hemoglobin S become permanently rigid and crescent shaped. The spleen recognizes the sickle-shaped cells as abnormal and destroys them. With fewer red blood cells, the person becomes anemic. (Anemia means having lower than the normal number of red blood cells or hemoglobin in the blood.)

The sickle cells create several problems for the body and can create a sickle cell "crisis." A crisis occurs when the blood is carrying low levels of oxygen such as happens with pneumonia (infection of the lung tissue) and septicemia (an infection traveling in the blood stream), when the blood does not have enough water in it such as in states of dehydration, and when the blood has too many acids in it such as in starvation acidosis, muscle exhaustion after extremely vigorous exercise (lactic acidosis), or diabetic ketoacidosis. In these situations, the sickle cells' shape and rigidity interferes with *microcirculation*, their passage through the smallest blood vessels in the body. Because these sickle cells are also stickier than normal red blood cells, they tend to clump together and form a single mass that can easily get stuck in the small blood vessels. When they get stuck, they can block blood flow to tissues and vital organs such as the spleen, kidney, lungs, and brain. Blocking blood flow to tissues such as muscles creates pain, and sickle cell crises often cause pain in the extremities, back, chest, and abdomen. When blood flow is blocked in the brain, a stroke may result.

The diagnosis of sickle cell anemia is made by examining the shape of the red blood cells under the microscope and testing the hemoglobin in the blood cells (this test is called *hemoglobin electrophoresis*). The health of people with sickle cell anemia must be carefully monitored. The treatment of sickle cell anemia generally involves trying to prevent a sickle cell "crisis." This term is used when there is a lot of "sickling" of the cells and the blood does not flow smoothly through the small blood vessels. It is not always possible to prevent a crisis, but if you have sickle cell anemia, talk with your doctor about how to avoid triggering a severe episode. Known triggers include

> low oxygen levels (which may occur if you travel to a mountainous region, for example);
> certain types of infections (people with sickle cell anemia should get the flu shot every year and receive the pneumococcal vaccine called Pneumovax);
> fever;
> dehydration (stay well hydrated at all times, including while exercising and during an illness);
> low folic acid (talk to your doctor about which vitamin supplements are best for you).

If your stroke was caused by sickle cell disease, you have an increased chance of having a second one with the same cause. Hydroxyurea is a medication used to treat sickle cell anemia. It works by increasing the body's production of a form of hemoglobin (hemoglobin F) that is not prone to sickling. As with every medication, hydroxyurea has side effects. These range from constipation and hair loss to severe infection and a tendency to bleed. This drug may not be tolerated by all sickle cell patients. If the side effects outweigh the benefits, then the drug should be discontinued. Research is ongoing into the effectiveness of hydroxyurea for preventing sickle cell crises as well as preventing stroke.

Other treatments for sickle cell anemia include *exchange transfusions,* during which blood is removed from the person with sickle cell anemia and replaced with blood from a donor who does not have the disease. Having regularly scheduled exchange transfusions, for years or even for life, can decrease the number of sickle cells in the blood and reduce the risk of a second stroke. With fewer sickle cells traveling in the bloodstream, the chance of them sticking together and blocking an artery is less. The goal of the transfusions is to keep the concentration of abnormal hemoglobin to less than 30 percent of the total. Research has shown that this treatment is effective in reducing the risk of stroke. However, chronic transfusion therapy has its own problems, including iron overload.

Another way to get rid of the sickle cells is to get rid of the bone marrow that produces the abnormal hemoglobin by performing a bone marrow transplant. This is a complex procedure. One of the biggest limitations for having this procedure is finding a donor with bone marrow that matches. Once there is a matched bone marrow donor, the person with sickle cell disease has to take toxic medications so that his body will not reject the new bone marrow. The procedure is expensive and there is no guarantee that it will work. Thus, the mainstay of treatment for sickle cell patients is managing their disease and trying to prevent sickle cell crises.

Polycythemia Vera

Ronald, a 65-year-old businessman, wasn't feeling right. He was tired, dizzy, weak, sweaty, and forgetful—not like himself at all. He was concerned that he might be developing Alzheimer's disease. Although Ronald avoided doctors and had not seen one in years, he felt this problem was significant enough to warrant a doctor's appointment. When the doctor asked him if he noticed any itching when he came out of the bath, Ronald was surprised. Indeed, he had been itchy coming out of the tub. His physician took a blood test and found that Ronald had *polycythemia vera.*

Polycythemia vera is a disorder of the bone marrow, the component of the bone responsible for creating new blood cells, including red blood cells (for carrying oxygen), white blood cells (for fighting infections), and platelets (for clotting). The bone marrow of people with polycythemia vera produces too many cells; so many that the blood becomes thick and tends to clot more easily. Thus, people with this disorder may experience a transient ischemic attack or stroke because of a thrombosis in an artery that supplies the brain. Clotting is a fairly common occurrence with this disorder, and up to one third of the people who have it experience stroke, heart attack, deep venous thrombosis, or pulmonary embolism.

Why did Ronald's physician ask about itchiness when coming out of the tub? There are cells in the body called *mast cells* that release a chemical called *histamine*. Histamine makes you itch. In polycythemia vera, people have an excess of mast cells and often experience itching. Like Ronald, people usually do not have problems or symptoms of polycythemia vera for many years, until they reach their sixties. Then they often experience generalized symptoms of weakness and fatigue. Tiny clots in the arteries in the brain may cause headache, dizziness, and blurred vision. They may not even visit a physician for these problems. Often the event that brings them into the office is a clot.

Polycythemia vera is easily diagnosed by a simple blood test, which is often done during a routine checkup. This blood test, called a *hematocrit level,* measures the concentration of red blood cells in the blood. In someone with polycythemia vera, the concentration is notably elevated (over 50 percent, whereas normal for a man is between 39 and 49 percent, and normal for a woman is between 33 and 43 percent). Other blood tests may show that the white blood cell count and the platelet count are higher than normal in a person with polycythemia vera. Treatment involves removing blood from the veins (*phlebotomy*) to decrease the red blood cell count. The amount of blood removed varies depending on how high the hematocrit level is and what problems the person is experiencing. For example, someone with a hematocrit level of 70 percent will most likely need phlebotomy twice a week, with a removal of one unit of blood (500 mL) weekly until the hematocrit level drops to lower than 45 percent. Once the hematocrit reaches 45 percent, the person will continue to have as many phlebotomy sessions as are needed to maintain that level. However, if a patient experiences severe cognitive problems or has blocked arteries secondary to the polycythemia vera, daily removal of a unit of blood may be required. A drug called *hydroxyurea,* which is used for people with sickle cell anemia, may also be prescribed for some people with polycythemia vera to help prevent or decrease any clotting problems that may arise.

Problems with the Blood Vessels

The blood vessels, arteries, and veins are transportation tubes for the blood, and they are the means by which nutrients and oxygen are carried throughout the body, including through the brain. To accomplish this critical job, these specialized tubes need to remain healthy and intact. Some medical conditions and injuries may prevent the arteries from doing their job and cause a stroke (see Table 11.2), either by creating blockages of blood flow in the artery or by weakening the arterial wall, making it more likely to burst open.

In Chapter 8 we discussed atherosclerosis, which is by far the most common cause of blocked arteries. Cholesterol buildup is not the only way to block blood flow in the arteries, however. In this chapter we discuss *arterial dissection* and *migraine headaches,* two other medical conditions that can lead to blocked arteries.

Table 11.2. **Problems with the Blood Vessels That May Lead to Stroke**

Arterial dissection

Migraine

Aneurysms

Arteriovenous malformations

Cerebral amyloid angiopathy

Cerebral venous thrombosis

Cavernous angioma

Dural arteriovenous fistula

Capillary telangiectasia

Fibromuscular dysplasia

Moyamoya disease

Pseudoxanthoma elasticum

Cerebral autosomal dominant arteriopathy with subcortical infarcts and
  leukoencephalopathy (CADASIL)

Sources: Wade S. Smith, Stephen L. Hauser, and J. Donald Easton, "Cerebrovascular Diseases," in *Harrison's Principles of Internal Medicine,* 15th edition, ed. Eugene Braunwald et al. (New York: McGraw-Hill, 2001); Timothy J. Counihan, "Cerebrovascular Disease," in *Cecil Essentials of Medicine,* 6th edition, ed. Thomas E. Andreoli et al. (Philadelphia: W. B. Saunders, 2004); H. A. Klausner and C. Lewandowski, "Infrequent Causes of Stroke," *Emergency Medicine Clinics of North America* 2, no. 3 (August 2002).

As we noted in Chapter 1, stroke can also result from bleeding in the brain, caused by a blood vessel bursting open. A burst blood vessel most commonly occurs due to high blood pressure, which we discussed in Chapter 9. Bleeding into the brain can occur for other reasons, however, including malformed arteries and arteries that are weakened by other medical conditions. In this chapter, we will discuss blood vessel malformation, called *aneurysm,* and *arterial venous malformations,* as well as a medical condition called *cerebral amyloid angiopathy,* as examples of how blood vessels are weakened and how these weakened vessels can lead to stroke.

Arterial Dissection

George, an otherwise healthy 47-year-old concert pianist, had been troubled by persistent neck pain. After seeing several physicians without obtaining relief, he went to a chiropractor. The chiropractor performed several maneuvers to alleviate George's pain, including a "high-velocity" manipulation of his neck. The next day, George awoke feeling a different type of pain in his upper neck. He also felt unsteady, as if the floor were tilted. He went to the hospital, where doctors performed two imaging tests—a magnetic resonance imaging (MRI) scan and a magnetic resonance angiogram (MRA) test—of his brain. A neurologist told George that he had a "dissection" of one of the arteries in his neck (the vertebral artery) and that he had suffered a stroke as a result. George was treated with anticoagulant medications for his stroke, and eventually he had a full recovery.

What is an arterial dissection, how does it happen, and how can it cause a stroke? An arterial dissection refers to the separation of the three neat layers of the arterial wall (the intima, media, and adventitia, which are described in Chapter 8). This separation can occur between the intima and the media or between the media and adventitia. Inside the arterial wall, there are tiny blood vessels, called the *vasa vasorum,* which supply oxygen and nutrients to the cells in the intima, media, and adventitia to keep them healthy and able to function. Sometimes spontaneously and sometimes in response to trauma to the neck involving twisting, these tiny blood vessels will hemorrhage and create a divide between the layers of the arterial wall.

The divide or dissection in the arterial wall can widen and fill with blood. If this dissected area becomes large enough, it can put pressure on the intima (the innermost layer whose cells are the closest to the bloodstream) from inside the arterial wall, pushing the intima into the lumen and decreasing the size of the lumen or even obliterating it. This is one way that the arterial dissection can cause a stroke. Stagnant blood sitting in the dissected area tends to clot (see Figure 3.5). With enough pressure created by the bleeding of the vasa vasorum, the area of dissection in the arterial wall can rupture, breaking through the intima layer of the arterial wall. This forms a connection between the dissected space and the blood flowing through the artery, which allows a piece of clot to escape from the area of dissection and travel to the brain. This is another way an arterial dissection can lead to stroke.

Arterial dissections occur most commonly in the carotid arteries in the neck, which feed the brain, and the vertebral arteries at the base of the head, which feed the brainstem and the cerebellum. The symptoms caused by the dissection vary depending on which artery dissects. For carotid artery dissections, the symptoms can include all or some of the following:

Face pain (on the same side as the dissection)
Neck pain (on the same side as the dissection)
Headache (on the same side as the dissection)

Weakness on one side of the body and face (on the side opposite the dissection)
Language problems
Visual disturbances

For vertebral artery dissections, the symptoms can include all or some of the following:

Face pain (on the same side as the dissection)
Facial muscle weakness (on the same side as the dissection)
Neck pain (on the same side as the dissection)
Headache (on the same side as the dissection)
Hoarseness
Hiccups
Vertigo (feeling that the world is spinning)
Ataxia (irregular and uncoordinated movements of limbs on the same side as the dissection)
Nausea and vomiting
Trouble swallowing
Weakness of one side of the body (on the side opposite the dissection)

People who have connective tissue disorders (such as Ehlers-Danlos syndrome or Marfan syndrome) and those with muscular thickening of the arteries (*fibromuscular dysplasia*) are at increased risk for dissection. Trauma such as motor vehicle accidents and activities that involve abrupt movement in the neck, including snow skiing, waterskiing, wrestling matches, football, chiropractic manipulation, violent coughing, and bar fights, put people at increased risk for dissection.

The diagnosis of arterial dissection is made by angiogram (see Chapter 3). Once the diagnosis is made, some physicians prescribe anticoagulants to prevent any further clots, and then follow up with a repeat angiogram to see if the arterial lumen is reopening. In most cases, the dissected artery does open up and heals within three to six months. During the recovery phase, it is recommended that people avoid vigorous activities known to increase the risk of dissection. Other physicians believe that performing surgery to open up the artery and remove the clot is the most effective treatment. Treatment decisions vary depending on each person's specific situation.

Migraines

Migraine headaches are very common and rarely cause any neurologic complications. In some cases, migraines are believed to involve spasms of the arteries in which muscle cells in the blood vessel wall contract and the blood vessel is temporarily narrowed. This blood vessel spasm, known as *vasospasm*, can temporarily decrease blood flow to areas of the brain. In a small number of cases, the vasospasm caused by migraine can be so severe that it results in a stroke. However, *stroke as a result of a migraine is rare.* The vast majority of people with migraines will never have a stroke from their headaches.

Migraine headaches cause pain that varies from mild to constant and excruciating. Migraines are often associated with other symptoms, including

sensitivity to light (photophobia),
nausea,
fatigue,
vomiting,
blurred vision, seeing flashing lights or experiencing some loss of vision, and
weakness and numbness, sometimes similar to a stroke.

Some people experience a strange smell, vision, or overall feeling (an *aura*) before the headache of migraine. Its presentation varies with each individual.

The cause of migraines is not fully understood, and research in this area continues. For years, there has been a "vascular theory" of migraines. This theory is one of several migraine theories and while probably not entirely accurate, it helps to explain why someone with a migraine headache may suffer a stroke. Migraines have been linked to narrowing of the blood vessels in the brain and widening of blood vessels outside of the brain, in the *meninges* (the membranes that surround the outside of the brain) in the scalp. This widening of the blood vessels outside the brain is thought to be the cause of the pain. It is the narrowing of the blood vessels inside the brain that we are most concerned about. The reduction in blood flow in the brain due to this narrowing is not believed to be substantial enough to cause damage in most cases. However, in some rare cases the low blood flow is severe enough to create brain problems, most commonly a transient ischemic attack with symptoms lasting less than twenty-four hours, and much less commonly a stroke. It has been reported that young women who experience migraine with aura, take oral contraceptives, or smoke have an increased risk for stroke from their migraines.

A doctor can diagnose a migraine during an office visit simply by listening to a person's report of headache and associated problems. There are no tests required to make the diagnosis. Treatment for migraines includes avoiding triggers such as red wine, hunger, sleep deprivation, perfumes, and stress. Migraine medications are broken down into two categories: those that treat an active headache (called *abortive treatment,* since you are trying to get rid of the headache) and those that prevent a migraine from ever occurring.

Aneurysms

Michelle, an active 38-year-old sociology professor, suddenly developed the worst headache of her life while enjoying a quiet dinner with a friend. Her friend called 9-1-1 and Michelle was taken to a nearby emergency room.

There, the physicians found that Michelle was a bit drowsy but that she had no weakness or difficulty speaking. A CT scan showed bleeding around the outside of her brain, and an angiogram showed that she had a sizeable aneurysm of one of the blood vessels in her brain as well as a second, smaller, aneurysm affecting another of the blood vessels.

Michelle had surgery to stop the bleeding of the aneurysm; this surgery involved attaching a tiny metal "clip" to the site of the aneurysm to pinch the outpouching shut. Michelle had a stroke as a complication of the surgery, however, and the stroke left her with weakness on her left side. After a long period of rehabilitation, she returned home to live with her husband.

Michelle's problems began with an *aneurysm,* an abnormal outpouching of a blood vessel. An *outpouching* is an area where the linear artery balloons out to form a pouch. No one knows why or exactly how an aneurysm forms. However, by studying them under the microscope, scientists have learned about their structure. In an aneurysm, some structural parts of the arterial wall are missing, such as the media (the middle layer in the wall which is composed of mostly smooth muscle cells) and the internal elastic lamina, which is a layer of flexible, elastic connective tissue that separates the media from the intima (the first layer of arterial wall cells that the blood touches as it flows through the arteries). Other parts of the arterial wall are disrupted in an aneurysm. For example, the intima is disrupted by the deposit of an extra material, called hyaline, which is produced in the body. Due to these structural changes, the blood vessel wall within the aneurysm is thinner than in the rest of the blood vessel. It is also weaker in this area. Thus, high pressures within the blood vessel may cause further expansion of the outpouching and further thinning of the wall in an aneurysm. These abnormalities make the arterial wall at the site of the aneurysm susceptible to rupture. Eventually, the blood vessel wall can become so thin that it bursts.

Rupture of an aneurysm produces bleeding, most commonly in the *subarachnoid space,* located between the meninges (the thin coating around the brain) and the brain itself. There are three membranes that make up the meninges: the *dura mater,* the *pia mater,* and the *arachnoid.* (This helps explains the term *subarachnoid,* which means "below the arachnoid membrane.") Bleeding into the subarachnoid space causes blood vessels in the area to constrict. The blood vessel vasoconstriction (*vasospasm*) after a subarachnoid hemorrhage can be severe enough to block the blood supply to part of the brain and cause a stroke.

The bleeding from a ruptured aneurysm may also occur within the brain itself, in which case it is called an *intraparenchymal hemorrhage.* An intraparenchymal hemorrhage is similar to a bleed in the brain due to hypertension (referred to as a hypertensive hemorrhage in Chapter 9). They are both strokes caused by bleeding into the brain tissue.

It is estimated that about 2 percent of the population have an aneurysm in their brain, and that 25 percent of the people with a brain aneurysm have more than one. Not everyone with an aneurysm will have a stroke, because most aneurysms don't burst. Women are slightly more likely than men to have an aneurysm. As with arterial dissections, people with connective tissue abnormalities, such as Ehlers-Danlos and Marfan syndromes, are at increased risk of having aneurysms. People with neurofibromatosis and autosomal dominant polycystic kidney disease also have an increased risk for this blood vessel abnormality. Aneurysms are congenital (meaning they are present at the time of birth). Most people are not aware that they have an aneurysm until it ruptures.

Rupture can occur at a quiet dinner, as it did in Michelle's case, but is more likely to happen during strenuous activities that create a rise in blood pressure. Size matters with aneurysms in the brain; the bigger they are, the more likely they are to rupture. Ten millimeters is the critical number; an aneurysm more than 10 mm in diameter has a much higher risk of rupturing than a smaller one.

Rupture of an aneurysm is extremely painful and can be life threatening. Most people report the most severe headache of their lives when an aneurysm bursts and causes a bleed. They often have a stiff, painful neck as well. Some people start vomiting, and some even lose consciousness. It is reported that about 30 percent of people with a rupture die before reaching the hospital, about 20 percent die in the hospital, 20 percent are left with some disability, and 30 percent recover with no major problems.

Diagnosis of ruptured aneurysm with subarachnoid hemorrhage is made by CT scan 90 to 95 percent of the time. If a CT does not reveal the bleed and the doctors still suspect that a person has a subarachnoid hemorrhage, the physicians will perform a *lumbar puncture* (spinal tap) to examine the *cerebral spinal fluid* (*CSF*) for blood. If a person has a ruptured aneurysm and subarachnoid hemorrhage, they require surgery. Neurosurgical care may include evacuating the blood from the brain as well as stopping the bleeding and sealing off the aneurysm from the rest of the circulation. By applying special clips, which work like tiny clothespins, to the neck of the outpouching where it connects to the artery, the neurosurgeon can stop blood from flowing into it. This is a way to seal off the aneurysm from the rest of the blood vessels and to prevent it from bleeding again. Another way to treat the aneurysm is to use coils. Similar to an angiogram, the coiling procedure uses a catheter and threads it through the artery in the groin up into artery in the brain with the aneurysm. Then a tiny coil is pushed through the catheter. When the coil arrives at the site of the aneurysm, it starts to fill the outpouching. By the end of the procedure, the aneurysm is entirely full of coils. The coils prevent blood from entering the aneurysm.

There are benefits and risks to every procedure. For clipping and coiling, the risks are similar. There is a risk of damage to blood vessels and rupture of the aneurysm during the procedure. Both of these could cause a stroke. For coiling, there is the added risk of the coil floating off into the main blood vessel and getting stuck in a different artery, which could cause a stroke. For this reason, the neurosurgeon considers every case carefully before operating. (Surgical treatment of aneurysms is discussed in Chapter 14.)

You may be thinking, "What if I have an aneurysm and I do not know about it?" If you have had a stroke, you have undergone extensive evaluation of your brain with CT scans, MRIs, and possibly angiograms. These studies would have revealed an aneurysm if you had one. If you do have one, you need to speak with a neurosurgeon about your options, because treatment varies with the size and location of the aneurysm. Surgery to fix an aneurysm that has not bled can be risky and can cause a stroke.

Arteriovenous Malformations

An *arteriovenous malformation (AVM)* is another type of a blood vessel malformation that can lead to a stroke. In fact, AVMs account for about 1 percent of all strokes. The blood vessels within an AVM are abnormal in several ways. For example, the blood flow within AVMs does not follow the usual pattern of moving from artery to smaller blood vessels, called capillaries, to vein. There are no capillaries in these malformations; instead, the arteries connect directly to the veins. Without the tiny capillaries slowing down the rate of blood flow from artery to vein, the pressure within the AVM and in vessels adjacent to it can rise. This increased pressure makes a rupture of an AVM more likely than a rupture in a normal vessel.

Another abnormality of AVMs compared to normal vessels is that the arteries may tangle around each other. Most normal blood vessels follow a fairly linear path, but AVMs have multiple turns and twists in them. They can even twist around themselves. These tangles vary in size from less than half an inch to two and a half inches in diameter.

The third way in which AVMs are abnormal has to do with the disruption of the neat organized layers of a normal artery in an AVM. Arteries in the AVM have a thickened middle layer (media) and may have deposits of an extra substance called *hyalinized connective tissue* inside this middle layer. Also, one of the most important structural linings of the artery, called the *internal elastic lamina* (the flexible, elastic connective tissue layer that separates the intima and media), is fragmented in some places yet duplicated in others. These disruptions to the normal layers of the artery weaken its walls and make it more likely to burst.

Most AVMs are present at birth, and they usually cause bleeding within the brain before age 40. These malformations are more common in men than in women. Since AVMs usually do not cause any symptoms until they cause a hemorrhage, most people with AVMs do not become aware of their condition until they have a stroke. When an AVM does bleed, the symptoms may be severe. The bleeding can occur in the subarachnoid space or in the brain itself. People usually experience a severe headache or a seizure when an AVM ruptures.

AVM is usually diagnosed with an MRI of the brain. The approach to treating a ruptured AVM depends on how much blood has leaked out into the brain; the amount can vary widely. Once an AVM has bled, the risk of another bleed within a year is about 7 percent. The risk for a bleed from an AVM that has not bled is about 2 to 4 percent per year. It appears that smaller AVMs have a higher risk of bleeding than larger ones. It is impossible to accurately predict what will happen to an AVM. Will it all of a sudden grow bigger? Will it stay stable? Will it get smaller and disappear on its own? Will it bleed or not? Researchers are trying to come up with some reliable parameters to help answer these questions.

AVMs must be managed on a case-by-case basis. When considering surgical treatment for people with AVMs, doctors weigh several factors, including their age, their overall health, the volume of blood within the AVM, and the location of the AVM. (The surgical treatment of AVMs is discussed in Chapter 14.)

Cerebral Amyloid Angiopathy

In the medical condition called *cerebral amyloid angiopathy* (CAA), the walls of arteries in the brain are weakened by deposits of a protein called *amyloid*. With weakened arteries in the brain, a stroke from a bleeding artery is more likely.

Who gets cerebral amyloid angiopathy? People over 60 years old are at increased risk for this condition. Men and women are equally affected. Almost all people with Alzheimer's disease also have cerebral amyloid angiopathy. However, if you have this condition, it does not mean that you have Alzheimer's disease or that you will develop it. About 50 percent of people with cerebral amyloid angiopathy have some degree of mental deterioration due to dementia. Of these, only 50 percent demonstrate the pathology of Alzheimer's. The dementia from cerebral amyloid angiopathy could also be multi-infarct dementia or dementia of another type.

While definitive diagnosis of cerebral amyloid angiopathy requires a brain biopsy, many cases can be presumptively diagnosed based on the pattern of bleeding within the brain and on evidence of prior asymptomatic (silent) hemorrhages. Angiography is not used to diagnose this disease, because the arteries that are affected are too small to be seen by this technique. People with CAA are more likely to have small bleeds that go undetected. These small bleeds are considered "silent" because they produce no symptoms. However, people with CAA are also at risk for major bleeds into the brain, and this possibility is the main concern with this disease. MRI scanning with special imaging techniques may aid in diagnosis by revealing tiny areas of "silent" hemorrhages.

Scientists have not yet developed specific treatments for cerebral amyloid angiopathy, so treatment focuses on factors that may contribute to an increased risk of another bleed in the brain. To prevent a second stroke from cerebral amyloid angiopathy, we suggest you focus on three things:

1. Controlling high blood pressure
2. Avoiding medications that can predispose to bleeding (such as aspirin and Coumadin)
3. Avoiding alcohol

As we have seen, high blood pressure alone can cause hemorrhagic strokes, so the risks of stroke are even higher for people with both elevated blood pressure and cerebral amyloid angiopathy. Keeping high blood pressure under close control can help reduce your risk of hemorrhage due to CAA.

Generally speaking, people with cerebral amyloid angiopathy should not use Coumadin or other blood thinners, which can contribute to bleeding in general and to brain hemorrhage in particular. Many other common medications can also increase your risk of a brain hemorrhage if you have CAA. Aspirin should only be used under the direction of a physician, and should never be used as an occasional treatment for headache, pain, or fever. Other anti-inflammatory medications such as ibuprofen (Advil, Motrin), or naproxen (Naprosyn), while not as hazardous as aspirin, are also best avoided. Acetaminophen (Tylenol) may be used without concern by individuals with cerebral amyloid angiopathy. Stronger prescription pain medications, such as Ultram, Percocet, and Oxycontin, are also safe in this condition, and may be available as an alternative to anti-inflammatory medications for people who cannot take medications that may interfere with blood clotting.

Many physicians advise people with cerebral amyloid angiopathy to avoid alcohol completely. Alcohol can contribute to bleeding within the brain, and can act together with cerebral amyloid angiopathy to increase your risk of stroke.

Uncommon Heart Conditions That Lead to Stroke

The heart is an incredible organ that keeps us alive by pumping blood throughout the entire body. Maintaining the health and integrity of the heart is critical for its ability to function. If the heart muscle is weakened, the electrical system fails, or the normal anatomy is damaged, disaster can strike in the form of a stroke. In Chapter 8 we discussed several different common problems with the heart that can lead to a stroke, including weak pumping action caused by a heart attack or congestive heart failure, rhythm problems like atrial fibrillation, malformed valves, and holes in the heart. One uncommon problem that we did not discuss is an abnormal growth inside the heart.

Atrial Myxoma

Fred had been feeling tired and feverish for a few days, so he made an appointment to see his physician. Fred was 45 years old and in good health, with no apparent medical problems. The day before the appointment, Fred collapsed to the ground. He could not move his right arm or leg and he was having difficulty speaking. His wife called 9-1-1. Fred had had a stroke. During the diagnostic work up to find a cause, an echocardiogram of Fred's heart revealed a golf ball–sized mass in his left atrium.

Fred had a very rare heart condition called *atrial myxoma* (*myxa* is Greek for mucus). This is a noncancerous growth (tumor) in the heart made of a slippery substance like mucus—hence the name. These growths are fragile, and a piece of one can easily break off and travel through the bloodstream to the brain. In fact, this occurs in 20 to 45 percent of people with atrial myxomas.

Symptoms vary depending on the size and location of the growth. An atrial myxoma may be the size of a dime, the size of an orange, or somewhere in between. If the myxoma is obstructing blood flow from the left atrium to the left ventricle, it will cause a backup of blood in the lungs. In this case, the person may experience shortness of breath due to the excess fluid in the lungs. If the myxoma is small and doesn't cause any obstruction, the person may not notice anything unless a piece of the tumor breaks off and causes a stroke. Many people with these tumors report nonspecific, generalized complaints like feeling tired and feverish. They may also report unexpected weight loss. While many people are happy to lose weight without really trying, nondeliberate weight loss is often a sign that something is wrong, so if this happens to you, be sure to let your doctor know.

Atrial myxoma is diagnosed by an echocardiogram. The growth is usually easily visualized with this test. Because of the high rate of recurrent strokes from atrial myxoma, the best treatment to prevent a second stroke is surgical removal of the tumor.

Infections or Inflammatory Conditions

When foreign organisms such as bacteria and fungi enter the body, they can wreak havoc. The body tries to fight the invaders with the *inflammatory cells*, the white blood cells that are its form of self-defense. Sometimes the

Table 11.3. Infections or Inflammatory Conditions That May Lead to Stroke

---

Giant cell arteritis
Takayasu disease
Polyarteritis nodosa
Wegener granulomatosis
Systemic lupus arthritis
Rheumatoid arthritis
Meningitis (resulting from syphilis, tuberculosis, fungi, bacteria, or zoster)
Cryoglobulinemia
HIV
Neurocysticercosis
Rhinocerebral mucormycosis

Sources: Wade S. Smith, Stephen L. Hauser, and J. Donald Easton, "Cerebrovascular Diseases," in *Harrison's Principles of Internal Medicine,* 15th edition, ed. Eugene Braunwald et al. (New York: McGraw-Hill, 2001); Timothy J. Counihan, "Cerebrovascular Disease," in *Cecil Essentials of Medicine,* 6th edition, ed. Thomas E. Andreoli et al. (Philadelphia: W. B. Saunders, 2004); H. A. Klausner and C. Lewandowski, "Infrequent Causes of Stroke," *Emergency Medicine Clinics of North America* 2, no. 3 (August 2002).

invaders prevail, and they spread throughout the body. The inflammatory cells keep fighting. In some cases, the body's own inflammatory cells damage it in this battle, and in rare cases, the cells cause a stroke by clogging up an artery.

There are medical conditions in which the body's inflammatory cells tend to collect in the arteries of the brain for no apparent reason. There are neither organisms to fight nor injuries to heal, but the inflammatory cells migrate to the walls of the arteries anyway. The cause of these inflammatory conditions remains a perplexing mystery that researchers are trying to solve. Infections and inflammatory conditions that may lead to stroke are listed in Table 11.3.

Inflammation of the Blood Vessels

A number of medical diseases involve inflammation of the blood vessels, a condition called *vasculitis.* The various types of vasculitis are listed in Table 11.4. As you can see from the list, different forms of vasculitis affect the blood vessels feeding different organs in the body. All of the types of vas-

Table 11.4. Types of Vasculitis and the Blood Vessels Each Attacks

Vasculitis	Blood Vessels
Giant cell arteritis	Branches of the carotid artery in the neck
Takayasu arteritis	The aorta and its branches
Polyarteritis nodosa	Blood vessels to the kidney, gastrointestinal, peripheral nervous system
Wegener granulomatosis	Blood vessels to sinuses and upper airway, the lung, and the kidney

culitis listed in Table 11.4 can lead to a stroke. Although the inflammatory process may be more pronounced in certain blood vessels of a person's body, the inflammation may also be taking place in other arteries, including those in the brain. Vasculitis is rare, and a stroke from vasculitis is even rarer.

Exactly what causes the inflammation in vasculitis and how it damages blood vessels is not well understood. Scientists have a number of theories, but they are still researching these questions. Vasculitis is thought to involve multiple processes and many different cells. One of the processes implicated is *immune complex deposition* in the blood vessel walls. When an antibody made in the body sees a foreign molecule (one that it does not recognize as part of the body), such as a bacteria or a virus, it attaches to it and forms an immune complex. In some cases, the antibody may mistake a molecule that is actually part of the body as a foreign molecule and attach itself to it. Immune complexes can travel in the bloodstream and then be deposited in the blood vessel walls.

The other processes that are thought to play a role in vasculitis all involve white blood cells and antibodies. A special type of white blood cell, called a T cell, may cause direct damage to the blood vessel wall, or antibodies may be directed against a specific molecule in the vessel wall. The different vasculidites (plural for vasculitis) may work by a combination of these mechanisms or by just one of them, and each type of vasculitis might work differently. However, they all have in common inflammation and damage in the blood vessel walls.

The activities of the white blood cells, the antibodies, and the immune complexes can weaken the blood vessel walls, making them more likely to develop a hole and leak, which could cause bleeding. The damage and

Table 11.5. Common Initial Symptoms of Different Types of Vasculitis

Vasculitis	Symptoms
Giant cell arteritis	Headache, scalp tenderness, jaw pain, visual disturbances, fatigue, pain in the joints
Takayasu arteritis	Lack of pulse in the arms, lightheadedness, fever, fatigue, pain in joints
Polyarteritis nodosa	Fever, fatigue, weight loss, pain in joints, muscle pain, abdominal pain, nausea and vomiting
Wegener granulomatosis	Persistent upper respiratory tract infections (sinusitis, nasal congestion, mastoiditis), cough, shortness of breath, coughing up blood, fever, fatigue, weight loss

buildup of many cells caused by these inflammatory activities may also block blood flow in the blood vessel. Inflammation can also lead to stroke because it remodels the vessel walls. After all this damage and destruction aimed at the blood vessel wall, it needs to build itself up again. This rebuilt wall often is not as strong as the original wall. Plus, there is often scar tissue around the area of inflammation, which can block blood flow even further.

The symptoms of vasculitis vary widely depending on the vessels it affects. Table 11.5 reviews the most common symptoms of giant cell arteritis, Takayasu arteritis, polyarteritis nodosa, and Wegener granulomatosis. Even though the blood vessels affected and the symptoms differ, the diagnosis and treatment of the various types of vasculitis are similar. In many of these diseases, blood test results are abnormal, indicating increased inflammation in the body. There are blood tests that look for the specific antibodies associated with some of these diseases. However, the gold standard for diagnosis is a tissue biopsy, in which a very small sample of bodily tissue is examined under a microscope. Depending on the vasculitis, different tissues are used. For example, in giant cell arteritis the temporal artery is biopsied, in polyarteritis nodosa, the kidneys are commonly biopsied, and in Wegener granulomatosis the nasal passages or lungs are often biopsied.

Doctors can determine the extent of inflammation in the cerebral arteries by using a test called an angiogram, in which a dye is injected into the artery and then an x-ray is taken to obtain a picture of the blood vessels (see Chapter 3). The outlines of the arteries can be seen and any narrowed or blocked arteries identified. The angiogram can miss vasculitis in the smaller blood vessels, so for some people diagnosis requires a biopsy of brain tissue. A microscopic examination of a biopsy of the arteries in the brain can demonstrate whether inflammatory cells are present in the vessel walls.

Treatment of vasculitis conditions involves anti-inflammatory drugs such as high-dose steroids. Other immunosuppressant medicines used to attack cancer cells are sometimes helpful in vasculitis to attack the inflammatory cells that have gone wild.

Meningitis

Meningitis is an infection of the *meninges,* the thin protective covering around the brain. This infection may be caused by bacteria, fungi, viruses, tuberculosis, or syphilis. Meningitis can lead to inflammation of the arteries in the brain by extending the infection through the bloodstream. Rarely, this inflammation can lead to stroke due to narrowing of the arteries involved.

Symptoms of meningitis are nonspecific and include fever, headache, lethargy, and confusion. People often seek medical attention after a high fever, persistent generalized headache, or confusion. Doctors may suspect from the symptom history people tell to them that meningitis is present, but the definitive diagnosis is made by obtaining cerebral spinal fluid via a lumbar puncture (spinal tap). During a lumbar puncture, the patient lies on her side while a physician inserts a tiny needle into the center of her lower back to access the fluid around the spinal cord. The treatment for this infection depends on its cause; that is, a person with bacterial meningitis would be given antibacterial medicine, and a person whose meningitis is fungal in origin would receive antifungal medication.

Stroke Resulting from Medications

Medications have the ability to fight infection, reduce inflammation, thin the blood, lower blood pressure, lower blood sugar, alleviate pain, and so much more. They can save lives. However, medications may also come with unwanted side effects such as fatigue, muscle pain, sun sensitivity,

Table 11.6. Medications That May Lead to Stroke

Estrogens
Phenylpropanolamine (no longer available in the United States)
Pseudoephedrine
Phenylephrine
Ephedrine
Vioxx (rofecoxib; no longer available in the United States)

---

and nausea, to name a few. The side effects vary depending on how the drug works. Some drugs in some people can create adverse reactions, such as bleeding into the gastrointestinal tract or stroke, that are severe enough to make it necessary to discontinue the medication (see Table 11.6). The risks and benefits need to be examined in each individual case before starting any medication.

Medications can cause strokes in several ways, for example by creating a tendency to form blood clots (a *hypercoagulable state*) within the body, or by increasing blood pressure. The mechanism by which some medications cause stroke remains a mystery. Research into how drugs may cause stroke is an active area of investigation. In this section we will discuss estrogen, which can make the blood more likely to form a clot, and medicines that are commonly sold over the counter, which contain ingredients that can increase blood pressure. We will also discuss Vioxx.

Estrogen

Estrogen is a natural hormone made primarily by the ovaries. It has several functions, starting with the development of the ovaries, fallopian tubes, uterus, vagina, and breasts. It also affects the bones, metabolism, fat deposition, hair distribution, skin, and platelets. The effect on the platelets is the most relevant to our discussion of stroke. Estrogen helps platelets stick together, increasing clotting in the blood. Because of this, estrogen can cause stroke.

For years, estrogen has been prescribed for postmenopausal women. Sometime between the age of 45 and 55, the ovaries stop producing estrogen and women go through menopause. Hot flashes, night sweats, sleeplessness, and vaginal dryness are all uncomfortable signs of menopause that for years have been treated with estrogen replacement therapy. Only recently have medical studies revealed the perils of this practice and the powerful effect of estrogen on clotting.

In the Women's Health Initiative (WHI), one of the largest studies researching the effects of estrogen replacement therapy on women's health, two important substudies were stopped early due to some surprising and disturbing results. Researchers wanted to examine the question of whether estrogen helped protect women against coronary artery disease, whether it decreased the risk of hip fracture, and whether it increased the risk of breast cancer in postmenopausal women. One of the substudies designed to help answer these questions looked at the effects of estrogen and progesterone (a hormone responsible for controlling the reproductive cycle), and another substudy looked at the effect of estrogen alone.

In this WHI substudy, researchers enrolled almost 17,000 women between the ages of 50 and 79. These women were randomly placed into two different groups. One group of women received estrogen in the form of conjugated equine estrogen at a dose of 0.625 mg a day and progesterone in the form of medroxyprogesterone acetate at a dose of 2.5 mg a day. The progesterone was used along with estrogen because it helps prevent uterine cancer. The other group of women received a *placebo* (a sugar pill). After a little over five years, the study was terminated because the women receiving estrogen experienced multiple adverse effects. It appeared that estrogen had the positive effect of decreasing hip fractures, but it also increased the risk of coronary artery disease, breast cancer, pulmonary embolism (a clot in the arteries of the lung), and stroke. In fact, there was a 41 percent higher incidence of stroke in the group taking estrogen and progesterone compared to the group taking the placebo. This study was reported in the *Journal of the American Medical Association*.[1]

In the other WHI substudy, researchers wanted to look at the effect of estrogen replacement therapy alone on women's health. Almost 11,000 women were enrolled in this study. These women were the same age as those in the estrogen and progesterone study, between 50 and 79, but unlike in the other group, all of them had had a hysterectomy. They, too, were randomly assigned to two different groups. One group of women received estrogen in the form of conjugated equine estrogen at a dose of 0.625 mg a day, and the other group received a placebo. (Because the women in this study did not have uteruses, there was no risk of endometrial cancer from estrogen replacement therapy and thus no need for progestins to be taken.) Over the course of almost seven years, these women were followed carefully and studied extensively. Again, the study was terminated early due to adverse effects. The women receiving the estrogen had an increased risk of stroke compared to those receiving the placebo. This study also revealed more risks: an increased risk of blood clots in leg veins (deep venous thrombosis, or DVT) and blood clots in the lungs (pulmonary embolism, or PE). Estrogen therapy was shown to decrease the risk of hip fracture. The results of this study were also reported in the *Journal of the American Medical Association*.[2]

As a result of these studies, the Food and Drug Administration (FDA) has made the following recommendations regarding estrogen hormone therapy (also available at www.fda.gov/cder/drug/infopage/estrogens_progestins/Q&A.htm):

1. Postmenopausal women should not take estrogen and progestin to protect the heart.
2. Estrogens and progestins may increase the risk of heart attack, stroke, blood clots, and breast cancer.
3. Although other doses of Prempro and other estrogens and progestins were not studied, it is important to warn postmenopausal women who take estrogens and progestins about the potential risks, which must be presumed to be the same.
4. When these drugs are being prescribed only to prevent osteoporosis, health care providers are encouraged to consider other treatments before prescribing estrogen or estrogen with progestin.
5. Estrogens and estrogen with progestin should be used at the lowest dose for the shortest duration.

The FDA continues to work with manufacturers to update their labeling of estrogen and estrogen with progesterone medications. Labels must include warnings about an increased risk of heart disease, heart attacks, strokes, and breast cancer.

Postmenopausal women are not the only ones taking estrogen. Women who take oral contraceptives are also taking estrogen and, not surprisingly, they are three times more likely to suffer from a stroke or a clotting problem, such as a DVT, than women who do not take contraceptives. Women on oral contraceptives are often young and healthy, and their risk of stroke is very low, though if they use this type of birth control they have a higher risk compared to women their age who do not use oral contraceptives. On the other hand, if you are reading this and you are a young or middle-aged woman who has already had a stroke and who uses oral contraceptives, your risk of another stroke is higher than for an otherwise healthy woman. Smoking increases the risk of clotting for women on oral contraceptives. If you smoke, you should definitely use a different form of birth control.

Better yet, if you smoke, you should quit smoking. We advise you to consult your doctor and discuss the best form of birth control for you.

Over-the-Counter Medications

Jane learned the hard way that a seemingly harmless diet pill she picked up at a local drugstore was not harmless at all. Jane was a 37-year-old mother of a 9-month-old boy. She was healthy but overweight after giving birth to her son. In an effort to lose weight, she started taking a diet pill that contained the drug phenylpropanolamine. Jane took the diet pill for several months and was successful at losing weight. Since she was getting good results with the diet pill, she kept taking it daily. One evening, while making dinner as her husband played with the baby, Jane suddenly fell to the ground. She could not get up. Jane was unable to move her left leg or left arm, and her speech was slurred. In a panic, her husband called 9-1-1. Jane was rushed to the emergency room, where a CT scan demonstrated a large bleed on the right side of her brain.

The doctors decided to treat Jane conservatively and not to operate, since the bleed was not causing her brain to shift its position in the skull, the bleed was not getting any bigger, and Jane's weakness was not getting any worse. She did have a full work up to try to find the cause of the stroke. Jane had no history of high blood pressure or other medical illness. In fact, she was in good health until this episode. Her MRI angiogram did not reveal any AVMs, aneurysms, or other blood vessel abnormalities. All her blood lab tests (platelets, clotting factors, bleeding time, inflammatory cells, glucose, and cholesterol) were normal. So what caused Jane's hemorrhagic stroke? The only possible cause that the doctors could find was that diet pill containing phenylpropanolamine. That "harmless" over-the-counter diet pill was responsible for her stroke. Unfortunately, Jane never regained full muscle strength in her left arm and leg. After inpatient and outpatient rehabilitation, her ability to function did improve. However, she could not walk on her own or perform many of her daily activities independently.

Common medicines such as nasal decongestants and diet pills that many people buy at the drugstore can potentially cause stroke. The stroke risk posed by these over-the-counter remedies is small, but it is important for someone who has already had a stroke to be aware of it. These medicines may contain phenylephrine or pseudoephedrine, both of which are *vasoconstrictors*—that is, they narrow the blood vessels—and they can suddenly raise blood pressure. These medications have been associated with both hemorrhages and blockages. In fact, one vasoconstrictor that was previously widely used, phenylpropanolamine, has been removed from the market because of these risks. If you already have high blood pressure, read the labels of over-the-counter medications and dietary supplements carefully before taking them. If you are not familiar with one of the ingredients, ask the pharmacist. It is best to consult your physician before taking any new medications, regardless of whether or not you need a prescription to obtain them.

In February 2004, the FDA prohibited the sale of dietary supplements containing *ephedra* (also known as *ma huang*), which were primarily used to enhance athletic performance and control weight. The FDA felt that ephedra alkaloids are too dangerous to include in dietary supplements, as they can raise blood pressure and stress the circulatory system, causing heart attack and stroke. Since the makers of dietary supplements are not required to prove the safety or effectiveness of their products, the FDA found that there was not sufficient control or regulation of the ephedra supplements. For example, manufacturers could add as much ephedra as they wanted to the supplement. Consumers could also combine the different ephedra supplements to further enhance their athletic performance or lose more weight, which would just increase their risk of adverse outcomes.

Rofecoxib (Vioxx)

Rofecoxib was a prescription drug, a selective COX-2 inhibitor, *non-steroidal anti-inflammatory drug* (NSAID), that was used to treat the pain and swelling associated with osteoarthritis and rheumatoid arthritis as well as pain associated with menstruation. It was approved by the FDA in May 1999 and then voluntarily withdrawn from the market by Merck Pharmaceuticals in September 2004, because of an increase in heart attacks and strokes in people who took the medication during an investigational study. The exact association between rofecoxib and stroke is not yet fully understood, but the evidence was strong enough that the drug is no longer available on the market.

Researchers designed a study to evaluate the effects of rofecoxib in preventing recurrent colon polyps. Part of the study was also created to examine the long-term safety of the drug. People in the study were given either a sugar pill (placebo) or rofecoxib. They were monitored closely for over eighteen months. For the first eighteen months of the trial, people taking the rofecoxib at a dose of 25 mg every day had no more heart attacks or strokes than those taking sugar pills. However, after eighteen months, the study showed that the people taking the rofecoxib had an increased risk, in fact double the risk, of heart attack and stroke compared to those people taking the sugar pill. The study was stopped.

The blood supply to the brain can be blocked and bleeding in the brain can occur for many different reasons. The cause may be common, such as one of the conditions—heart problems, high blood pressure, or diabetes—described in previous chapters. It also may be a rare disorder like those described in this chapter. Although the likelihood that you will experience any of these less common disorders is slim, we hope that you will use this chapter as a resource should you or someone you love develop one of these conditions that can lead to stroke.

• •

Chapter 12

Genetics and Stroke

The daughter of one of our patients told us about her concerns: "Ever since my father's stroke, I've wondered if I will have one, too. Is there something in my family's genes that makes us susceptible to strokes? After all, my father's father also had a stroke. I've read everything I can find about stroke, and I'm determined to do everything possible to avoid one."

Most people who suffer a stroke want to know what caused it. Their family members are also curious about genetic factors that may influence their own chance of having a stroke. Some rare conditions that can lead to stroke *are* caused by a single gene, but most strokes appear to have many causes, with genetic factors and environmental factors both playing a role. Even so, if your first-degree relative (that is, a parent or a sibling) has had a stroke, you are about two times more likely to have a stroke than someone who has no family history of stroke. This increased risk certainly does not mean that you *will* have a stroke. And since most strokes are caused by a combination of factors, many of them within your control, there is plenty you can do to help avoid having a stroke.

Parents who carry genes for disorders such as cystic fibrosis, sickle cell anemia, and Marfan syndrome have a high likelihood of passing these genes on to their children. These disorders are considered genetic. Knowing your family's medical history can give you insight into your risks of having or developing a genetic disease. Other health problems such as malnutrition, pneumonia, and spinal cord injury are not genetic. Rather, they are the result of environmental factors such as diet, infections, and accidents. Genes do not play a major role in these disorders.

Most diseases appear to be the result of a combination of genetic *and* environmental factors. Rheumatoid arthritis, skin cancer, and osteoporosis are examples of these. With skin cancer, for example, genes play a part in the onset of the disease, but environmental factors such as sun exposure throughout one's life and a history of sunburns play an important role in the development of the disease. In many disorders, the cause may be related to more than one gene as well as to the influence of more than one environmental factor. Stroke falls into this category.

The genetics of stroke is an area of medicine that is getting more attention from researchers. For years, physicians have known that family history plays a role in many of the most common risk factors for stroke, such as high blood pressure, diabetes, and high cholesterol. That these diseases—and strokes themselves—tend to run in families is a clue that genes are involved in some way. Over the past few years, researchers have gained insight into which genes are responsible for certain rare types of stroke. They have isolated a gene that may be associated with stroke as well as a potentially protective gene that guards against stroke.

Stroke is a heterogeneous disease, meaning there are many different causes of stroke, from atherosclerosis to cocaine use. Also, there are different kinds of stroke, those caused by a clot (ischemic) and those caused by bleeding within the brain (hemorrhagic). All of these complexities make the study of the genetics of stroke difficult. Furthermore, each type of stroke needs to be considered individually.

Family History and Stroke

If a first-degree relative (parent or sibling) of yours has had a stroke, you should keep your family's medical history firmly in mind. To best understand your own risk of stroke, you need to know what kind of stroke your relative had and what caused it. For coronary artery disease (CAD), it is important to know if your father had a heart attack before age 55 or if your mother had a heart attack before age 65. If so, you are considered to have a family history of coronary artery disease and to be at increased risk of heart attack and stroke from atherosclerosis. If your first-degree relative had high blood pressure, you are at increased risk for hypertension, which is one of the main risk factors for stroke. The same is true for Type I diabetes.

Knowing your family medical history will help you to take precautions early to prevent a stroke. For example, a 30-year-old man may not feel any symptoms of his high cholesterol and may not even have high blood pressure. But, if he knows that his father had a history of hypertension and a heart attack at age 45, then he may be more inclined to check his cholesterol level at a young age. Lowering his intake of saturated fats is even more important. Making healthy food choices starting from a young age and exercising daily could help slow down and even prevent the process of atherosclerosis. Exercising and keeping his weight in check will also help him avoid high blood pressure.

A family history free of risk factors for stroke does not mean that you are completely safe from the disease. You should still eat properly and exercise daily, because anyone can develop atherosclerosis, hypertension, and diabetes by being overweight, eating saturated fats, eating carbohydrates with a high sugar load (like candy and white bread), and leading a sedentary life. Although family history is important, it is not the *only* factor to consider when it comes to stroke.

Specific Genes and Rare Disorders

In some people genetic inheritance plays a prominent role in the development of a stroke. In autosomal dominant diseases, if one parent has the disease, each child has a 50 percent chance of receiving the gene that causes it and inheriting the disease. The autosomal dominant disorders that are associated with stroke include the following:

> A disorder of the arteries in the brain causing strokes and degeneration of the brain, called *CADASIL* (*cerebral autosomal dominant arteriopathy with subcortical infarcts and leukoencephalopathy*)
> Abnormal enlarged blood vessels in the brain that can bleed (*cavernous angiomas*)
> Abnormally high cholesterol levels in young adults associated with lumps or nodules (*xanthomas*) on the ankles and hands (*familial hypercholesterolemia*).

Researchers have identified the genes associated with these conditions. Table 12.1 lists these genes. In this section, we will discuss these diseases and describe the genetics of each.

CADASIL

CADASIL stands for cerebral autosomal dominant arteriopathy with subcortical infarcts and leukoencephalopathy. What does all that mean? *Cerebral* means pertaining to the brain. *Autosomal dominant* refers to the genetics of the disease and how it can be passed from parent to child. *Arteriopathy* means disease of the arteries. *Subcortical* means the abnormalities are seen below the cortex of the brain, deep within the tissues of the brain. *Infarct* is a term used to describe an ischemic stroke caused by lack of blood to the

Table 12.1. **Genes Associated with Conditions That Predispose a Person to Stroke**

Condition	Associated Gene(s)
CADASIL	NOTCH3
Cavernous angiomas	CCM1 (KRIT1), CCM2, CCM3
Familial hypercholesterolemia	LDL receptor
Familial defective apolipoproteinemia	Apolipoprotein B-100 gene

brain. *Leukoencephalopathy* means a disease affecting the white matter of the brain. CADASIL is a much easier name to use for this rare disease. Susie's story demonstrates how this disease typically affects people.

Susie was a 30-year-old woman with a history of migraines and depression. She did not have high cholesterol, high blood pressure, or diabetes. She exercised regularly, ate a healthy diet, and did not smoke. Since her senior year in college, Susie had suffered from migraines with an aura of flashing lights. A few months after her migraines were diagnosed, she became depressed. Then one day, Susie suddenly felt weak in her left hand and arm. Her arm also felt "funny," as if there were pins and needles all over it. She could not pick anything up or carry anything. The weakness and strange sensations lasted a few hours.

Even though Susie was back to normal, the experience was so scary that she sought medical attention. A neurologist told her that what she had experienced was a TIA (transient ischemic attack). The neurologist ordered an MRI (magnetic resonance image) to get a picture of her brain and found several spots on it that represented old, small infarcts. After a full diagnostic work up that included a skin biopsy and genetic testing, she was diagnosed with CADASIL, the same disease her mother had. Her mother was 65 and suffered from dementia.

When a relatively healthy young adult or middle-aged person who has no history of high cholesterol, high blood pressure, diabetes, or smoking has a TIA or a stroke, physicians consider CADASIL as a possible cause of the event. If the person has a parent with CADASIL, this diagnosis is all the more likely.

This very rare genetic disorder is associated with two common disorders: migraine and depression. Few people with migraines have CADASIL. However, about a quarter of the very small number of people who have

CADASIL suffer from migraines. People who have CADASIL usually have migraines with an aura. An aura is an unusual experience that foreshadows the headache of a migraine. It is a type of warning sign and can be anything from a strange feeling, visual changes with flashing lights, or strong smell. It is certainly possible for someone with this disease to experience migraines without an aura, but this type of migraine is less commonly associated with CADASIL. Depression is a common disorder in our country and around the world. Few people with depression have CADASIL. Of the very small number of people who have CADASIL, approximately 20 percent also have a mood disorder such as depression. Again, keep in mind that migraines and depression are very common and that CADASIL is very rare.

People with CADASIL may have no symptoms until their first stroke. Most people with this disease suffer their first stroke or TIA in their thirties or forties. Some of the ischemic strokes may be "silent," meaning no symptoms accompanied the loss of blood supply to that particular part of the brain. However, approximately two-thirds of people with CADASIL suffer permanent neurologic damage as a result of the disease. By the time people with CADASIL are in their sixties, they usually have suffered a significant loss in their cognitive abilities, including a loss of memory, abstract thinking ability, and judgment, and perhaps even a change in personality. At this point, all of their little infarcts have led to dementia.

CADASIL can be identified on CT and MRI because the infarcts (ischemic strokes) the disease creates show up on the images as spots in specific locations in the brain. There is a specific pattern of abnormalities that radiologists (doctors who read x-ray films and radiological images) recognize as being consistent with CADASIL.

What causes the infarcts? The answer is abnormalities in the arteries. In this disease, a granular material is deposited in the small arteries all over the body, including the brain. This extra granular material of unknown origin thickens the walls of the arteries and diminishes the size of the lumen. With a smaller lumen, less blood can travel through the artery to feed the brain and an infarct is more likely.

The abnormalities in the arteries are generalized, meaning they are found in many different organs in the body, including the skin. A simple skin biopsy is often enough for a doctor to make the diagnosis of CADASIL. A special microscope called an electron microscope is used to identify the granular material in the arterial walls. If the skin biopsy is conclusive, there is no need to biopsy the arteries of the brain, which is a more complicated and risky procedure than a simple skin biopsy.

Scientists have discovered the gene that causes this disease. It is called the *NOTCH3 gene* and it is located on chromosome 19 at site q12. The NOTCH3 gene directs the formation of a protein that acts as a receptor on a membrane. To understand receptors we can use a lock and key analogy. Proteins called *receptors* act as the lock, and proteins called *ligands* act as the key. When the right key gets into the right lock, the door opens. When the right ligand protein binds to the right receptor protein on the membrane, this interaction "opens the door" for a chain of reactions that help the cells to develop and function normally. Examples of these important reactions that occur when the "key fits the lock" include forming other proteins, regulating the development, size, and number of cells, and performing functions such as clearing away cholesterol from the bloodstream. If there is a change in the NOTCH3 gene, the receptor protein (the lock) is not made correctly. If the receptor protein is not made correctly, the protein that acts as the key will no longer fit into it. There will be a buildup of improperly made receptor proteins and a lack of other proteins necessary for the proper functioning of the cell. The normal balance of proteins is mixed up.

There is evidence that the mutation in the NOTCH3 gene creates multiple changes that damage the cells in different ways, including allowing an extra granular material to form within the cells. This granular material interferes with the cells' ability to obtain their nutrients, and this lack of cell nutrition causes damage to the tissues in the area. The mutation in the NOTCH3 gene is thought to directly damage endothelial cells, which are found in the innermost layer of cells in the arterial wall. It also damages smooth muscle cells, which are found in the middle layer of the arterial wall. (The wall of a normal artery and its neat, organized layers are described in Chapter 8.) Scientists are still investigating the details of how the defective NOTCH3 gene causes the abnormalities that lead to CADASIL.

Genetic testing is available for diagnosing CADASIL. Family members of people with CADASIL are eligible for this test. Counseling before and after the genetic test is essential. The person being tested must be prepared to handle the psychological issues associated with the diagnosis of a genetic disease. People may be angry and blame their mother or father, and they may feel guilty if they have children to whom they have given the disease. They need help dealing with these feelings.

Currently, there is no cure for CADASIL, nor are there many treatment options. Treatment of CADASIL is an area of active research and controversy. Some physicians prescribe aspirin or other anti-platelet medications, although this treatment remains controversial because of concerns of causing bleeding within the brain. Many physicians recommend that people with CADASIL not take any blood thinners such as Coumadin and heparin. Acetazolamide has been found to help with the migraines.

Cavernous Angioma

Familial cavernous angioma is another rare autosomal dominant disease that causes stroke. Most people with cavernous angiomas get them randomly and not from their parents. In the familial type, the cavernous angiomas are passed on from generation to generation, from parent to child. (Either type causes an increased risk of stroke.)

What is a cavernous angioma? Basically, it is a malformation of a blood vessel. *Cavernous* means hollow and *angioma* refers to an abnormal swelling of a blood vessel. Basically, a cavernous angioma is a collection of large, thin-walled, vascular tubes. They are not arteries or veins. They are cavity-like channels with a wide diameter found in the brains of people with this disorder. The blood inside them is not propelled forward as it would be in a normal artery, and some of it may not move much at all. Instead, it may gel or clot. The size of these vascular channels ranges from a few millimeters to a few centimeters. Their walls are thin and prone to rupture and cause bleeding into the brain. Cavernous angiomas are found in about 0.5 percent of autopsy cases. Many people with the familial form of cavernous angioma have more than one angioma in their brain.

Most people with cavernous angiomas do not even realize that they have them. In fact, they could live their entire life without knowing, die of some other disease, and only have their cavernous angioma discovered incidentally upon autopsy. However, some people suffer from headaches, seizures, or localized problems like weakness in the right foot or numbness and tingling in the right arm. Some people find out they have a cavernous angioma after it bleeds and causes a stroke. The symptoms or problems a person experiences as a result of a bleeding cavernous angioma vary. The location of the cavernous angioma determines the symptoms the person would have if it bled. An MRI or CT scan helps to identify a cavernous angioma.

Cavernous angiomas that have not bled yet have a 0.6 percent annual risk of bleeding. If the cavernous angioma has already bled, then the annual risk of bleed increases to 4.5 percent. If someone's angioma has bled, it is recommended that they be evaluated for surgical removal. Surgery is also an option if a person is experiencing seizures that are hard to control and are debilitating. The neurosurgeon will need to consider each case individually. If the cavernous angioma is located in an easily accessible part of the brain, then surgery will be less challenging than if it were located deep within the tissues of the brain. What structures lie next to the cavernous angioma is also a factor. If the center for controlling breathing or the center for controlling movement of the leg is right next to the cavernous angioma, the surgery becomes trickier and riskier. There are a number of factors to consider before going forward with surgical removal. The risks and benefits of surgery need to be carefully considered for each person.

Scientists have identified three genes responsible for causing cavernous angiomas. Ongoing research is helping to answer questions about how mutations in these genes lead to malformed vessels. One gene, called *CCM1 (cerebral cavernous malformation 1)*, is located on chromosome 7 in the specific region of the chromosome known as q11.2-q21. This gene is also sometimes referred to as the *KRIT1 gene,* which stands for the *Krev interaction-trapped 1 protein.* The KRIT1 or CCM1 gene directs the formation of a protein called KRIT1. The exact actions of this protein are unknown, and researchers are analyzing many possible functions. There is evidence that the KRIT1 protein is important in creating the shape of the endothelial cells and creating their communication system with other cells. When there is a mutation in the KRIT1 gene, the KRIT1 protein does not function properly and endothelial cells are not formed correctly. This problem leads to the creation of large cavity-like vessels instead of normal arteries. Although many questions about this gene remain unanswered, there is enough information to allow for the use of genetic diagnostic testing.

The two other genes that are known to cause familial cavernous angiomas are *CCM2* and *CCM3*. Much less is known about these genes, and to date there is no genetic testing available for them. Like CCM1, CCM2 has been located on chromosome 7, but at a different specific site, p15-p13. The CCM2 gene normally is responsible for creating a protein called *malcavernin*. The function of malcavernin and its relation to cavernous angioma are areas of active research. The least is known about the CCM3 gene. It has been isolated to chromosome 3. However, scientists do not even know what protein it is responsible for creating. There is much to be learned about the genetics of familial cavernous angiomas.

Familial Hypercholesterolemia

Jeff was a 20-year-old college student with no health concerns. He had noticed some lumps in his elbows and on the back of his leg around his Achilles tendon, but they were not painful and really did not bother him. So he ignored them. One afternoon, he was playing soccer when he experienced crushing chest pain. He went to the nearest emergency room, where he was told that he was having a heart attack. His father had died from a heart attack at age 42, and his mother, who was 50 years old, just started taking medication for her high cholesterol.

While Jeff was in the hospital, his cholesterol was found to be 750 mg/dL. (Normal is less than 200 mg/dL.) With this extremely elevated cholesterol and his family history of both parents having high cholesterol, the diagnosis of familial hypercholesterolemia was strongly considered. His genetic testing revealed that he did indeed have this rare disease. His mother was subsequently tested for familial hypercholesterolemia and was also found to have the disease.

Given that Jeff had an extremely elevated cholesterol level, the physicians taking care of him were not surprised to find that he had two genes for this disease, one from his mother and one from his father. At age 20, Jeff started on cholesterol-lowering medications. From that day forward, he monitored his diet religiously and avoided foods high in cholesterol and saturated fats. He continued exercising regularly.

Familial hypercholesterolemia (*FH*) is the most common genetic disease that causes high cholesterol levels. This disease leads to severe atherosclerosis (cholesterol plaque formation in the arteries) at an early age. People with familial hypercholesterolemia have high cholesterol levels at one year of age. One of the main complications of these high cholesterol levels in childhood is a heart attack at an early age. People with familial hypercholesterolemia have a much higher risk for coronary artery disease, up to twenty-five times the risk compared to people without this disease. The process of atherosclerosis occurs throughout the arteries of the body, including those in the brain, so stroke at an early age is also a possibility with familial hypercholesterolemia.

In 1985, Michael Brown and Joseph Goldstein received the Nobel Prize for discovering that a mutation on the LDL (low density lipoprotein) receptor gene caused familial hypercholesterolemia. The mutation disrupts the body's ability to make LDL receptors, which are responsible for clearing LDL out of the bloodstream. With fewer LDL receptors, there is more LDL in the blood to form atherosclerotic plaques. LDL is made of cholesterol, protein, and triglycerides. It is one of the main transportation devices for cholesterol. (LDL is discussed in detail in Chapters 8 and 15.)

We now know that there are over two hundred different mutations of the LDL receptor gene that can cause familial hypercholesterolemia. Approximately 1 in 500 people who live in North America has one LDL receptor gene with a mutation that gives them familial hypercholesterolemia. This means that they have one LDL receptor gene that is mutated and is not functioning properly. This mutated gene is not creating normal LDL receptors. However, each person has two LDL receptor genes. People with one mutated gene have half the number of functional LDL receptors that someone with two normal genes has.

People with familial hypercholesterolemia who have one mutated gene are known as *heterozygotes* for the gene. They tend to have cholesterol levels two times greater than normal. A normal cholesterol level is below 200 mg/dL. People with one gene for familial hypercholesterolemia have cholesterol levels somewhere between 275 and 500 mg/dL. Many men with this disease have heart attacks in their forties and fifties, while women with this disease often have heart attacks in their fifties and sixties. In this disease, LDL also accumulates in parts of the body other than the arteries. For example, it can accumulate under the skin in the form of painless, moveable, soft lumps or nodules, sometimes called *xanthomas*. These cholesterol nodules typically appear on the elbows, knees, and buttocks. Cholesterol can also build up in tendons (which connect a muscle to a bone). The Achilles tendon in the back of the lower leg around the ankle and the tendons on the back of the hand that extend the fingers are common sites for xanthomas. In some people with familial hypercholesterolemia, a yellowish ring called *corneal arcus* develops around the cornea of the eye. This yellowish ring is composed of deposits of cholesterol.

It is possible to inherit two mutated LDL receptor genes, one from a mother and one from a father, as Jeff did. If someone inherits two mutated LDL receptor genes, they are known as *homozygotes* for the gene. This form of the disease is rarer and occurs in one in a million people. People with two mutated LDL receptor genes have a more severe form of familial hypercholesterolemia. This makes sense if you consider that they have no normal LDL receptor gene, and thus no LDL receptors to function normally to help clear out the LDL cholesterol from the bloodstream. Cholesterol levels in these people run higher than 500 mg/dL and can reach 1,000 mg/dL. People with this type of familial hypercholesterolemia may experience heart attacks in their twenties. They also have more deposits of cholesterol throughout their body. Their xanthomas are bigger and more numerous, because there is more LDL floating around in the bloodstream looking for a place to lodge, since it cannot attach to a normal LDL receptor and be cleared from the body.

Treatment for familial hypercholesterolemia is aggressive. People with this disease usually die of coronary artery disease. Because high cholesterol and atherosclerosis are the problems, the treatment is to lower cholesterol in any way possible. Strict diets that limit cholesterol and saturated fat intake, daily exercise, weight loss, smoking cessation, and medications to lower cholesterol levels are all part of the treatment regimen.

Familial Defective Apolipoprotein B-100

Familial hypercholesterolemia is not the only disease known to cause abnormally high cholesterols, nor is the LDL receptor gene the only gene that influences cholesterol levels. Mutations in the apolipoprotein B-100 gene have a similar effect on cholesterol levels and create similar symptoms of cholesterol nodules in the ankles and hands of people with the disease called *familial defective apolipoprotein B-100*. The gene is different, but the outcome is the same.

The mutation in the apolipoprotein B-100 gene does not affect the LDL receptors. Instead, it decreases the likelihood that LDL cholesterol will bind to its receptors in the liver. Apolipoprotein B-100 is made in the liver and is an important structural part of the LDL molecule. The apolipoprotein B-100 part of LDL is the component that interacts with the LDL receptor to ensure proper binding in this lock and key relationship. Without the correct apolipoprotein B-100, the LDL molecule does not bind to its receptor and there is more LDL in the bloodstream, which puts a person at increased risk for atherosclerosis of the coronary arteries as well as arteries throughout the body, including the brain. Genetic testing is available for this disease; the treatment is the same as for familial hypercholesterolemia: limited cholesterol and saturated fat intake, exercise, weight loss, smoking cessation, and medication for lowering cholesterol.

Familial hypercholesterolemia and familial defective apolipoprotein B-100 are two examples of rare diseases that create high cholesterol levels and are caused by mutations in one specific gene. However, most people with moderately elevated cholesterol (in the 240 to 350 mg/dL range) have elevated cholesterol because of multiple factors: the influence of a number of different genes, not just one, and the influence of a number of environmental circumstances such as diet, exercise, and smoking.

Studies have revealed some of the genes linked to disorders associated with stroke, and genetic testing is available for people who may be at risk of developing them. If you know that you have a gene that puts you at risk, you can better prepare for your future and take all precautions necessary to try to avoid a stroke. For example, if you have a mutation in the gene that encodes the LDL receptor associated with familial hypercholesterolemia, you can stay on a strict diet and take medications to lower your cholesterol starting at an early age. By doing so, you may avoid a heart attack or stroke.

New Research into Genes and Stroke

A group of researchers, Søren Bak, David Gaist, Søren Hein Sindrup, Axel Skytthe, and Kaare Christensen, looked at the Danish Register of Causes of Death and the National Discharge Register to identify sets of twins in which one had died of a stroke. They followed the surviving twin to see if he or she would also suffer a stroke. Twins may be either identical (*monozygotic*), from the very same egg, or fraternal (*dizygotic*), from two different eggs. Identical twins are *genetically* identical, whereas fraternal twins are genetically no more similar than any other pair of siblings. (Siblings normally share 50 percent of their genetic makeup.) This study compared the rate of stroke among identical twins and among fraternal twins. According to the study, the risk of stroke death for an identical twin after the co-twin had died of a stroke was twice the risk for a fraternal twin after the co-twin had died of a stroke. The results of this study were published in the medical journal *Stroke*.[1] Identical twins, who share more of their genetic makeup, had a greater shared risk of stroke than fraternal twins, who share less of their genetic makeup. These results suggest that something in the genetic makeup predisposes a person to stroke.

There is also some evidence of a susceptibility gene for stroke, a gene that may lead to stroke but does not appear linked to a single specific cause of it. In fact, according to an Icelandic study, patients with atherosclerosis that affects the large arteries in the neck (the carotid arteries) and patients with blood clots in their hearts that break off and travel to their brain seem to have the same gene, which scientists have pinpointed on chromosome 5 at site q12. This landmark study was published in the *American Journal of Human Genetics* in 2002, and has not yet been duplicated in another population.[2] For this reason, the results are considered preliminary and more research needs to be performed to confirm the findings. Nonetheless, we now have evidence that the connection between a particular gene and a person's risk of stroke is significant, and these studies may lead to further useful investigations in the future.

Current research also points to a possible protective gene for stroke. An Italian research group identified a certain gene (−765G to C polymorphism of the COX-2 gene) as an inherited protective factor against both heart attack and stroke, and the group's results were published in the *Journal of the American Medical Association* in 2004.[3] Exactly how this protection works is not understood. One theory is that the protective gene may decrease the risk of rupture of an atherosclerotic plaque. When a plaque ruptures and breaks away from the vessel wall, it sends small pieces of plaque into the bloodstream. These pieces can flow through the blood vessels until they get stuck and block blood flow, causing a heart attack if the blockage is in a coronary artery or a stroke if the blockage is in the cerebral arteries. The protective gene may decrease the number of active substances (called *metalloproteinases*) in the blood that are involved in causing atherosclerotic plaques to rupture. The implications of this research are very exciting. We may one day devise a genetic test that can predict one's risk of stroke, and we may develop gene therapy for stroke survivors and their families. After assessing the risk of stroke, the next step is to find a way to prevent a stroke from happening if the risk is high.

Most strokes occur because of a combination of factors; they usually cannot be blamed on one gene or one environmental factor alone. If you are a stroke survivor or if you are related to someone who has had a stroke, however, you need to know about the genetic causes of stroke. If you have a family history of risk factors for stroke, be sure to tell your doctor, because this information will help to guide your therapy. The information may also prove invaluable to your first-degree relatives, some of whom may well have the same condition. If you do share genetic risk factors for stroke with your loved ones, read on. We are going to tell you about the many things that you and your family can do to reduce your chance of stroke. We will also discuss research into new treatments for stroke that hold great promise for those who may be at risk.

●●●

Chapter 13

Medications That Help Prevent Stroke

Medications are a key element in the prevention of stroke. New medications continue to be developed to help prevent stroke, and our understanding of the risks and benefits of existing medications continues to expand. In order to decide which medication or medications might best help you or a loved one, you will want to consult a physician who is an expert on preventing strokes and who is up to date on the evolving scientific literature on this subject.

If you have already had a stroke or TIA, it is essential to identify the underlying cause of the stroke if possible. This helpful piece of information will guide a doctor in prescribing the best medical treatment to prevent another stroke. In this chapter we discuss medications designed to help prevent stroke and how these medications are used in primary and secondary stroke prevention. Taking a drug to prevent an event (such as a stroke) is often called *prophylactic treatment* or *preventive treatment.*

Medications That Prevent Blood Clot Formation

Aspirin

Aspirin partially blocks the function of *platelets,* small particles in the blood that play a key role in forming blood clots. The ability to form blood clots helps the body control bleeding. For example, if you cut your finger, your platelets help your body form a scab. The same mechanism that keeps us from bleeding to death when we have a minor injury also contributes to the development of a stroke. By interfering with the function of platelets, aspirin helps to prevent the formation of blood clots, which may lead to a stroke.

Aspirin and its predecessors have been used for medicinal purposes for centuries. In 1763, the Royal Society received a communication from Reverend Edward Stone of Oxfordshire that stated, "Among the many useful discoveries which this age has made, there are very few which better deserve the attention of the public than what I am going to lay before your Lordship. There is a bark of an English tree, which I have found by experience to be a powerful astringent and very efficacious in curing." The tree Stone referred to was the willow, whose bark contains a substance similar to modern aspirin. Today, of course, we are able to produce aspirin in mass quantities in a laboratory, rather then relying on tree bark. Though Stone is given credit for this discovery, much earlier, in the fourth century BC, Hippocrates advised chewing willow leaves to relieve the pains of childbirth; Pliny (first century) and Galen (second century) referred to the pain-relieving properties of an aspirin-like substance, as well.

In modern times, aspirin has been used for decades to prevent strokes. Although it is well tolerated by most people, some people get an upset stomach from aspirin, and, more rarely, ulcers or stomach bleeding can occur due to aspirin treatment. In recent years, lower doses of aspirin have been used for stroke prevention, and the risk of side effects has been reduced. Doses for stroke prevention typically range from 80 mg daily (one baby aspirin) to 325 mg daily (one regular aspirin tablet). Coated aspirin (such as Ecotrin) may cause less stomach upset than standard aspirin.

Plavix (Clopidogrel)

Like aspirin, Plavix partially blocks the function of platelets, but through a different mechanism than aspirin. It is often used in place of aspirin and appears to be about as effective overall for stroke prevention. Some physicians will switch individuals to Plavix who have had a stroke despite taking prophylactic aspirin, though there is not currently much evidence to support this practice. Aspirin and Plavix are sometimes prescribed in combination, with the assumption that the two will be more effective than either one alone. Limited research exists to support this practice at present, and there is some evidence that the combination may increase the risk of bleeding.

Plavix is usually very well tolerated, causing few or no side effects. Rarely, Plavix causes thrombotic thrombocytopenic purpura (a blood disorder), and in that case its use must be discontinued.

Ticlid (Ticlopidine)

Ticlid is very similar in its effects to Plavix and in the United States has been available longer than Plavix. While it appears to be as effective as Plavix, it is more likely to cause serious blood abnormalities. For this reason, periodic blood count monitoring is recommended for anyone taking this medication.

Because of the similar benefits and higher risk of complications, doctors do not prescribe Ticlid as often as they prescribe Plavix.

Aggrenox (Aspirin/Dipyridamole)

Aggrenox is a combination of two medications in a single pill: aspirin and dipyridamole. Dipyridamole also reduces platelet function, and there is some evidence indicating that the combination of the two medications may be more effective than aspirin alone. It is possible to obtain dipyridamole in a pill that does not contain aspirin. While it might seem reasonable to take a dipyridamole tablet together with an aspirin tablet, most physicians do not recommend this as a substitute for Aggrenox, which contains both of these medications in a sustained-release formulation.

Coumadin (Warfarin)

Coumadin (warfarin) acts as a powerful anticoagulant or blood thinner. (The term *blood thinner* is misleading. The blood is not truly thinner in someone taking warfarin, but it does have less of a tendency to form clots.) As noted throughout this book, many strokes are caused by blood clots that may develop in one place (for example, the heart) and then break off and travel to the brain, or else develop directly within the blood vessels supplying the brain. Preventing blood clot formation can be a powerful way of preventing strokes.

Coumadin is the most effective treatment available for the prevention of stroke due to atrial fibrillation or mechanical heart valves; it may also be appropriate in individuals with other sources of embolism, such as a dilated heart (*cardiomyopathy*) or severe inoperable blood vessel narrowing.

Sensitivity to Coumadin varies substantially from person to person. Its potency can be affected by specific foods. Vitamin K is a normal and necessary component of a healthy diet, but when people who are taking Coumadin eat foods that provide a great deal of vitamin K, they may lose the protection provided by Coumadin. While larger doses of Coumadin can overcome the effects of vitamin K, the most prudent course is to limit intake of foods or supplements providing this vitamin. Table 13.1 is a list of foods known to contain high amounts of vitamin K.

Alcohol can also diminish the effect of Coumadin, as can be seen in the results of the *protime test,* the blood test used to monitor the drug. This test provides a measurement called the *international normalized ratio* (INR). A higher INR indicates that the blood is slower to clot. Alcohol can raise your INR, and can also cause stomach inflammation, which may result in bleed-

Table 13.1. Foods Rich in Vitamin K

Kale	Brussels sprouts
Parsley	Watercress
Endive	Scallions
Turnip greens	Cabbage (moderate amount of vitamin K)
Swiss chard	Broccoli (moderate amount of vitamin K)
Collard greens	Pistachios (moderate amount of vitamin K)
Spinach	

Note: This is not a complete list, but it includes some of the more commonly consumed foods that are rich in vitamin K. If you have questions about any foods, consult a nutritionist.

ing. For these reasons, we generally recommend avoiding alcohol if you are taking Coumadin.

Another problem with Coumadin is that its potency can be affected by several medications. Antibiotics, including erythromycin and sulfonamides, may increase its effects. These medications deplete the intestinal bacteria inside the large intestine. These bacteria normally produce vitamin K, which partially counteracts the effects of Coumadin. When antibiotics suppress the bacteria, there is less vitamin K and Coumadin has a stronger effect, raising the INR. This does not mean that you cannot take antibiotics if you are taking Coumadin, but you may need more frequent blood tests to monitor your INR. The amount of Coumadin you take may need to be adjusted during your course of antibiotics. Table 13.2 is a list of other medications that can interfere with the effect of Coumadin in the body. The story that follows illustrates how diet and medications can interact with the effects of Coumadin, with serious consequences.

Nancy, a 69-year-old grandmother, lived alone in her apartment. A few years ago she was feeling extremely fatigued and short of breath, and she was waking up at night feeling she needed to run to the window to get air. She was diagnosed with severe narrowing of one of the heart valves, the aortic valve, a condition known as *aortic stenosis* (see Chapter 8). Nancy needed surgery to replace her aortic valve with a mechanical heart valve. After that, she had to take Coumadin every day to reduce her risk of developing blood clots.

When Nancy developed a sinus infection, her doctor prescribed antibiotics. During her illness, she lost her appetite and no longer ate her usual green salads for lunch. Nancy went to the emergency room one night with a severe stomachache. During her evaluation, her doctors discovered that her INR was 8 instead of her target of 3. This meant that she was in danger of suffering a hemorrhagic stroke or bleeding elsewhere in her body. She was admitted to the hospital for monitoring and received an injection of vitamin K to reverse the excessive anti-coagulation and prevent internal bleeding. She was advised about the importance of watching her diet and checking with her doctor about interactions between any new medications and Coumadin.

Coumadin is generally well tolerated. Most people experience few side effects, with easy bruising being the most common side effect. In a small number of people, more serious bleeding can result from Coumadin, in-cluding bleeding into the urine or bowel movements, severe nosebleeds, and internal bleeding. Rarely, Coumadin can cause bleeding inside the brain—a hemorrhagic stroke. Symptoms that may indicate an excessive level of anticoagulation include bleeding in the urine, severe or persistent nosebleeds, black and tarry stools (due to blood turning black in the intes-tines), and vomiting blood. Severe bleeding can occur due to an accidental injury, such as falling and hitting your head or a car accident, but bleeding can sometimes occur without any traumatic event. While all of the medica-tions we have discussed thus far in this chapter can cause abnormal bleed-ing, the risk of serious abnormal bleeding is highest with Coumadin. For this reason, Coumadin is sometimes not used as a treatment in someone who is believed to be at high risk of bleeding due to medical conditions (such as a recent stomach ulcer) or at high risk of injury (such as an elderly person with a history of repeated falls).

Coumadin therapy needs to be monitored closely by the physician to make sure that the level of anticoagulation is within the therapeutic and safe range. INR levels are generally checked weekly, using the protime test, once a Coumadin dose is determined, and the dose is adjusted based on the result. In individuals with a stable INR level, monitoring is often reduced to once every few weeks. Most commonly an INR range of 2 to 3 is the target, though in people with mechanical heart valves and in certain other situa-tions, higher levels may be desirable.

Low Molecular Weight Heparins

Low molecular weight heparins are a group of related medications, includ-ing Fragmin (dalteparin), Lovenox (enoxaparin), and Innohep (tinzapa-rin). Like Coumadin, these medications are all anticoagulants and reduce

Table 13.2. Selected Medications That Interfere with Coumadin

Tylenol (acetaminophen)	Antabuse (disulfiram)
Zyloprim (allopurinol)	Flagyl (metronidazole)
Cordarone (amiodarone)	Anturane (sulfinpyrazone)
Tagamet (cimetidine)	

Note: This is not a complete list. Tell your physician if you are taking Coumadin before you begin taking any new medication.

the blood's tendency to form clots. Low molecular weight heparins are given via injection once or twice daily, and are used primarily for short-term treatment for stroke prevention. In certain circumstances, however, they may be used as a longer-term treatment in place of Coumadin.

Complications of low molecular weight heparins are similar to those of Coumadin, with bleeding being the greatest concern. Bruising or bleeding at the site of injection is a common, though generally not serious, complication.

Medications Used to Treat Conditions Related to Stroke

Some medications that are used to treat other medical conditions also reduce the risk of stroke. For example, taking medication to control high blood pressure treats the high blood pressure and also reduces the risk of stroke. In this section, we will cover only the medications that have particular application to people who have had a stroke.

Statin Medications

As discussed in Chapter 8, statins are medications used to reduce the risk of stroke and heart disease by lowering the levels of LDL cholesterol (the "bad" cholesterol) and raising the levels of HDL cholesterol ("good" cholesterol). Commonly used statins include pravastatin (Pravachol), atorvastatin (Lipitor), rosuvastatin (Crestor), fluvastatin (Lescol), lovastatin (Mevacor), and simvastatin (Zocor). Scientific studies have found that people taking statin medications have a lower risk of stroke than people who do not take these medications. The benefits of this treatment are seen even for people who do not have elevated cholesterol levels. This finding had led to speculation that statin medications may have effects other than their cholesterol-lowering properties, which may be responsible for some of this benefit. Doctors are increasingly using statin medications as part of a regimen of preventing a second stroke, even in individuals with minimally elevated or borderline cholesterol levels. It is quite possible that in the future we will be recommending statin medications for secondary stroke prevention in people who have completely normal cholesterol levels.

Recent evidence suggests that some statin medications may be more effective than others, and that cholesterol should be maintained at a level that is substantially lower than earlier recommendations suggested. The PROVE-IT study found that in patients who had recently had heart attacks, high doses of atorvastatin (Lipitor) were more effective than standard doses of pravastatin (Pravachol) in preventing death or major cardiac problems. This benefit did not extend to reducing the risk of stroke, and the implications of this study for stroke prevention are still under debate. Further studies are planned to determine the best strategy for reducing the risk of stroke and other cardiovascular disease using statin medications.

Statins are usually well tolerated, but side effects can occur. Among the more common side effects are muscle abnormalities, which can lead to muscle pains and weakness. These abnormalities can become serious if the medication is continued, and they should be reported promptly to your doctor. Blood tests can check for muscle inflammation and monitor muscle-related side effects of the statin drugs.

Blood Pressure Medications

Many different medications are used to lower blood pressure; they are known broadly as *anti-hypertensive medications*. Because elevated blood pressure is well known to be a major risk factor for primary stroke and recurrent stroke, many physicians and others have assumed in the past that differences among blood pressure medications would not matter for the purposes of preventing a stroke. In other words, they assumed that the blood pressure accurately reflected the risk of a stroke, and that if one could lower the blood pressure, it didn't really matter which medication accomplished this—the result would be the same.

Surprisingly, this idea has been proven to be false in large, well-designed studies using blood pressure medications to reduce the risk of stroke. In particular, some blood pressure medications seem to be *significantly more effective* in reducing the risk of stroke than others. Due to the complexity of these research studies, the results are not always clear about the "best" or "worst" medications, but rather provide some general direction. Generally speaking, these studies have suggested that the use of blood pressure–lowering medications known as ACE inhibitors (including captopril, lisinopril, enalapril, and ramipril) and diuretics (sometimes known as "water pills") such as hydrochlorthiazide and others are most effective at reducing stroke risk in individuals with elevated blood pressure. Alpha-blockers, such as doxazosin, and calcium channel blockers, such as nifedipine (Procardia), verapamil, amlodipine (Norvasc), and diltiazem (Cardizem), appear to be less effective in reducing the risk of stroke. Finally, other blood pressure–lowering medications such as beta-blockers, including atenolol (Tenormin) and metoprolol (Lopressor, Toprol), are intermediately effective for stroke prevention.

Many people with high blood pressure require more than one, and often several, medications to achieve good control of their blood pressure. Another important consideration is that other factors may influence the choice of medications used to control blood pressure. For example, for someone with heart disease, a beta-blocker may reduce blood pressure, control angina symptoms, and reduce the risk of sudden death from cardiac causes. Someone with *benign prostatic hypertrophy* (an enlarged prostate gland) may benefit from an alpha-blocker such as doxazosin for treatment of the prostate. Having this medication serve "double duty" by treating both high blood pressure and an enlarged prostate simultaneously makes good sense.

Another consideration is the side-effect profile of these medications. For example, a man who experiences erectile dysfunction (difficulty in achieving or sustaining an erection during sexual activity) due to a beta-blocker may need to switch to an alternative blood pressure medication. Every blood pressure medication (indeed, every medication) can have side effects, and these side effects play a part in the selection of blood pressure–lowering medications.

The bottom line is that physician and patient need to work together to select a blood pressure–lowering medication or medications for the patient's individual circumstances and other medical considerations. Thankfully, there are so many effective blood pressure medications that almost everyone can achieve good control of their blood pressure and reduce their risk of stroke.

Taking Your Medication Regularly

Doctors are frequently surprised to learn that a patient under their care is not taking their medications as prescribed. There are many reasons why patients fail to take their medications. Side effects are a common reason.

When they experience side effects, some patients mistakenly assume that there are no alternative medications that could be substituted. Side effects vary and can include almost any symptom, including stomach upset, diarrhea, loss of appetite, loss of sexual desire, problems with sexual function, depression, or sedation (feeling sleepy or drugged). If you think you may be experiencing side effects from a medication, you should discuss this situation with your doctor to see if switching to another medication could reduce or eliminate these side effects. *Do not stop taking a prescribed medication without informing your physician.*

Another common reason for failing to take medication as prescribed is cost. For individuals without prescription coverage from their insurance company, medication costs can add up quickly. Some people who are trying to stretch their financial resources take reduced doses of medications (taking half of a pill instead of a whole pill as prescribed, for example) or skip doses of medication. These strategies can be dangerous and expose you to the risk of stroke. A better strategy is to let your physician know that the cost of the medications is problematic. In some cases, less expensive but equally effective medication choices exist. And some drug companies have programs to provide free or reduced-cost medication to individuals who cannot afford the full price for a medication.

Some people have difficulty remembering to take their medications. Working with your doctor to select medications that are taken only once a day rather than multiple times during the day may be the simplest solution. If this does not solve the problem, you might use one of the commercially available alarms to help, perhaps one that is inserted into the top of the medication bottle or one of the pill cases with built-in alarms. Or you could use a hand-held computer programmed with alarms throughout the day.

Another common reason people fail to take their medications as prescribed is that they do not see the point. Many physicians do not provide enough information about why they are prescribing a medication; alternatively, patients may be overwhelmed with excessive amounts of information at a doctor's office visit. There are several sources of helpful information to supplement that provided by your physician. Many pharmacies provide information sheets on common medications. (If you don't receive one, you should ask the pharmacy to give you one.) Pharmacists are trained to provide medication education, and they are an often underutilized source of more personalized information. Finally, there are now drug information resources available on the Internet that are designed for consumers and that can provide straightforward information about specific medications (see Resources).

In this chapter we have described medications that reduce the risk of stroke either directly or by treating a condition that can lead to stroke. In the next chapter we discuss surgical procedures that can help reduce the risk of stroke.

•••

Chapter 14

When Surgery Is an Option

Surgery and other invasive procedures can play an important role in preventing stroke. We recognize that surgery is a scary proposition for many people, including stroke survivors, and we know that having adequate information about the risks, benefits, and alternatives to any surgical procedure is critical before making a decision about this type of treatment. In this chapter we seek to provide this information about procedures that are currently in use, and we also discuss some newer procedures that are not yet widely used but that are either under study or that appear likely to become more common.

Carotid Endarterectomy

In a procedure called *carotid endarterectomy,* the inner lining of the carotid artery is surgically removed. This procedure is done when a moderate or severe blockage to this artery has developed in the neck, leading to an increased risk of stroke or of recurrent stroke. The blockage is usually due to gradual buildup of atherosclerosis—the fatty deposits that occur within the blood vessel wall over many years (see Chapter 8).

Surgeons have performed carotid endarterectomies for many years, and the procedure has been proven to reduce the risk of a stroke or second stroke when used in the correct circumstances. Carotid blockages are complex, as discussed in Chapters 3 and 8. Knowing what percentage of the blood vessel is blocked is very important, but it is not the only determinant of whether carotid surgery is recommended or not. We will review several common scenarios in this chapter; these scenarios can serve as a general guide to understanding who will require surgery. Keep in mind that surgical treatment of blocked arteries is an evolving area of medical practice and that there is no universal agreement about guidelines for making these decisions.

Carotid blockages are often divided into two broad categories: *symptomatic* and *asymptomatic*. Doctors often discover asymptomatic blockages when listening with a stethoscope over the neck of a patient during an exam. A carotid artery narrowing in the neck will often make a swooshing sound (called a *bruit*) as the blood flows past the partial blockage caused by atherosclerosis. Doctors often find these bruits during routine examinations, such as a yearly physical examination. A bruit is an indication that the flow within the blood vessel is turbulent, usually due to a partial blockage of the carotid artery. A symptomatic blockage might be discovered when someone has symptoms of a transient ischemic attack, such as temporary loss of the ability to speak. If the evaluation of the TIA reveals a blockage in the corresponding carotid artery (that is, the one that supplies blood to the area of the brain affected by the TIA), this is considered a "symptomatic" carotid artery blockage. There is also a common "gray area" of people who have had TIAs or strokes in one area of the brain (for example, the right hemisphere) and who are found to have a blockage in a carotid artery that does not supply blood to the area of the brain where the stroke or TIA occurred. Most physicians consider a blockage that doesn't match the stroke or TIA "asymptomatic" for the purpose of deciding the best treatment.

Doctors generally recommend a carotid endarterectomy for individuals who have a symptomatic carotid artery blockage of 70 percent or greater (that is, when 70 percent or more of the diameter of the blood vessel is blocked). If you have a blockage in the range of 30 to 69 percent, your doctor might recommend carotid surgery, but the benefits need to be carefully weighed against the surgical risks. For blockages of less than 30 percent, the majority of doctors will not recommend surgery. Some physicians will recommend an endarterectomy for individuals with an asymptomatic carotid artery blockage of greater than 60 percent, after careful consideration of the risks and benefits. Carotid endarterectomy is considered major surgery. It requires general anesthesia and close monitoring. Patients undergoing this surgery typically stay in the hospital for a day or two, but they have a fairly rapid recovery and return to their usual activities. Some local soreness, swelling, and bruising of the neck is common, but these symptoms generally resolve over a few weeks.

While it is true that the greater the degree of narrowing (also called *stenosis*) in the carotid artery, the greater the risk of a stroke or TIA, many people will not have a stroke even if they have substantial narrowing. Thus, even if you have significant narrowing of your carotid artery, it is impossible to determine precisely how likely it is that you will have a stroke. Statistically, for people with symptomatic carotid stenosis of 70 to 90 percent, it is estimated that there is a 13 percent net reduction in the risk of stroke over a twenty-year period after carotid endarterectomy. For stenosis from 50 to 69 percent, the net reduction is approximately 5 percent. These statistics mean that many people undergo this serious surgery to prevent stroke even though they might never have had a stroke even if they didn't have the surgery. Because medical science cannot yet predict exactly who will have a stroke without surgery, the only rational approach is to work with a physician to review his best estimates of your personal risks of a stroke versus the risks of the surgery. Once the odds are estimated, the decision becomes a matter of personal choice.

What about a complete blockage of the carotid artery? These blockages are not usually surgically treated. Since the artery is completely blocked, it is assumed that whatever damage (if any) is going to occur has already occurred, and that reopening the artery will not serve any purpose. In some cases the other blood vessels supplying the brain are able to compensate for the blockage, although the degree to which they can compensate varies from person to person.

The timing of carotid endarterectomy remains somewhat controversial. Recent studies have suggested that "sooner is better than later" in individuals with a recent TIA or stroke, and that surgery within two weeks after a TIA or stroke is preferable. Many physicians prescribe anticoagulant medications (such as warfarin or enoxaparin) from the time the carotid narrowing is found until the surgery is performed in order to minimize the risk of a stroke while awaiting surgery.

Ironically, the major concern with carotid endarterectomy is that a stroke can occur as a complication of this surgery. It is estimated that between 2 and 10 percent of endarterectomies are complicated by stroke and that between 1 and 3 percent of endarterectomies result in death. Scientific studies have shown that one significant factor in the risk of this type of complication is the experience of the surgeon. In general, the more carotid endarterectomies a surgeon performs each year, the lower the rate of complications. This is only a general statement, since some surgeons are particularly gifted despite having handled a small number of cases, whereas others may have performed many surgeries but lack the technical skills to be an outstanding surgeon. This relationship between the number of cases and complications does mean that it is important to obtain information about the surgeon's experience and add that information to the other factors considered when choosing a hospital and a surgeon for this procedure.

Some carotid artery blockages regrow after a carotid endarterectomy and may also occur on the other side of the body. Periodic (perhaps yearly) monitoring of the carotid arteries by carotid ultrasound after this type of surgery is usually recommended. If a blockage should reoccur, surgery can sometimes be performed a second time to reopen the artery.

Carotid and Basilar Artery Stenting

Stenting is an intriguing new treatment for blocked arteries. This technique, which is now widely used for blockages of blood vessels in the heart, consists of threading a thin flexible tube through the blood vessels and then inflating a balloon in the area of blockage. The expanding balloon opens up the area that is severely narrowed and allows blood flow to be restored. A thin metal mesh tube is inserted into the area where the blockage had been and then is expanded to hold the blood vessel open (see Figure 14.1). The metal mesh tube, known as a *stent,* keeps the blood vessel from returning to its blocked condition. Newer stents (known as *drug-eluting stents*) are impregnated with medication to prevent return of the blockage over time. These medications interfere with the regrowth of the blockage.

Stent placement does not usually require general anesthesia, though sedation may be used. It is normally performed in a procedure room on an outpatient basis, rather than in an operating room. It takes one to two hours in most cases. There is usually little pain associated with the procedure.

While stents are widely used and medically accepted treatments for blockages of blood vessels in the heart, they remain innovative and largely experimental treatments for blood vessels supplying the brain. Research studies are ongoing comparing the benefits of this treatment for the carotid arteries compared with more traditional endarterectomy surgery. Stents are also being used for blood vessel blockages where surgery is not technically feasible.

Similar to carotid endarterectomy, the greatest risk in stenting the arteries in the neck is the possibility of sustaining a stroke as a complication. A stroke can occur when a piece of material is dislodged from the blood vessel wall and ends up traveling down the blood vessel to cause a blockage. The walls of the blood vessels may be damaged during this procedure, and the damage can lead to stroke. Also possible are allergic reactions to the material (*intravenous contrast*) injected so the surgeon can visualize the blood vessels during the procedure. Kidney damage can occur but is usually temporary. The potential benefit of this procedure is the prevention of stroke, though it is still unclear how this benefit compares with endarterectomy

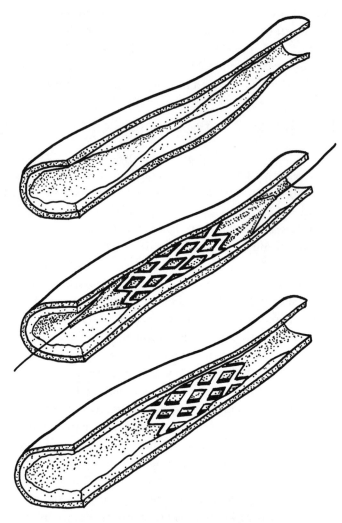

Figure 14.1. Stent placement in an artery. An atherosclerotic narrowing is shown in the top figure. In the middle figure, a balloon has been passed over a wire through the narrowing and is being inflated. Note that the mesh stent is surrounding the balloon and is expanded as a result of the balloon inflation. In the bottom figure, the balloon has been deflated and removed, and the stent is left in place to keep the blood vessel wall open.

or treatment with medications. Stenting is a promising new procedure that is still being evaluated in relation to the more established surgical carotid endarterectomy to determine which approach is safer and more effective.

External Carotid–Internal Carotid Bypass

Bypassing a blockage in a blood vessel is a theoretically appealing way of dealing with a blockage. This technique involves rerouting blood flow around a severe blockage through another blood vessel. To some extent, the brain does this naturally. The blood vessel connections at the base of the brain provide blood flow with alternate routes in case of blockage or damage to a blood vessel. But this natural system is often incomplete, inadequate, or not situated correctly to address many of the blockages that may develop. Surgically connecting blood vessels that are not normally connected is one way of creating bypasses.

One technique to address blockages in the blood vessels supplying the brain is known as *external carotid–internal carotid bypass.* This technique creates a connection between a key artery supplying blood to the brain, known as the *internal carotid artery,* and a second, nearby, artery that does not normally supply blood to the brain, known as the *external carotid artery.* The connection between these two is made "downstream" from a blockage in the internal carotid artery, permitting the external carotid artery to supply blood to the portion of the brain that is at risk for a stroke.

Despite its conceptual appeal, this procedure has largely fallen out of favor among physicians caring for stroke survivors. Studies of outcomes after this procedure failed to show the hoped-for benefit, and even showed an increased risk of stroke after this procedure. This surgery has largely disappeared from the list of options for stroke prevention.

Arteriovenous Malformation Embolization and Resection

Arteriovenous malformations (commonly known as AVMs; see Chapter 11) are abnormal blood vessels within the brain that connect the high-pressure arteries directly with the low-pressure veins. The fragility of the walls of these abnormal blood vessel growths means that arteriovenous malformations may bleed spontaneously, causing a hemorrhagic stroke.

Several approaches have been taken to shrink or eliminate AVMs, and these approaches are often used in combination. Many AVMs are removed surgically, but this procedure can be technically challenging. AVMs are frequently lodged deep within the brain, and surgeons need to consider the damage they may cause to the adjacent brain tissue when they attempt to remove them. As a result, surgery often does not remove the entire AVM, and some risk of bleeding remains. In addition, the surgical procedure usually causes some damage to the brain, resulting in stroke-like aftereffects. AVMs can also regrow over time, requiring subsequent surgeries.

Another technique for dealing with AVMs involves attacking the AVM from the inside. Using a thin flexible tube (*catheter*) threaded through the blood vessels, a physician can inject small pellets into the bloodstream so that they lodge within the AVM and block the blood vessels providing blood to the AVM. This technique, known as *embolization*, can shrink the AVM and reduce the risk of bleeding, though it does not usually eliminate the AVM entirely. This procedure may be used as the primary treatment for the AVM, or it can be used before surgery to make the surgery more manageable.

Lastly, radiation therapy can be used to treat AVMs. The radiation causes the blood vessel cells to become less active and also stabilizes and often shrinks the AVM. Damage to surrounding brain tissue can occur, and this possibility limits the dose of radiation that can be provided.

The major risks of surgery involve the damage caused by the procedure itself, and the risk of bleeding of the residual parts of the AVM after surgery. Bleeding can also complicate the embolization of an AVM, though the risk is generally lower than bleeding associated with surgery. Embolization can cause stroke if the pellets block a blood vessel that is providing blood to a portion of the brain. The threading of the catheter through the blood vessels also carries a small risk of stroke on its own. The immediate risks of radiation therapy are relatively minor, though there may be long-term effects of radiation on the brain, including memory loss in some cases.

Aneurysm Clipping and Coiling

Aneurysms are abnormal, thin-walled outpouchings of blood vessels; these outpouchings can burst and cause bleeding within or around the brain (see Chapter 11). Aneurysms may affect multiple blood vessels in some individuals, though typically only one of these aneurysms causes the symptoms that bring a person to seek medical attention.

Aneurysms may be surgically corrected, most commonly by placing a surgical "clip" across the opening from the blood vessel into the aneurysm (see Chapter 11 and Figure 14.2). This clip causes blood flow to cease within

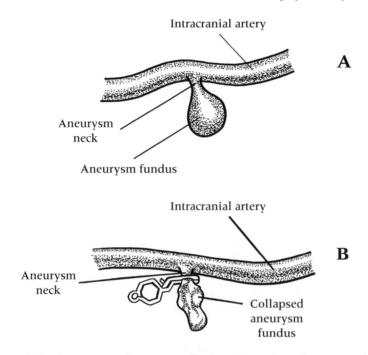

Figure 14.2. Aneurysm and aneurysm clipping. (A) A "berry" aneurysm is shown as a balloon-like outpouching of a blood vessel wall with a narrow connection to the main blood vessel. (B) A clip has been placed across the narrow "neck" of the outpouching, interrupting blood flow to the aneurysm. The collapsed aneurysm appears "deflated" compared to the balloon-like aneurysm in figure (A).

the aneurysm, making it no longer at risk for rupture. While this surgery is very effective, some aneurysms are not amenable to this type of treatment, due either to the shape of the aneurysm or to its location. For this treatment to work, the aneurysm must have a well-defined "neck" where a clip can be placed; such a neck is commonly but not always present.

Another approach to treating aneurysms is similar to the approach described for AVMs, treating them from the inside of the blood vessel. A long thin flexible tube (catheter) is threaded through the blood vessels into the aneurysm, and one or more detachable *coils* (small spring-shaped devices) are placed within the aneurysm. These coils cause the blood flow to be disrupted within the aneurysm and a blood clot to form. The blood clot fills the aneurysm by "sealing" it and prevents it from rupturing. This procedure can be performed on an outpatient basis and does not require general anesthesia in most cases.

The risks of aneurysm clipping include damage to adjacent blood vessels and stroke, rupture of the aneurysm during the procedure, and failure to fully block the opening into the aneurysm. Risks of using coils to clot the aneurysm include the coil floating into the main blood vessel and causing a stroke, or the blood vessel being damaged with the catheter, causing a stroke. Rupture of the aneurysm can also occur during this procedure, requiring emergency surgery. Studies have shown that some small aneurysms may be better left untreated, whereas larger ones have a high risk of rupturing and therefore should receive surgery or coil placement.

Closure of Patent Foramen Ovale

A *patent foramen ovale* (PFO) is an abnormal opening between the two sides of the heart that can allow blood or other material to travel from the right atrium into the left atrium (see Chapter 11). Many individuals have an asymptomatic patent foramen ovale, and the value of surgical treatment in these individuals is not clear. For individuals who have had a stroke due to a patent foramen ovale, however, closure of the PFO may be advised.

In the past, treatment of a PFO involved open-heart surgery and was a major and rarely undertaken procedure. In recent years, however, catheter-based treatment has been developed, which allows closure of the PFO without the need for open-heart surgery. In this procedure, a catheter is threaded into the right atrium, the heart chamber that has an abnormal opening, into its counterpart on the left side (the left atrium). The catheter is used to pierce the thin wall between these two chambers, and an umbrella-like device is opened on both sides of the wall. This device, known as an *Amplatzer device,* covers both sides of the opening and holds itself in place after the catheter has been removed.

This procedure does not always provide complete closure of the PFO, though it typically at least reduces the size of the PFO and reduces the risk of recurrent stroke. Other risks of the procedure include stroke (in rare cases) or damage to the heart requiring open-heart surgery.

Surgery is a critical tool for the prevention of stroke in some people. While surgery has its risks, it can be a very powerful method of reducing stroke risk for the long term. Newer, less invasive procedures hold the promise of achieving the same benefits with less risk and easier recovery.

••

Part IV

PREVENTING STROKE: LIFESTYLE ISSUES

Chapter 15

•••

Diet and Stroke

In the preceding chapters we described the medical conditions that can lead to stroke and how these conditions are treated. These treatments can help reduce the risk of someone having a stroke. In this part of the book, we turn to lifestyle issues—how you can reduce your risk of stroke by making specific decisions about how you live your life. Watching what you eat is a smart place to start. Everyone knows that they should eat a healthy diet, but that is certainly easier said than done. Bill Cosby's mother had a number of strokes, but her experience didn't convince her son to eat healthy foods. In fact, just the opposite was true, until one day his doctor told him that his cholesterol level was too high. Then he panicked. (That's how he tells it in his book *I Am What I Ate . . . and I'm Frightened!!!*)

If you have had a stroke, thinking about how what you have eaten in the past might affect your current health can be frightening. However, dietary changes can have a tremendous impact on your health, and you *can* make these changes. For our purposes, there are two main issues to consider when it comes to eating a healthy diet. The first is simply motivation. Trying to change old habits and form new ones takes time and energy, and it can be difficult to remain motivated. But if you have suffered a stroke, now is a time when you are likely very motivated to make lifestyle changes that can include embracing a healthier diet.

The second issue is more of a problem. This issue has to do with the conflicting messages, some from the media and some from the medical community, about what exactly constitutes a healthy diet. A famous example is the Atkins diet developed by the now deceased Dr. Robert C. Atkins. This diet, embraced by many consumers and some health care providers, also has its critics. Some say the diet helps people lose weight and live a healthier life, while others claim it is too high in animal fats and cholesterol. In this chapter, we are not going to propose that you follow any specific formula or dietary regimen. Rather we want you to embrace some simple guidelines that will help you to improve your nutrition.

Eating healthy foods in the proper amounts can improve your cholesterol level, lower your blood pressure, help you to maintain a more stable blood sugar level, and assist you in losing weight. *Nearly everyone who has had a stroke can make dietary changes that will lower their risk of having another stroke.* Eating nutritiously is important for everyone, but if you have already had a stroke, a healthy diet is a critical component of recurrent stroke prevention.

The Stroke Savvy Diet

Many of us can vividly recall the television images of Popeye eating his can of spinach and flexing his muscles. Our parents reminded us of Popeye's prowess to inspire us to eat our vegetables at the dinner table. In Popeye's heyday, there weren't many research studies to support the importance of eating a diet rich in vegetables, but many of our parents passed this message along to us anyway, and we did the same to our children. Now, however, we know *for a fact* that eating a diet rich in vegetables is good practice. Scientists have proven that a good diet can help to prevent many diseases and stop the progression of many others, including stroke. Eating more vegetables isn't enough, however. There are many other nutritional considerations, especially if you have had a stroke. In this chapter, we'll discuss what we call the "Stroke Savvy Diet." Our recommendations are in line with the American Heart Association's guidelines. However, you should discuss your diet with your doctor or nutritionist, particularly if you have an underlying condition such as diabetes or high blood pressure.

Our Stroke Savvy Diet consists of six basic principles that we encourage everyone to follow. These general guidelines apply to most people and will improve the health of almost anyone who adheres to them. As we explain more about the Stroke Savvy Diet, we'll give specific advice about preventing another stroke. These guidelines are a great starting point, however, and they are easy to follow once you get in the habit of considering them before choosing what food you will eat. They are:

1. Eat 5 to 7 servings of fruits and vegetables daily.
2. Eat food that is low in fat and cholesterol.
3. Choose whole grains over white flour.
4. Limit the amount of refined sugar you eat.
5. Eat no more than 2,400 milligrams of salt per day, and don't add salt to your food.
6. Avoid tobacco and limit your alcohol intake.

Fats: Public Enemy Number One?

Fats have a bad reputation, and rightly so. We'll tell you why in a minute. First, though, you need to know that some fat is good for you. In fact, your body needs fat. Fat is an important source of energy and is the primary component of cell membranes and the *myelin sheath* (the fat that coats and protects nerves in your brain, your spinal cord, and your peripheral nerves). Also, four vitamins (A, D, E, and K) are fat soluble—they won't work for you unless some fat accompanies them. Fat helps the body produce necessary hormones such as estrogen and testosterone, as well. It often gives food flavor and texture. On a weight management note, fat is digested slowly, so a little fat in your meal can make you feel full more quickly. The bottom line? Don't cut all fat out of your diet.

Too much fat in the diet can cause you to gain weight. If your body does not use the fat you eat, then it is stored as *adipose tissue* (a technical name for fat). Again, fat is important in your diet; about 20 to 30 percent of your calories should come from fat. Most people who live in industrialized countries where food is plentiful consume much more fat than this. And, as we shall see, not all fats are the same.

Fats and Lipids

Before we discuss which fats are good for your arteries and which ones are bad, we need to discuss the terms *fats* and *lipids*. In most people's minds, fat is a greasy substance like butter or oil. Many different medical words are used when talking about fats: *lipids, triglycerides, fatty acids, saturated fats, monounsaturated fats, polyunsaturated fats, lipoproteins,* and *cholesterol,* to name a few. We will discuss each of these terms.

What is a lipid? The Greek root *lipos* means *fat,* and *eidos* means *form.* Lipids are fat and fat-like substances that do not dissolve in water. There are three main classifications of lipids:

1. Simple lipids, such as fatty acids and triglycerides
2. Complex lipids such as lipoproteins, including low density lipoproteins (LDL) and high density lipoproteins (HDL)
3. Sterol lipids, such as cholesterol

Physicians routinely test the blood of their patients for the level of lipids in all three categories. You may have heard people talk about their "lipid profile," or perhaps your physician has ordered a lipid profile for you. This is a simple blood test that checks the levels of the three main types of lipids in your blood. Low levels of triglycerides, cholesterol, and LDL and high levels of HDL are ideal for healthy arteries. You will see why as you read on.

Simple Lipids: Fatty Acids and Triglycerides

The simplest lipids are called *fatty acids.* A fatty acid is a molecule made up mostly of hydrogen and carbon atoms attached to each other by bonds. When fatty acids combine with one another and connect with a glycerol molecule, they form *glycerides.*

Triglycerides are made of three fatty acids connected to a glycerol. They are another example of simple lipids. Most often, the term *triglyceride* is used to describe fats found in our arteries or in the food that we eat. The terms *fats* and *triglycerides* are sometimes used interchangeably.

The body stores fatty acids primarily in the form of triglycerides. High levels of triglycerides together with high levels of cholesterol in the blood can accelerate atherosclerosis. That is why you should have your levels of cholesterol and triglycerides checked and get these levels within a safe range.

Complex Lipids: Lipoproteins

When fatty acids connect with other molecules such as sugars and proteins, they are considered complex. An example of a complex lipid is a *lipoprotein,* which is made up of triglycerides, cholesterol, and protein. The main function of lipoproteins is to transport triglycerides and cholesterol through the bloodstream. Since triglycerides and cholesterol are insoluble in water, they do not move freely in the bloodstream, which is predominately water. They need special transportation vehicles—lipoproteins. Lipoproteins have protein in them, which allows them to navigate easily through the bloodstream. There are four main types of lipoproteins:

1. Chylomicrons
2. Very low density lipoproteins (VLDL)
3. Low density lipoproteins (LDL)
4. High density lipoproteins (HDL)

As their names suggest, categorization of the lipoproteins is based on density. The least dense compounds are the *chylomicrons,* made mostly of triglycerides from your diet. They have the least amount of protein and

Table 15.1. **Lipoproteins**

Lipoprotein	Source	Predominant Ingredient
Chylomicrons	Diet	Triglycerides
VLDL	Liver	Triglycerides
LDL	VLDL	Cholesterol
HDL	Liver	Protein

cholesterol. The VLDL, made in your liver, is composed mostly of tri-glycerides (but fewer triglycerides than chylomicrons contain), some cholesterol and small amounts of proteins (more than chylomicrons contain). The much talked about LDL is made from the breakdown of VLDL and has the most cholesterol in it of all four lipoproteins. LDL is considered the "bad" lipoprotein because it transports the majority of the cholesterol to the different cells and tissues in the body, including the arteries. HDL has the most protein and the least triglycerides and is thus the heaviest lipo-protein. The HDL is the "good" lipoprotein that helps clear away cholesterol. LDL is often called LDL cholesterol, and HDL is often called HDL cholesterol. Table 15.1 lists lipoproteins, their sources, and their predominant ingredients.

Sterol Lipids: Cholesterol

In addition to simple and complex lipids, there is a third category of lipids known as the *sterols*. Cholesterol is an example of a lipid in this category. Like the simple lipids, the sterols are predominately made of carbon and hydrogen bonds. Unlike the simple lipids, the sterols have complicated rings in their biochemical structure.

Our bodies make cholesterol in the liver. We also eat cholesterol in our food. Cholesterol can be used by the body to make other substances, such as estrogen, testosterone, and vitamin D, or it can remain in the bloodstream. The buildup of cholesterol contributes to the creation of the atherosclerotic plaques that block the arteries (as we discussed in Chapter 8).

Like triglycerides, cholesterol is transported through the bloodstream by lipoproteins. Low Density Lipoprotein (LDL) carries the most cholesterol. The HDL is the helper lipoprotein that works to clear away the cholesterol. Reducing LDL cholesterol and achieving high levels of HDL can help prevent the development of atherosclerotic plaques.

Saturated Fatty Acids Are Bad and Unsaturated Fatty Acids Are Good

Let's return to good and bad fats. There are four different types of fatty acids in food: saturated, monounsaturated, polyunsaturated, and partially hydrogenated. All of these fatty acids look fairly similar in structure, but there are small differences that can have a big impact on the body.

What does *saturated* mean? Saturated refers to the number of bonds between the carbon atoms of the fatty acid. Fatty acids are basically carbon and hydrogen atoms connected together by double or single bonds.

A saturated fatty acid has no double bonds in its biochemical structure, which means there is no room for another hydrogen atom. It is saturated, meaning it is full of hydrogen atoms. An unsaturated fatty acid has double bonds in its biochemical structure, which means there is room to add more hydrogen atoms. It is unsaturated, meaning it is not full of hydrogen atoms. Unsaturated fatty acids are good for you and saturated fatty acids are not, so you should always be aware of what type of fat you are eating.

Knowing the meaning of saturated and unsaturated paves the way to understanding the terms *partially hydrogenated, monounsaturated,* and *polyunsaturated fats.* Partially hydrogenated fats have had hydrogen atoms added to them in a chemical process. They are sometimes referred to as *trans-fats.* Monounsaturated fats have one double bond in the structure of their fatty acid, and polyunsaturated fats have more than one double bond in the structure of their fatty acid. The monounsaturated and polyunsaturated fats are the "good" fats; saturated and partially hydrogenated (trans-fats) are the bad ones.

The good fats—the polyunsaturated and monounsaturated fatty acids— are considered good because they do not increase low density lipoprotein (LDL) levels in the body. In fact, some even increase high density lipoproteins (HDL), the lipoproteins responsible for clearing out cholesterol. On the other hand, the bad fats—saturated fatty acids and partially hydrogenated fatty acids—are considered bad because they increase LDL and cholesterol, perhaps by encouraging the body to make its own cholesterol.

All the foods we eat contain combinations of different fatty acids. Some foods are higher in saturated fatty acids than unsaturated fatty acids. How can you tell which fats are high in unsaturated fatty acids and are thus the good ones? Read on!

Good fats. The good fats are derived primarily from plants and fish. They are polyunsaturated and monounsaturated fatty acids. Polyunsaturated fatty acids come in two basic forms: *omega 3 fatty acids* and *omega 6 fatty acids.* The

Table 15.2. **Oils Rich in Omega 6 Fatty Acids**

Corn	Sunflower
Safflower	Walnut
Sesame	Wheat germ
Soybean	Flaxseed

Table 15.3. **Sources of Monounsaturated Fats**

Avocado
Most nuts (such as peanuts, hazelnuts, Brazil nuts, cashews, and almonds)
Olives
Olive oil
Rapeseeds (most commonly eaten as canola oil)

omega 3 fatty acids are considered the best because there is scientific evidence that they decrease LDL and increase HDL. Omega 3 fatty acids are found naturally in some types of fish, including salmon, herring, mackerel, sardines, and tuna. Fish is not the only natural source of these good fatty acids; certain plants have also been found to have high quantities of *alpha linolenic acid,* which is transformed into omega 3 fatty acids in the body. These plants include flaxseeds, rapeseeds (from which canola oil is made), walnuts, almonds, and beans. The omega 6 fatty acids also lower LDL, but there is no evidence that they raise HDL. Oils rich in omega 6 fatty acids are listed in Table 15.2. Monounsaturated fatty acids are also good for you. A well-known source of monounsaturated fatty acids is olive oil, which is frequently used in the Mediterranean diet and is becoming more and more popular in the United States. Good sources of monounsaturated fatty acids are listed in Table 15.3.

Bad fats. The saturated fatty acids are derived primarily, though not always, from animal sources. There are some plant oils that are loaded with saturated fatty acids, such as coconut oil, palm oil, and palm kernel oil. See Table 15.4 for a list of foods high in saturated fatty acids. Other bad fats to watch out for are *partially hydrogenated fats,* also known as trans fatty acids, or *trans-fats.* These trans-fats are found primarily in man-made products such as margarine, packaged desserts (cookies, cakes, pastries, and doughnuts) and fast foods. Check the labels of the foods you purchase and look out for the term "partially hydrogenated." This bad fat can sneak into just about any packaged food.

Table 15.4. **Sources of Saturated Fats**

Coconut oil
Dairy products (such as butter, cheese, ice cream, and yogurt)
Egg yolks
Fatty chicken meat with skin
Palm kernel oil
Palm oil
Red meat

Recommendations on Fats

With all of this knowledge about fatty acids, you will now be able to understand the rationale behind the recommendations made by the American Heart Association regarding your daily intake of fat. These recommendations are summarized in Table 15.5. The American Heart Association suggests that you limit your intake of all fats to five to eight teaspoon-sized servings per day for cooking, baking, and in salad dressings. A teaspoon serving is considered one teaspoon of vegetable oil, one tablespoon of seeds or nuts, one-eighth of a medium-sized avocado, or ten small olives.

Fat in dairy products is saturated and should constitute a small portion of your diet. The AHA recommends using low-fat (1 or $1/2$ percent) or no-fat (skim) versions of milk, yogurt, and cheese. Three to four servings of milk products a day are recommended, mostly for the protein and calcium these foods provide. A serving is considered one cup of milk, one cup of yogurt, one ounce of cheese, or one-half cup of cottage cheese.

Limit foods high in saturated fat, trans-fats, and cholesterol, including full-fat dairy products, fatty meats, tropical oils (palm oil, palm kernel oil, and coconut oil), partially hydrogenated vegetable oils, and egg yolks. As a guideline, the American Heart Association recommends using fats and oils that contain two grams or less of saturated fat per tablespoon, such as canola, olive, soybean, and safflower oil.

Saturated fat should account for no more than 10 percent of the total daily calories for a healthy person and no more than 7 percent for a person who has heart disease, high LDL cholesterol, or diabetes. Cholesterol should be limited to three hundred milligrams a day in a healthy person and less than two hundred milligrams for someone with heart disease. To follow these guidelines, you must check food labels carefully.

Table 15.5. **The American Heart Association's Dietary Guidelines for Fat**

Limit fat to 5 to 8 teaspoon servings per day for cooking, baking, and in
salad dressings
Use 1% fat or no-fat dairy products
Use fats and oils with 2 grams or less of saturated fat per tablespoon
Limit fat to no more than 10% of the total daily calories for a healthy person
Limit fat to no more than 7% of the total daily calories for a person with
heart disease, high LDL cholesterol, or diabetes
Limit cholesterol to 300 milligrams a day in a healthy person
Limit cholesterol to less than 200 milligrams a day for someone with
heart disease

Sources: The American Heart Association (www.americanheart.org); *The New American Heart Association Cookbook* (New York: Clarkson Potter, 2001).

Carbohydrates: Public Enemy Number Two?

Carbohydrates are the latest "no-no" of the American grocery store. Some breads and even candy packages are labeled "low carb!" Like certain diet books, these foods are selling like hotcakes. You don't need to banish all carbohydrates from your diet, however, because not all carbohydrates are bad for you. In fact, they are the body's main source of energy. Here's the rub: if your body does not need the carbohydrates that you consume, these unused carbohydrates will be stored in your body as fat, leading to weight gain. About 45 to 65 percent of your total calories should come from carbohydrates. Just as with fats, there are good carbohydrate choices and bad carbohydrate choices. Why are some good and some bad? The answer lies in the nutrient value of the carbohydrate, the amount of fiber it contains, and its glycemic load.

Nutrient Value

First you should look at the nutrient value of the carbohydrate you are about to ingest. A candy bar provides virtually no vitamins or minerals and a significant amount of saturated fat. A candy bar is nutrient poor but fat and calorie rich. In contrast, a carrot has an abundance of vitamin A with no fat and relatively few calories. It is considered nutrient rich but fat and calorie poor. Both a carrot and a candy bar contain carbohydrates, but they have very different nutrient values.

Table 15.6. **Sources of Soluble Fiber**

Apple pulp	Oranges
Barley	Pears
Beans	Peaches
Grapefruit	Peas
Oat bran	Strawberries
Oatmeal	

Table 15.7. **Sources of Insoluble Fiber**

Apple skin	Green beans
Brussels sprouts	Potato skin
Beets	Turnips
Carrots	Wheat bran
Cabbage	Wheat cereals
Cauliflower	Whole wheat breads

Amount of Fiber

Fiber is a good guy in the diet. Most people are aware of the benefits of fiber on the gastrointestinal tract; it helps to regulate bowel movements. But fiber also helps to lower cholesterol. Fiber combines with cholesterol in your gastrointestinal tract and helps the body eliminate cholesterol.

There are two types of fiber, soluble and insoluble. Foods containing both of these kinds of fiber are good choices. For example, the apple's skin is a form of *insoluble fiber,* and the apple's pulp is a form of *soluble fiber.* Soluble fiber lowers cholesterol and is found in a variety of foods, a sampling of which are listed in Table 15.6. Insoluble fiber helps to regulate the bowels. Sample foods in this category are listed in Table 15.7.

Glycemic Load

All the carbohydrates you ingest are broken down into smaller pieces in your body. Your body digests some carbohydrates more easily and thus more quickly than others. This is another factor that distinguishes the good carbohydrate from the bad. Simple carbohydrates like the sugars in a candy bar have the fewest chemical bonds and are the easiest to digest, so they create the fastest and sharpest rise in blood sugar level. The effect a carbohydrate has on the blood sugar level is also known as its *glycemic load.* Simple

Table 15.8. Good Carbohydrate Choices

Vegetables (including asparagus, beets, broccoli, cauliflower, celery,
    cucumbers, eggplant, spinach, turnips, lettuce, peppers, green beans,
    snow peas, squash, zucchini, tomatoes, and peas)
Fruits (including cherries, grapefruit, peaches, apricots, oranges, pears,
    apples, grapes, and raisins)
Legumes (such as soybeans, kidney beans, lentils, and lima beans)
Breads (including oat bran, wheat, and pumpernickel)
Pasta (such as protein-enriched spaghetti and whole grain spaghetti)

carbohydrates have high glycemic loads. They are the bad guys. Complex carbohydrates like wheat bread have more chemical bonds and take longer to digest. They have low glycemic loads. They are the good guys.

Good carbohydrates. The *complex carbohydrates* are digested slowly, providing a slow release of glucose into the bloodstream. For this reason, they have the lowest glycemic load. Good choices for carbohydrates are listed in Table 15.8.

Of the foods listed in Table 15.8, the fruits and vegetables not only have a low glycemic load but are also nutrient rich, with plenty of vitamins and minerals, and high in fiber. The high fiber has the added benefit of helping to lower cholesterol. Oat bran bread is another good source of fiber that also has a low glycemic load. Legumes are good choices because they contain fiber and protein.

Bad carbohydrates. Less healthy are the simplest carbohydrates. These are also known as *refined carbohydrates*. Because they are the easiest to digest, they have the highest glycemic load. For example, carbohydrates like doughnuts, waffles, white bread, cornflakes, baked potatoes, and cookies are readily digested and create a quick, sharp rise in sugar levels in the bloodstream. This high blood glucose calls for an insulin surge to help clear the glucose from the bloodstream and bring it into the cells of the body. Shortly after the surge of sugar from a high glycemic load, the insulin clears the glucose and the person is left with a low blood sugar level that once again signals hunger. These highs and lows create a vicious cycle.

With this cycle of high blood sugar quickly followed by low blood sugar, it is easy to see how a person can overeat by eating carbohydrates with a high glycemic load. That's why many diet plans recommend skimping on the carbs. We recommend a compromise: avoid carbs with a high glycemic load, but continue to enjoy appropriate amounts of carbs with a low glycemic load

Table 15.9. **Examples of One Serving Size of Fruits and Vegetables**

$^1/_2$–1 cup of cooked vegetables

4 ounces of fruit juice

$^1/_2$ cup of fresh fruit

1 medium-size piece of fruit

Sources: National Heart, Blood, and Lung Institute (http://hin.nhlbi.nih.gov/ portion/servingcard7.pdf); The American Heart Association (www.americanheart .org/presenter.jhtml?identifier=4774).

Table 15.10. **Examples of One Serving Size of Whole Grains**

---

1 slice of wheat bread

$^1/_2$ cup of hot cereal

$^1/_2$ cup of cooked whole grain pasta

1 cup of cereal flakes

Sources: National Heart, Blood, and Lung Institute (http://hin.nhlbi.nih.gov/ portion/servingcard7.pdf); The American Heart Association (www.americanheart .org/presenter.jhtml?identifier=4465); The Harvard School of Public Health (www .hsph.harvard.edu/nutritionsource/carbohydrates.html).

that are rich in vitamins, minerals, and fiber. Choose your carbs wisely, and monitor your overall caloric intake.

Recommendations on Carbohydrates

The AHA recommends eating a variety of fruits and vegetables every day, giving five or more servings as their guideline. Examples of one serving for fruits and vegetables are listed in Table 15.9. You should also eat a variety of grain products, including whole grains, which are a good source of fiber. The AHA recommends eating six or more servings of whole grains a day. The size of single servings of whole grains is described in Table15.10.

What about Proteins?

When you eat foods that contain protein, the protein is digested into smaller molecules called *amino acids*. These amino acids are the building blocks for the body's proteins. The important functions of proteins are listed in Table 15.11.

Table 15.11. **Proteins Our Bodies Make**

Enzymes to help facilitate biochemical reactions like digestion of food

Antibodies to help fight infection

Growth factors to help regulate the growth of many different cells and tissues

Collagen to help provide structural support to many different tissues, including the blood vessels

Hormones to help regulate bodily functions, like insulin, which brings glucose into cells

Transportation molecules to help carry molecules that cannot travel in the blood, like lipoproteins, which carry cholesterol, and hemoglobin, which carries iron

Actin and myosin, which are essential for muscle movement

There are twenty-two amino acids, ten of which are considered "essential" to obtain through food because our body does not produce enough of them on its own or does not produce them at all. We need to get these amino acids from dietary sources such as meat, fish, eggs, beans, and nuts. Humans need dietary protein to function. However, too much protein can cause problems. There is evidence that consuming a high-protein diet for months or years may lead to osteoporosis, because the body takes calcium out of bone to neutralize the acids created by digesting high-protein meals. Protein should make up about 10 to 35 percent of your total daily calories. The AHA recommends no more than six ounces of high-protein foods a day. Table 15.12 lists examples of what a serving size of three ounces looks like.

There are good and bad choices for protein. Good protein choices are low in saturated fat. The best choices contain polyunsaturated fats such as omega 3 fatty acids, which are found in fish. Bad protein choices are high in saturated fat and thus increase cholesterol, specifically LDL cholesterol.

We recommend eating fish about twice a week, with an average meal consisting of 6 ounces of fish. Salmon, herring, mackerel (Atlantic or chub,

Table 15.12. **Examples of One Serving Size of Protein**

---

3 ounces of red meat or chicken is about the size of a deck of cards.

3 ounces of cooked fish is about the size of a checkbook.

Sources: National Heart, Blood, and Lung Institute (http://hin.nhlbi.nih.gov/portion/servingcard7.pdf).

Table 15.13. **Good and Bad Food Choices**

Food Type	Good	Bad
Fats and oils	Polyunsaturated	Saturated
	Monounsaturated	Partially hydrogenated
Carbohydrates	Vegetables	Candy
	Fruits	Packaged pastries
	Whole grains	White breads
Proteins	Fish	Red meat
	Beans	Egg yolks
	Low-fat or no-fat dairy	Animal organs (such as
	Tofu	liver and brain)
	Lean chicken	
	Egg whites	
	Nuts	

not king), sardines, and tuna (light canned white tuna, not albacore) are all good choices due to the high concentrations of omega 3 fatty acids in them. As with many foods, eating fish is not without its problems. High levels of mercury and other contaminants have been found in certain types of seafood. Avoid fish with the highest levels of mercury, including king mackerel, shark, swordfish, and tilefish. Examples of fish with the lowest levels of mercury include catfish, cod, canned white tuna (not albacore), flounder, haddock, pollock, salmon, scallops, shrimp, and sole. The FDA website www.cfsan.fda.gov/~frf/sea-mehg.html is a good source of information on fish and mercury levels. We encourage you to vary your diet and to choose from fish with the lowest levels of mercury. Table 15.13 summarizes the good and bad food choices in the three categories of foods discussed in the past several pages: fats, carbohydrates, and proteins.

So far in this chapter we have highlighted the importance of making good food choices. We now turn to several topics of special interest for people concerned about stroke. At the end of the chapter we tell you how you might get started on your path to a "healthier you" by following the Stroke Savvy Diet.

The Battle of the Bulge

The first question is: are you overweight? You cannot always tell just by looking in the mirror, and weight alone does not give you the answer. The *body mass index* (*BMI*) is used to define weight categories based on height,

Table 15.14. **Body Mass Index Calculations**

Weight in pounds divided by height in inches × height in inches, all multiplied by 703.

$$\frac{\text{Weight in Pounds}}{\text{Height in inches} \times \text{Height in inches}} \times 703 = \text{BMI}$$

Example:
Multiply your height of 68 inches by your height of 68 inches = 4624 inches.
Divide your weight of 150 pounds by 4624 = 0.0324.
Multiply this number by 703 = 22.80

$$\frac{150}{68 \times 68} \times 703 = 22.80$$

A BMI of 22.80 puts you in the normal range in the chart in Table 15.15.

Table 15.15. **Body Mass Index for Adults over 20 Years of Age**

BMI	Weight Category
<18.5	Underweight
18.5–24.9	Normal
25–29.9	Overweight
>30.0	Obese

and can be easily calculated with the formula shown in Table 15.14. Or, you can use the Internet: log on to the National Heart, Lung, and Blood Institute website at nhlbisupport.com/bmi/bmicalc.htm, and enter your weight and height to find your BMI. After calculating your BMI, refer to Table 15.15 to see whether you are currently underweight, normal, overweight, or obese.

If you fall into the overweight or obese categories, do not panic. You are not alone. According to the AHA, 136.5 million Americans over the age of 20 are overweight (with a Body Mass Index equal to or greater than 25). If you are overweight, one of the most important things you can do for your health is to lose weight by eating less and exercising more.

To lose weight, you need to eat fewer calories than you are currently eating and increase your level of activity to burn more calories. "Eat less and exercise more" sounds simple and yet it sometimes seems impossible to accomplish. The advice is too vague for most people, because most people need structure to accomplish a goal. That's why diet plans are very popular. There are plenty of plans to choose from—the no-fat diet, the high-protein diet, the low-carb diet, and so on.

Many people experience initial success when trying one of the many popular diet plans but then plateau (stop losing weight) or even regain the weight they have lost. This often happens because they do not continue on any type of maintenance diet. Diet plans are often strict and hard to follow, especially over the long term, and many people do not make lifestyle changes that they can continue after their initial weight loss program. A weight maintenance program, meaning maintaining a healthy lifestyle and nutritious diet that keeps your weight in check, is just as important as the initial weight loss. A common dieting cycle is to lose weight on a diet, gain the weight back (plus more sometimes), and then pick a new diet to follow. This cycle of serial dieting does not result in lasting weight loss.

To achieve lasting weight loss, you need to make permanent healthy lifestyle changes. The key changes are:

1. Exercise at least five times a week.
2. Avoid junk food.

By junk food we mean food that has a negative impact on your health (the foods listed in the bad choice column of Table 15.13). Junk food is food that is made mostly of saturated fat, partially hydrogenated fat, or sugar. You can tell when this is the case because a saturated fat such as coconut oil or palm oil, a partially hydrogenated fat, or a sugar such as high fructose corn syrup, will be listed on the food label of ingredients. Junk foods like candy, packaged pastries, and doughnuts are also high in calories. Check food labels and nutrition facts to find the number of calories and the amount of fat in the food. In the category of junk food, we also include fast foods such as hamburgers, french fries, and pizza. Even those seemingly nutritious muffins can fall into the junk food category if they are loaded with saturated fat, sugar, and calories.

Think we're taking away all the good stuff? The fact is, eating a lot of "tasty" junk foods is not going to help you prevent another stroke. These foods will only clog up your arteries with cholesterol and add pounds to your body. If you have had a stroke and can follow these two simple instructions—avoid junk food and engage in exercise—you will have a great chance of adding years to your life. We know that it can be difficult to exercise five times a week and avoid junk food, but what better motivation can

Table 15.16. **Calculating Basal Metabolic Rate**

Men   1.0 × weight in kilograms × 24 hours in a day
Women 0.9 × weight in kilograms × 24 hours in a day
(1 kg = 2.2 pounds; to convert pounds to kilograms, divide your weight
  by 2.2)

Examples:
1. A 110-pound woman would have a BMR of 1080.
110 pounds / 2.2 = 50 kg; 50 kg × 0.9 = 45
45 × 24 hours per day = 1080 calories a day

2. A 200-pound man would have a BMR of 2182.
200 pounds / 2.2 = 90.91 kg; 90.91 kg × 1.0 = 90.1
90.91 × 24 hours per day = 2181.8 calories a day

there possibly be than to avoid the potentially devastating or even deadly effects of another stroke?

Burn More Calories

If you are overweight, we want to help you lose weight by expanding on our advice to eat less and exercise more. We want to talk about calories: calories you consume and calories you burn. The bottom line is that to lose weight, you need to use more calories than you consume. Estimating the calories you use every day can be helpful to your diet plan. There are several different formulas for estimating daily energy expenditure. We've found a useful and user-friendly formula in the book *Basic Nutrition and Diet Therapy,* by Sue Rodwell Williams. The following discussion draws from principles, formulas, and charts found in Chapter 5, titled "Energy Balance," in this excellent nutrition textbook. [1]

Your body expends energy (burns calories) every day in three different ways:

1. Just being alive, also called your basal metabolic rate (BMR)
2. Physical activity during the day
3. Digesting your food, also called the thermic effect of food (TEF)

Just being alive, your lungs moving air, your heart pumping blood, your liver producing cholesterol, your brain thinking, your kidney filtering sodium, and your hair growing, accounts for the majority of calories you

Table 15.17. **Calories Burned by Physical Activity**

Activity	Calories Burned per Hour
Walking 2–3 mph	150–300
Bicycling 5½ mph	150–300
Light gardening	150–300
Washing car	150–300
Walking 3½–4 mph	300–420
Walking up and down small hills	300–420
Dancing (waltz, square)	300–420
Doubles tennis	300–420
Golf (no cart)	300–420
Climbing up and down big hills	420–600
Bicycling 11–12 mph	420–600
Jogging 5 mph	420–600
Cross-country skiing	420–600
Singles tennis	420–600

Source: Adapted from Sue Rodwell Williams, *Basic Nutrition and Diet Therapy,* 11th edition (St. Louis: Mosby, 2001), p. 65. Reprinted with permission from Elsevier.

burn each day. This is called your basal metabolic rate (BMR), the number of calories your vital organs burn in a day. The simple calculation for estimating your BMR is shown in Table 15.16.

You can burn a significant amount of calories through activity, depending on the amount and intensity of exercise you do. Even simple activities, such as getting dressed, writing, or playing the piano, can burn between 120 to 150 calories each hour. More rigorous activities, such as cross-country skiing, chopping wood, or jogging 5 mph burn more calories (between 420 and 600 calories each hour). See Table 15.17 for examples of various activities and the approximate number of calories they burn. There is a range of calories for the different activities because the number of calories you burn doing them depends on your weight and your current level of fitness. A sedentary person burns more calories walking up ten steps than a person who is fit.

There are Internet websites that will calculate the number of calories you expend during a specific activity. You simply enter your weight and the time you plan to spend on a certain activity, and they calculate the calories you will burn. The website www.healthstatus.com/calculate/cbc will calculate the number of calories you burn during a wide variety of activities, including aerobics, bicycling, brushing teeth, bowling, dancing, showering, sitting, walking, and writing.

Depending on how active you are throughout the day and how much you exercise, the calories you expend through activity could equal 20 percent to 50 percent of your basal metabolic rate (BMR). Activity levels are often divided into four broad levels of intensity:

1. Sedentary: minimal activity, very little to no exercise in the course of a week; minimal activity throughout the day such as sitting on the couch, watching TV
2. Very Light: some exercise, two days a week or less; some activity throughout the day such as dressing, bathing, sweeping, light gardening, mowing the lawn, and bowling
3. Moderate: regular exercise, five days a week; moderate activity throughout the day such as digging in the yard
4. Heavy: regular heavy exercise, six days a week or more; heavy activity throughout the day such as climbing mountains, bicycling 11 mph, jogging, playing singles tennis

These activity levels are used to get a rough estimate of how active a person is on an average day. After determining which category of exercise best fits your daily life, you can estimate the number of calories you burn through physical activity each day. See Table 15.18 for the different categories of activity levels and the estimated number of calories they burn. For example, if you exercise two times a week and engage in some activity throughout the day such as light gardening, you are in the very light activity category. On an average day, the number of calories you burn through physical activity equals your basal metabolic rate (BMR) multiplied by 30 percent. There are other formulas that are used to estimate the number of calories burned through daily physical activity. None of them is precise. They give a ballpark figure you can use when trying to estimate your total energy expenditure in a day. A more precise number could be obtained if you identified all the activities you did in a given day and then calculated the calories you burned in each activity.

The first two ways of burning calories are living and exercise. The third way to burn calories each day is digesting and metabolizing your food. Your food has an effect on your metabolism called the *thermic effect of food* (*TEF*), also sometimes referred to as the *specific dynamic action* (*SDA*) of food. Your body needs to spend time and energy breaking down the food you eat and

Table 15.18. **Physical Activity Levels and Average Calories Burned**

Activity Level	Calories Burned
Sedentary	Basal metabolic rate × 20%
Very light	BMR × 30%
Moderate	BMR × 40%
Heavy	BMR × 50%

transporting it to its final destination. This process is known as the thermic effect of food, and it burns approximately 10 percent of the calories you ingest. You may be thinking, "That sounds good! The more I eat, the more calories I burn." Ten percent, however, is a very low percentage, and this is certainly no way to lose weight. For example, the average adult eats 2,000 calories daily, and only 200 of these are used for digestion (the TEF of a 2,000 calorie diet is 200). If you increase your intake to 3,000, you only burn an extra 100 calories, for a total of 300. The TEF of a 3,000 calorie diet is 300.

In order to increase the number of calories you burn in a day, you need to know the average number of calories you use each day. To calculate this number, refer to Table 15.19. The figure you get is an estimate of the total number of calories you use each day by simply breathing and being alive (BMR), physical activity (BMR × % activity level), and digesting your food (TEF). Total energy output (calories burned) = BMR + physical activity + TEF.

Table 15.19. **Calculating Average Number of Calories Burned in a Day**

Your total energy output for the day in calories equals:
BMR + average physical daily activity (as a percentage of BMR) + TEF
   (10% of calories eaten)

Example:
For a woman who weighs 135 pounds (61 kg), who walks about 5 miles a day, 5 days a week (a moderate level of activity), and who eats an average of 2,000 calories a day:

Basal metabolic rate (BMR) = 0.9 × 61 × 24		= 1,318 calories
Activity	= BMR × 40%	= 527 calories
TEF	= 2,000 × 10%	= 200 calories
Total energy output		= 2,045 calories

If you are more interested in the numbers and calculations of calories burned throughout the day, we suggest you refer to *Basic Nutrition and Diet Therapy* by Sue Rodwell Williams, which can be borrowed from the library or purchased through a bookstore or Amazon.com. However, if you are not inclined to make calculations for yourself, there are a number of websites that will do these calculations for you (such as www.thedietdiary.com/diet/nutrition/RestingEnergy.html). You simply enter your height, weight, age, and activity level and they do the numbers.

Eat Less Food

If you are trying to lose weight, your total energy output for the day should be greater than your energy input. You are in control of your energy input—it is the amount of food you eat. Looking at labels and counting calories helps you to figure out if you are taking in or using more calories in a day. To lose a pound of fat, you need to burn 3,500 calories. If you decrease your calorie intake by 500 calories a day, after one week you could lose a pound. To achieve the same result of a one-pound loss, you could also choose to keep your diet the same and jog at a 5 mph pace for an hour a day. A combination of less food and more activity is also possible; eat 250 calories less each day and walk at a 2 to 3 mph pace for an hour a day. Do both for one week. The net result is the same: a decrease of 3,500 calories.

You can be creative and develop your own diet plan, or you can work with a dietician to develop a plan. You may choose to use these numbers and calculations in your diet plans, or you may not. You may just try to eat three-quarters of what you would normally eat at a meal and exercise as many days of the week as you can, aiming for at least five days. Find out how well that works by monitoring your weight weekly.

When you are trying to lose weight, you should make healthy food choices. By cutting down on saturated fats, trans-fats, and simple carbohydrates, you will be cutting down on calories. Taking a few moments to count the calories of the food you are about to ingest can often encourage you to make a healthy choice.

Food calorie counters are available at bookstores and grocery store check-out lines. *The Complete Book of Food Counts,* by Corinne T. Netzer, is useful because it not only lists calories but also the fat, cholesterol, sodium (salt), fiber, and protein content of each item of food. *The T-Factor 2000 Fat Gram Counter,* by Jamie Pope and Martin Katahn, lists calories, cholesterol, sodium, fiber, and fat. The advantage of this book is that it lists saturated fat as well as total fat.[2]

Table 15.20. **Number of Calories in Selected Foods**

Food	Quantity	Calories
Apple (2¾" diameter)	1	34
Apple pie (¹/₆ of pie)	1	427
Applesauce (unsweetened)	½ cup	52
Bacon (pork)	1 slice	36
Bagel (white, 3" diameter)	1	157
Banana (8" long)	1	96
Bologna (pork)	1 slice	56
Bread (white)	1 slice	70
Brownie (2½" square)	1 square	310
Cake (yellow, 3" × 3" × 2")		
With chocolate frosting	1 slice	551
Without frosting	1 slice	296
Chicken (light meat)	1 ounce	47
Doughnut (cake, 3" diameter)	1	145
Grapefruit (4" diameter)	½ fruit	47
Hot dog (beef)	1	141
Hot dog (turkey)	1	102
Ice cream (vanilla)	½ cup	143
Lettuce (romaine)	½ cup	4
Lobster	3 ounces	83
Muffin (corn, 2¼" diameter)	1	138
Nuts (peanuts)	¼ cup	212
Orange (2⅝" diameter)	1	62
Pancakes (plain, 4" diameter)	1	66
Peanut butter (regular)	1 tbsp	96
Potato (baked)	½ cup	57
Potato chips (plain)	1 ounce	161
Soup (black bean)	1 cup	168
Tomato (raw)	½ cup	19
Tuna (canned, in water)	3 ounces	99
Turkey (light meat, no skin)	3 ounces	140
Veal (trimmed)	3 ounces	139
Waffle (frozen, 4" square)	1	82

Source: "Your Game Plan for Preventing Type 2 Diabetes," www.ndep.nih.gov/diabetes/pubs/GP_FatCal.pdf.

Table 15.21. Dietary Focuses for People with Different Health Concerns

Problem	Limit	Recommendations
CAD/Stroke	Cholesterol	<200 mg a day
HTN	Salt	<2,400 mg a day
Diabetes	Sugar	Choose low-glycemic-load carbohydrates
Weight Loss	Calories	Take in fewer calories than you burn

Calorie counters are available on the Internet. Through a joint program, the National Institute of Health and the Centers for Disease Control and Prevention, the National Diabetes Education Program, and the U.S. Department of Health and Human Services have put together a calorie counter called "Your Game Plan for Preventing Type 2 Diabetes." You can download this document free from the Internet by logging on to www.ndep.nih.gov/diabetes/pubs/GP_FatCal.pdf. It lists many different food items, from fudge syrup to octopus. (Refer to Table 15.20 for a partial list of the caloric content of common foods, taken from the "Your Game Plan for Preventing Type 2 Diabetes" fat and calorie counter.) By becoming aware of the different calorie values of two food choices—such as an apple (34 calories) and a piece of apple pie (427 calories), or a piece of cake with no frosting (296 calories) and a piece of cake with chocolate frosting (551 calories)—you may be more likely to select the lower-calorie food choice. You do not have to become an avid calorie counter to lose weight, but it might help you to become aware of food choices that come with a very high calorie count.

If you think in terms of the calorie input and output balance, you may find that avoiding that 551-calorie piece of cake with chocolate frosting is worth it to you to avoid the one-hour jog you will need to take to burn it off. If the average person requires 2,000 calories in a day, and a piece of cake contains 551 calories, then a big chunk of the day's total calories have already been used by eating a food that has very little nutritional value. To lose weight for the long term, you need to make lifestyle changes that involve eating fewer calories, eating healthy foods, exercising more, and exercising regularly. Making these changes may very well translate into fewer doctor visits and a longer, fuller, and healthier life.

If you have heart disease, high blood pressure, or diabetes, or you are trying to lose weight, this chapter is full of dietary recommendations for you. Table 15.21 highlights the dietary concerns for each of these problems.

Table 15.22. **High Cholesterol Foods**

Red meat
Egg yolks
Packaged baked goods
Full-fat diary foods including

Butter	Yogurt
Cheese	Ice cream
Milk	Cream

In the next sections we will discuss dietary tips for people with coronary artery disease, hypertension, and diabetes, before turning to a section on swallowing difficulties.

Tips for People with Coronary Artery or Cerebrovascular Disease

Limit Cholesterol

If you have coronary artery disease (CAD) or cerebrovascular disease, focus on your cholesterol intake. Limit the amount of cholesterol that you eat to less than 200 mg each day. Foods that are high in cholesterol are listed in Table 15.22. To attain the goal of consuming less than 200 mg of cholesterol a day, avoid these foods.

We do not recommend a *no-fat* diet. As we discussed in the section on fats, some fat (omega 3 fatty acids) may in fact be beneficial to people with CAD. Fish is not the only source of omega 3 fatty acids. As we discussed, alpha linolenic acid is turned into omega 3 fatty acids inside the body. Foods high in alpha linolenic acid include beans, canola oil, walnuts, almonds, and flaxseeds. We do recommend a *low-fat* diet, keeping daily ingestion of fat to below 30 percent of total calories. For people with coronary artery disease, it is best to use those fats that are considered good for the blood vessels and heart (polyunsaturated or monounsaturated), and to avoid saturated fats and partially hydrogenated fats. For people with CAD, the AHA recommends that saturated fat be less than 7 percent total calories.

Eat Foods that Contain Fiber

Fiber is good not only for the digestive system but also for the blood vessels as it can help to lower LDL cholesterol. Foods that are high in fiber and low in fat and cholesterol are listed in Table 15.23.

Table 15.23. **Foods High in Fiber and Low in Fat and Cholesterol**

Whole wheat	Whole fruits
Oatmeal	Whole vegetables
Whole grains	

Eat Nuts

Research suggests that foods, such as nuts, that are rich in nitric oxide can be beneficial for people with cerebrovascular disease. Nitric oxide acts as a *vasodilator,* which means it widens the artery. This is beneficial to people suffering from arteriosclerosis (hardening of the arteries), which narrows the arteries, most frequently because of cholesterol buildup. *L-arginine* is an amino acid that the body transforms through a series of biochemical reactions to form nitric oxide. L-arginine rich foods are listed in Table 15.24.

Eat Foods that Contain Folic Acid

Some people with stroke have a high *homocysteine level.* To find out your homocysteine level, you just need a simple blood test. Homocysteine is a precursor of the amino acid called *cysteine.* Homocysteine promotes atherosclerosis in a number of ways: by damaging the cells in the blood vessel that separate it from the blood, the endothelial cells; by transforming LDL into a form that is more readily able to contribute to an atherosclerotic plaque (also known as *oxidizing* LDL); and by increasing the ability of monocytes to stick to the arterial wall, again aiding the process of atherosclerosis.

While there does seem to be a relationship between homocysteine levels and stroke, it is not yet known if lowering homocysteine levels will protect against stroke. While this issue is being studied, many physicians recommend taking some basic steps to lower your homocysteine level. If you

Table 15.24. **Foods Rich in L-Arginine**

Soy	Egg whites
Beans	Milk
Legumes	Nuts (especially almonds, cashews,
Fish	peanuts, pistachios, and walnuts)
Meat (especially red meat and chicken)	Seeds

Table 15.25. **Foods Rich in Folic Acid**

Asparagus	Liver
Baked potatoes	Mustard greens
Beans (especially pinto, navy, kidney, and chickpeas)	Nuts (especially almonds and peanuts)
	Oranges
Beets	Romaine lettuce
Broccoli	Spinach
Brussels sprouts	Sweet potatoes
Cabbage	Whole eggs
Collard greens	Wheat grain breads and cereals
Corn	

have high homocysteine levels, there is an easy dietary cure: Eat foods rich in folic acid or take a folic acid supplement (400 micrograms a day). Folic acid is helpful because it works to lower levels of homocysteine in the body. Foods rich in this nutrient are listed in Table 15.25.

Limit Alcohol

Alcohol is another dietary concern for people with stroke. If you do not drink at all, don't start. If you are accustomed to drinking, the AHA recommends that you limit your intake of alcohol to no more than one drink a day if you are a woman and two drinks a day if you are a man. The definition of one drink matters, because the alcohol content of different types of drinks can vary widely. According to the AHA, one drink has no more than one-half ounce of pure alcohol. Table 15.26 provides some general information on the alcohol content of various drinks. (Please see Chapter 17 for a full discussion of the pros and cons of alcohol use after stroke.)

Tips for People with High Blood Pressure

One of the most important ways to manage high blood pressure is to lose those extra pounds if you are overweight. Many (though not all) people with hypertension are overweight. Of course, losing weight is easier said than done, but with some effort and dedication, you can do it. Understanding healthy food choices in each food group, as we have discussed in this chapter, will help you cut calories without cutting valuable nutrients. As

Table 15.26. **Examples of One Drink of Alcohol**

12 ounces of beer

4–5 ounces of wine

1½ ounces of 80 proof spirits

1 ounce of 100 proof spirits

Sources: The American Heart Association (www.americanheart.org/presenter .jhtml?identifier=4422); The Harvard School of Public Health (www.hsph.harvard .edu/nutritionsource/alcohol.html).

noted above, to lose weight, you need to take in fewer calories than your body uses each day, and the easiest way to do this is to combine diet and exercise. (Exercise is discussed in Chapter 16.)

Eat Less Salt

Reducing salt (sodium) intake is the main dietary change to make if you are hypertensive. Salt is sneaky. It is found in almost every food we eat. Check the ingredients and you will see. If you eat frozen dinners or canned goods such as soups, beans, chili, pasta sauces, or vegetables, you are eating a lot of salt. Fast food is also loaded with salt. In fact, most chefs at restaurants add salt to their entrees. When you place your order, request "no added salt." And whatever you do, do not add salt to your food at the table at home or at a restaurant. If you find that your food tastes bland without salt, purchase a healthy salt substitute like Mrs. Dash.

Our bodies only need a small amount of salt to function properly—about 500 mg each day, which is a little less than one-quarter of a teaspoon. The average American eats about 15 grams of sodium a day, thirty times what we really need. While table salt, also known as sodium chloride or NaCl, is the most common form of sodium in the diet, sodium comes in other forms as well, such as sodium bicarbonate. Check your food labels for any ingredients with sodium or Na. If sodium is restricted to 2.4 grams (2,400 milligrams) per day, which is equivalent to one teaspoon of salt, blood pressure can be significantly reduced in many people.

Not everyone is "salt sensitive," meaning that for some people with high blood pressure, lowering their salt intake won't help lower their blood pressure. It is estimated that about 30 percent to 50 percent of people with hypertension are salt sensitive. People with high blood pressure are more likely to be salt sensitive than people with normal blood pressure. Salt sensitivity increases with age; people over 60 years old seem to be more salt sensitive than younger people. About 15 percent to 25 percent of people without hypertension are probably also salt sensitive, so even if you are not hypertensive, your salt intake may significantly affect your blood pressure. So watch that salt!

Salt draws water with it wherever it goes. You have probably noticed that after eating a bag of salty potato chips, you are very thirsty. Your body wants water to add to all the salt. Inside your body, the water follows the salt. More salt in the bloodstream means more water in the bloodstream. Increasing the amount of water in the bloodstream increases the amount of blood being pumped out of the heart each minute and thus increases the pressure on the walls of the arteries. This increases blood pressure (Chapter 9 discusses blood pressure in detail).

If you have congestive heart failure (discussed in Chapter 8), it is extremely important to control your salt and water intake. A weak heart has more difficulty handling the added blood pressure created by excess salt and water. The extra water is likely to leave the bloodstream and end up in the body's tissues in a gravity-dependent manner. For example, if you have stood upright most of the day, water can end up in the tissues around your ankles and feet, which will create swelling (*edema*). For people with congestive heart failure, this type of fluid retention often requires the use of a diuretic medicine to rid the body of the excess water.

Eat Foods that Contain Calcium, Potassium, and Magnesium

The DASH (Dietary Approaches to Stop Hypertension) research study brought the minerals calcium, potassium, and magnesium to the forefront of blood pressure management. This study was published in the *New England Journal of Medicine* in 1997.[3] In this study, 459 people ate a diet low in fruits, vegetables, and dairy, with fat content typical of the average American diet, for three weeks. Then they were randomly assigned to one of three diets:

1. The control ("regular") diet (the same diet they had eaten for the first three weeks)
2. A diet rich in fruits and vegetables
3. A combination diet rich in fruits, vegetables, and low-fat dairy products and low in saturated and total fat content

Table 15.27. Age-Based Recommendations for Dietary Calcium

Age	Calcium
19–51 years	1,000 mg
Over 51 years	1,200 mg

They stayed on these diets for eight weeks. During this time, their sodium intake and their body weight were maintained at constant levels.

At the end of the study, the researchers found that the people on the combined diet had a markedly reduced blood pressure. For subjects with high blood pressure (defined by a systolic pressure greater than 140 and a diastolic pressure greater than 90), the combination diet dropped blood pressure by much more than the control diet. Even the non-hypertensive subjects experienced a drop in their blood pressure on the combination diet. These findings suggest that a diet rich in fruits, vegetables, and dairy products and low in saturated and total fat can make a significant difference in your blood pressure. It is believed that the nutrients in these diets helped make the difference, because weight and salt were maintained throughout the study. This combination diet was high in calcium, potassium, and magnesium. The DASH study suggests that these minerals may play an important role in blood pressure, most likely through a *diuretic* effect (meaning that the calcium, potassium, and magnesium help the kidney get rid of sodium and water and hence lower blood pressure).

Calcium may be a beneficial mineral for people with high blood pressure. If you are a "salt sensitive" person with hypertension and you are also low in calcium, consuming more calcium may reduce your blood pressure. Calcium is necessary in the diet for other reasons as well—in particular, for preventing *osteoporosis* (thinning of the bones). It may not help lower blood pressure in everyone, however, so we do not recommend that all people with high blood pressure take in more calcium. Discuss your optimal calcium intake with your physician. The Food and Nutrition Information Center's recommendations for dietary calcium are shown in Table 15.27, and are also available at www.nal.usda.gov/fnic/etext/000105.html. To reach the goal of 1,200 mg of calcium, a person would need to drink about three to four eight-ounce glasses of milk a day. Other foods that are good sources of calcium are listed in Table 15.28.

Potassium is another mineral that may affect blood pressure. In hypertensive individuals who have low potassium levels, increasing potassium intake can indeed lower blood pressure. Potassium may help lower blood

Table 15.28. **Foods Rich in Calcium**

Artichoke	Molasses
Broccoli	Mustard greens
Cheese	Nuts (especially almonds, Brazil nuts,
Chinese cabbage (bok choy)	pistachios, peanuts, walnuts)
Collards	Orange juice (fortified with calcium)
Hummus	Sardines (canned with bones)
Kale	Spinach
Legumes (especially chickpeas,	Squash
navy beans, pinto beans, and	Turnip greens
soybeans)	Yogurt
Milk	

pressure by helping the kidneys excrete sodium. Note that taking diuretic medication for your blood pressure may encourage your kidneys to waste potassium into your urine, creating a potassium deficit in your body. Be sure to ask your doctor to check your potassium level if you are on diuretics. Depending on your level, your doctor may prescribe potassium supplements.

The human body needs between 2,000 mg and 4,000 mg of potassium a day. Increasing potassium intake is as easy as eating an extra banana a day. Other good sources of potassium are listed in Table 15.29. As with calcium, we do not recommend that all hypertensive people increase their potassium. Ask your doctor to check your potassium level and discuss the test results with her.

Table 15.29. **Foods Rich in Potassium**

Apricots	Milk
Avocados	Nuts (especially peanuts)
Baked potato	Orange juice
Bananas	Peaches
Cantaloupe	Prunes
Dates	Raisins
Fish (especially halibut, cod,	Spinach
clams, and sardines)	Tomatoes
Honeydew melon	Winter squash
Kiwi	Yogurt

Table 15.30. Recommended Daily Allowances for Magnesium

For Men	Magnesium mg	For Women	Magnesium mg
19–30 years	400 mg	19–30 years	310 mg
Over 30 years	420 mg	Over 30 years	320 mg

Table 15.31. Foods Rich in Magnesium

Baked potato	Halibut
Black-eyed peas	Milk
Beans (especially soybeans, kidney beans, and pinto beans)	Nuts (especially almonds, cashews, peanuts, and walnuts)
Green leafy vegetables (especially spinach and kale)	Whole grains

Because magnesium is involved in many different chemical reactions in the body, including the breakdown of carbohydrates and the building of proteins, it may also contribute to controlling blood pressure. The recommended dietary allowance of magnesium differs for men and women and with age. See Table 15.30 for details. Magnesium is found in many places, including hard water. Other sources of magnesium are listed in Table 15.31.

We do not recommend routinely taking supplements of calcium, potassium, or magnesium. These minerals are plentiful in healthy foods such as fruits, vegetables, whole grains, dairy products, fish, and chicken. It is important to note that either a deficiency or an excess of any of these minerals can cause problems, heart problems in particular. For this reason, we recommend eating foods rich in these minerals rather than taking supplements. One exception is if you are taking a diuretic such as Lasix (furosemide) and your doctor has prescribed potassium supplements. More research on the DASH diet and these minerals needs to be completed before the AHA will make any specific recommendations regarding them. For now, the DASH diet results are just more evidence pointing to why it is important to make healthy food choices, including fruits, vegetables, whole grains, and low-fat dairy in your diet while restricting the amount of saturated fat and total fat you eat.

Limit Alcohol

Alcohol may be beneficial in preventing atherosclerosis when used in small amounts, but it can raise blood pressure if used to excess. (See Chapter 17 for a further discussion of the use of alcohol after stroke.)

Tips for People with Diabetes

For people with diabetes, sugars and simple carbohydrates are the essential nutrients to monitor. If you have diabetes, you probably check your blood sugars after meals. The target blood sugar one and one-half to two hours after a meal is 180 or less. Healthy food choices are critical for maintaining steady blood sugar levels in people with diabetes. For this reason, carbohydrates with a high glycemic load—those that create a quick, sharp rise in blood sugar—should be avoided. As we discussed in the section on carbohydrates, candy, cakes, cookies, white bread, baked potatoes, and white rice are quickly digested and almost immediately create a high blood sugar level that is rapidly countered by a high insulin level. The insulin clears the glucose from the bloodstream and often leaves the person with low blood sugar. This causes signals to be sent to the brain, telling it that it's time to eat again. A person with diabetes must avoid this cycle in order to maintain a steady blood sugar and to prevent weight gain.

Carbohydrates are the main food of concern for a person with diabetes, but protein and fat must also be monitored. Even though the protein content of a meal does not usually alter the blood sugar level after a meal, if a meal contains a large amount of protein (more than about four ounces), it can increase blood sugar levels. You may be wondering how this happens. The answer is *gluconeogenesis* (making new glucose). As mentioned earlier in the chapter (in the section on protein), protein is digested into amino acids. The liver can use these amino acids to make glucose, raising the blood sugar level.

Why should a person with diabetes be concerned about fat content? The extra calories from consuming too much fat are stored in the body as fat. People with diabetes need to try to control their weight, not add to it. Also, saturated and partially hydrogenated fats can increase cholesterol. Remember that there is a close association between diabetes and stroke. It is prudent for people with diabetes to follow the diet we recommend for people with stroke and heart disease.

Just as with people who have high blood pressure, many people with Type II diabetes are overweight. One of the best ways to control your blood sugar is to lose weight by eating less and exercising more. Exercise can increase your body's response to insulin. A person who has insulin-resistant Type II diabetes may become more sensitive to insulin after regular exercise. With more exercise in his daily schedule, a person with diabetes may be able to lower the amount of insulin or medication that he takes. In some cases, diet and exercise can even eliminate the need for medication.

When Swallowing Is a Problem

After a stroke, some people have difficulty swallowing (*dysphagia*). While you were in the hospital recovering from your stroke, you probably had a number of tests. One of these tests was a swallowing test. Proper swallowing is critical to avoid aspirating food into your lungs, where it can cause pneumonia. If you had difficulty swallowing, you most likely worked with a speech pathologist on different techniques to insure proper swallowing. Depending on the cause and severity of your problem, you may require a modified-texture diet.

Some patients require thickened liquids after a stroke, due to difficulty swallowing thin drinks. In this case, cornstarch is generally used to thicken the liquids. However, the cornstarch often takes away from the taste of the drink. Palatability is a concern, as is maintaining adequate hydration, which can be assessed by examining the mucus membranes in the mouth to check for moisture, by checking the amount of urine made each day, and by monitoring the person's weight. With regard to solids, some patients require softer foods, or even purees, after a stroke. Again, palatability and adequate intake are concerns. This type of diet makes getting enough fresh fruits and vegetables difficult, and may lead to overuse of salt in an attempt to make the food more palatable. Creative cooking strategies are needed to insure that the food is both nutritious and tasty. If you have difficulty swallowing after your stroke, we suggest you work closely with a speech pathologist and a nutritionist to develop a healthy diet plan that you can enjoy.

When we eat, it is helpful to consider what our body needs and how we can fuel it so that it can function at its maximum level. We should not have to give up taste to eat nutritious foods. Healthy eating can be very flavorful with the right creativity and planning. Above all, consider the good and bad choices for fats, carbohydrates, and proteins with every meal and snack. Think about creating your own diet plan to fit your personal needs, and then discuss your plan with your physician or a nutritionist.

The American Heart Association has published several heart-healthy cookbooks that provide the recipes for delicious meals that are low in salt, fat, cholesterol, and calories. The calorie, fat, cholesterol, and sodium counts are listed for each recipe. A cookbook such as this can be helpful in creating your own healthy diet plan.

Getting started on lifestyle changes such as diet can be daunting. The Stroke Savvy Diet can help. If you take small steps and tackle one area at a time, the process of changing your diet may be easier. To get started, we suggest that you look again at the list of six principles on page 218 and consider your overall health. Begin with the one principle that you think will help you the most. For example, if you have high blood pressure and you are accustomed to putting table salt on your food, the first thing you can do is cut out the excess salt. After a week or so on that modified diet, tackle another principle and concentrate on it. For example, make an effort to eat more fruits and vegetables the next week. Keep incorporating the principles into your diet one at a time until you embrace all six changes and your food choices reflect these six principles every day.

Improving your diet and concentrating on making dietary lifestyle changes is hard work. The rewards for this hard work are well worth it. By changing your diet and making healthy food choices like those outlined in the Stroke Savvy Diet, you have the ability to make positive changes to your body. If you are overweight, you can lose weight. If you have high cholesterol, you can lower it. If you have hypertension, you can lower your blood pressure. And if you have diabetes, you can get your blood sugar in better control. You may still need medication to treat these medical conditions, but you will probably need less of it.

Chapter 16

●●●

Exercise and Stroke

Like the Stroke Savvy Diet described in Chapter 15, the Stroke Savvy Exercise Plan is a general plan for reducing the likelihood of stroke. We all need to talk with our doctors about how to exercise safely and effectively. This advice applies especially to anyone who has had a stroke. In this chapter we will share general information about exercise and how it can help you prevent stroke.

If you have recently had a stroke, you may be ready to start a walking program, or you may be wondering how you are going to exercise when you feel exhausted and weak. You may have difficulty getting out of a chair, let alone walking. This chapter aims to help you regardless of where you are in terms of physical conditioning and regardless of your current limitations. We also take into account the fact that people have different exercise habits. Some of you are avid exercisers and others are exercise avoiders. Maybe you are somewhere in between. Regardless of how you approached exercise in the past, we hope that after reading this chapter you will exercise regularly—it will help you to prevent another stroke.

In this chapter, we begin by discussing the general benefits of exercise and how exercise can help to prevent stroke. Then, we cover the many different possibilities for cardiovascular exercise after a stroke. We address the needs of people with different levels of function after stroke:

Those with severe difficulty functioning due to stroke
Those with moderate difficulty functioning due to stroke
Those with mild difficulty functioning due to stroke
Those without residual functional problems after stroke

Next, we address the risks of exercise and point out specific circumstances where the risks outweigh the benefits. The most important part of this chapter is our Stroke Savvy Exercise Plan, with suggestions on how to start an exercise program and how to exercise if you have other underlying medical problems.

We strongly recommend that you check with your physician before starting any exercise program. In a book like this, we certainly can offer some insight on how stroke survivors can safely exercise; however, we can't take the place of your doctor, who knows you and your medical history. *Exercise is safe only when your physician says it is safe.*

A final note before we begin: although it may sound as if we think taking up and continuing with an exercise program is easy, we know that it can be very difficult. But we also are very aware of how beneficial exercise can be for almost everyone, and perhaps particularly for someone who has had a stroke or is at risk of stroke. Exercise nearly always makes you healthier and happier. But, again, check with your physician before beginning an exercise program.

Benefits of Cardiovascular Exercise

To begin, we need to define *exercise*. It means different things to different people. To doctors and other health care providers, the generic term *exercise* really breaks down into five broad categories: strengthening, flexibility, cardiovascular conditioning, balance, and coordination exercises. All of these types of exercise are extremely important for someone who is recovering from a stroke. However, research has shown us that cardiovascular exercise has the greatest impact in preventing a second stroke. For this reason, we will focus on cardiovascular, also called *aerobic,* exercise in this chapter. The simple way to think of cardiovascular exercise is as any sustained method of exercise that significantly increases your heart rate.

To Prevent a Second Stroke

What is so special about cardiovascular exercise when it comes to preventing another stroke? Regular cardiovascular exercise can have a positive effect on some of the major risk factors for stroke by:

Lowering your LDL cholesterol level
Raising your HDL cholesterol level
Decreasing your blood pressure (if you have hypertension)
Reducing excess weight (if you are overweight)
Improving your blood sugar levels (if you have diabetes)

Exercise helps to protect your arteries from cholesterol buildup. As we discussed in Chapter 8 and Chapter 15, the LDL cholesterol is the "bad" cholesterol that gets incorporated in atherosclerotic plaques and the HDL is the "good" cholesterol that helps remove cholesterol from the bloodstream so that it will not be incorporated into an atherosclerotic plaque. Exercise lowers the levels of LDL and raises the level of HDL in the bloodstream. The combination of less bad cholesterol and more good cholesterol greatly reduces the likelihood of atherosclerosis progression.

Exercise directly affects your heart muscle. Just as our leg muscles get stronger with regular exercise, so does our heart muscle, which is arguably the most important muscle in the body. A stronger heart muscle means more efficient pumping of blood throughout the body. With regular exercise, blood pressure drops and resting heart rate slows down.

Exercise helps control diabetes. Regular exercise has been shown to increase insulin sensitivity in people with Type II diabetes. This means that your blood glucose may not rise as high or as often, which translates into less damage to the endothelial layer of the arteries. With less damage to the arterial walls, cholesterol plaque formation is less likely (see Chapter 8).

Apart from helping you modify stroke risk factors and prevent a second stroke, there are many other benefits to cardiovascular exercise that will help improve your quality of life.

For Your Mind

Most runners have experienced the "runner's high." After about twenty minutes of jogging, the brain releases its own euphoric chemicals called *endorphins*. These endorphins are natural opioids that make people feel good. Runners may set out for their run stressed and distressed, but most return feeling exhilarated and energized.

Other forms of exercise can create the same positive psychological effect. In fact, walking routinely has been shown to reduce the symptoms of depression for healthy people as well as those with chronic disease. Many people use exercise as a form of stress reduction. It can even help alleviate symptoms of anxiety. People find that after their workout, they feel more relaxed and the problems that were plaguing them before exercising don't seem as serious. Exercise seems to have the ability to clear the mind. Others report that their best ideas come to them while they are exercising. Whether because exercise is a break from the stress of daily life or because of the effect of endorphin release, most people feel happier and less stressed after exercising. Instead of feeling exhausted, many people feel as though they have more energy for the rest of the day.

For the Rest of You

Other health benefits of a regular cardiovascular exercise program include protection against osteoporosis, reduced back pain, more restful sleep, and increased endurance and strength, which translates into an improved ability to perform activities of daily living with ease.

If you are not a regular exerciser, we hope the discussion of the benefits of exercise have convinced you to start exercising. If you are already a regular exerciser, we applaud your efforts and hope this information serves as encouragement for the future.

One moment Jack was going about his normal routine as an accountant, and the next moment he collapsed while getting up from his desk. He had suffered a stroke that left him with weakness in his left arm and leg. His whole world was turned upside down. With high LDL levels, low HDL levels, elevated blood pressure, and excess weight all working in favor of a second stroke, Jack knew he had to fight hard to regain his health. Although he was sad about having had a stroke, he realized that it was a wake-up call and that his future depended on his ability to form new health habits.

Before his stroke, Jack did not exercise regularly. In fact, physical activity was a whole new world for him. Now, after his stroke, exercise seemed almost impossible with a weak leg and arm. Initially, Jack got much of his cardiovascular workout through using his wheelchair. He worked hard with physical therapists on strengthening his muscles and relearning how to walk. These therapy sessions often provided Jack with a significant cardiovascular workout. As he gained strength and mobility, he started to use a recumbent stepper for his cardiovascular exercise. This gave him a good workout and increased the strength in his legs.

After several months, Jack regained strength and control of his movements enough to walk with the assistance of a cane and a foot brace. At this point, he felt ready to consider a different cardiovascular program. He talked with his rehabilitation team who recommended a stationary bike with hand levers as well as pedals to propel the wheels. In the beginning, Jack needed his wife to help him keep his leg on the pedal. Later on, he was able to wrap an ace bandage around both his leg and the pedal to keep his foot from slipping off.

Jack got into a regular exercise routine. He rode the bike for thirty minutes five times a week and noticed remarkable results. After a few weeks of regular exercise, he felt better all over—even his mood improved. His left leg got stronger, and his body felt more toned. He was losing weight. After a few months of regular exercise combined with his low-salt, low-fat, reduced-calorie diet, Jack's LDL was down and his HDL was up. The amount of blood pressure medicine that Jack required also went down. He lost ten pounds, which made it easier for him to move around. Jack continued his diet and exercise routines religiously for years to follow. The stationary bike remained a favorite for him, but he also enjoyed thirty-minute walks with his wife around the neighborhood on good days or in the malls on foul weather days. Ten years after his stroke, he is still working, exercising, and feeling good.

Different Exercise Options for Different Functional Levels

If you have had a stroke, exercise is good for you no matter where you are in your stroke recovery. Regardless of whether your stroke was one week ago or one year ago, exercise will almost certainly help. However, if you were recently discharged from the hospital, you are probably feeling run down and tired. This is because most people leave the hospital deconditioned. After lying around in a hospital bed for a week or more, your muscles start to lose their power and get smaller (*atrophy*). You feel weak and your endurance is low. The best remedy for this situation is to exercise.

On top of this generalized weakness, your stroke might have left you with specific limitations such as the inability to move an arm and leg. You may have increased muscle tone (*spasticity*) in an arm or leg that makes it difficult to control. Some stroke survivors will have visual problems and difficulty with balance, as well. You may be reading this right now and thinking, "How can I possibly exercise?" Remember these facts:

1. Cardiovascular exercise is *any* activity that significantly increases your heart rate for a sustained amount of time.
2. People can exercise in many ways, even if they have physical limitations.

Problem solving and creativity come into play when someone who has had a stroke is left with physical problems that impede his functioning. The rehabilitation team of physiatrist, physical therapist, and occupational therapist are an excellent source for exercise guidance and suggestions. They will be able to work with you and tailor a program that will suit your specific needs.

To give you an idea of the exercise possibilities for people who have had a stroke, we will discuss four broad categories of functional limitations and provide general exercise suggestions for each one. These categories may not exactly reflect your own personal physical condition, but you can use them as a guide when considering different exercise options. You may not fit neatly into one category, and with time you may move into a different category. As you read this section, you will probably come up with a list of exercise questions that you want to discuss with your doctor or your physical or occupational therapist.

Severe Functional Limitations

Right now you may be lying in bed, unable to get up by yourself. You may not be able to move your right arm or leg. You may need a lot of help with the activities of daily living: eating, grooming, bathing, dressing, and toileting. Transferring from the bed to a wheelchair may require the help of two people. You may be able to help with wheelchair propulsion using your strong arm, but your endurance may be very low and you may tire after helping to propel the wheelchair a few feet. You may also need help sitting at the edge of the bed. If you find yourself in this situation, you can still exercise.

Some physical activity is better than none. The more active you can be, the better. Sitting at the edge of the bed and practicing sitting balance with the help of a friend or therapist requires the use of many muscles and can be exhausting. While you are sitting, you can work on exercising other parts of your body; leg lifts, knee extensions, and ankle movements, and shoulder rotations, arm circles, elbow extension (straightening) and flexion (bending), and wrist extension/flexion can be part of the workout, with weights added as you are able to tolerate them. You do not have to be sitting to get a cardiovascular workout. You can exercise the various parts of your body even while lying down. Moving each joint is critical to avoid *contractures* (the inability to move a joint due to the formation of fibrous tissues around it), and for this reason range-of-motion exercises should be completed daily (with assistance as necessary). In range-of-motion exercises, the joint is moved through its full range of bending (flexion) and straightening (extending), or as far as possible. If you cannot move the joint yourself, a therapist can move it for you. At home, a trained caregiver

Table 16.1. Cardiovascular Exercise Options for People with Severe Functional Limitations

Sitting exercises
Leg lifts
Ankle movements
Shoulder rotations
Arm circles
Range-of-motion exercises in all joints (with assistance for affected joints)

can perform these range-of-motion exercises with you. Table 16.1 lists cardiovascular exercise options for people with severe functional limitations.

Moderate Functional Limitations

You may not be able to move your arm and leg at all, or you may have significantly increased tone in an arm or leg, making movement difficult. Despite these limitations, you may be able to perform many of the activities of daily living on your own because you have endurance and strength in the unaffected muscles of your body. You may not be able to walk independently, but you may be working on doing so. If you can tolerate sitting for thirty minutes or so with some support, then you may have a number of exercise options.

The swimming pool may be a good choice for cardiovascular exercise. Movement in your extremities is much easier with the help of flotation devices and a therapist or friend. (Special flotation belts can be worn to help you stay upright while exercising in a pool.) Because the water provides buoyancy, aquatic exercise is often easier for stroke survivors than land-based exercise. Supervised aquatic exercise programs are now available at a reasonable cost at many locations, including YMCAs and community pools.

Another good exercise option for someone with paralysis is to use recumbent exercise machines such as a recumbent stepper or a recumbent stationary bicycle. See Figure 16.1. With these machines, you can utilize your strong leg and possibly your arm, depending on the machine. If you use a recumbent bicycle with both pedals and arm levers, your strong arm can help propel the wheels. The recumbent machines are angled slightly backward and are easier to use than upright machines because they provide support while sitting. A therapist or friend may need to help you stabilize your paralyzed leg and arm.

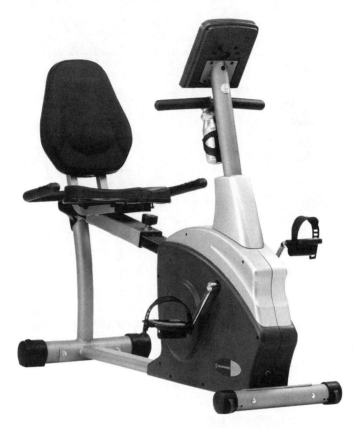

Figure 16.1. Recumbent stationary bicycle. Photo courtesy of Nautilus, Inc., Vancouver, Washington.

Exercise machines built to provide a cardiovascular workout, or upright stationary bicycles with arm levers and pedals may also be cardiovascular exercise options for you, depending on your sitting balance and strength. Upper extremity exercise machines are essentially stationary bicycles for the arms. These machines exercise the arms while the person is sitting down. You can use a strap or an ace bandage to help hold a weakened hand on the "pedal." Even stroke survivors with significant weakness are often able to use recumbent stationary bicycles. Again, if you have difficulty keeping your weak foot on the bicycle pedal, a strap or an elastic ace bandage can be used, and the inertia of the bicycle will help you complete the bicycling movement, even if the weak leg cannot contribute much. Figure 16.2 shows an upright stationary bicycle with arm levers and pedals.

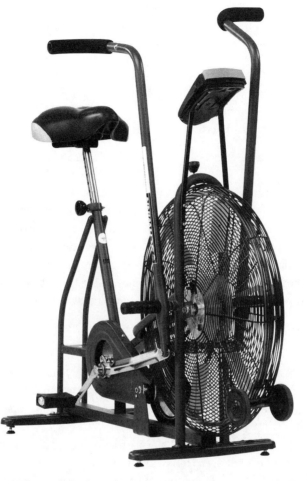

Figure 16.2. Stationary bicycle with arm levers and pedals. Photo courtesy of Nautilus, Inc., Vancouver, Washington.

After a stroke, you may find that your affected arm or leg seems more stiff or rigid than the other one. This stiffness and lack of control over movement may affect certain types of exercise but should not prevent you from finding an appropriate form of cardiovascular exercise that makes minimal demands of the affected limb. For example, if your left arm has limited movement, you could walk or use a stationary bike or treadmill, leaving the work to your legs. Alternatively, if your left leg has limited function, you may be able to use a stationary bike with both arm levers and foot pedals,

Table 16.2. **Cardiovascular Exercise Options for People with Moderate Functional Limitations**

Exercises in the pool
Recumbent stationary bicycle
Recumbent stepper
Upper extremity exercise machine
Stationary bicycle (with assistance from friend or family member, or with
  Velcro strap)

---

letting your arms and your right leg do the work. This would require more assistance from a friend or therapist, and the recumbent (leaning backward instead of sitting upright) version of the stationary bike may make this exercise easier. For people with *hemiparesis,* weakness affecting both the arm and the leg on one side, recumbent exercise machines that combine arm and leg activities may be the most practical. Table 16.2 lists cardiovascular exercise options for people with moderate limitations after a stroke.

Mild Functional Limitations

If you have weakness on one side or in one limb but you are still able to use both of your arms and your legs, you are probably able to perform most of the activities of daily living on your own. You are probably walking independently, perhaps with the aid of a cane or an *AFO* (*ankle-foot orthosis*—a foot brace).

With only mild weakness in a leg or arm, you have several options for cardiovascular exercise. The swimming pool may be your first choice. Choose a pool that is well heated and has easy entry, with railings and a nonskid surface on the deck. Even with these safety features, you may still need assistance getting in and out of the water, depending upon how strong you are. A stationary bike with modifications is another good option. If your leg is weak or hard to control, you can have a friend or therapist help stabilize it or use an ace bandage or a Velcro strap to keep it in place. You may pick a stationary bike with both foot pedals and arm levers (such as the Schwinn Airdyne), so you can use your strong arm or arms to help propel the wheels. Another stationary bicycle option is a recumbent version in which the user can sit in a more supportive chair, which is helpful if sitting balance is a problem. Recumbent steppers (such as the NuStep) are also an option.

Table 16.3. Cardiovascular Exercise Options for People with Mild Functional Limitations

---

Stationary bike (with assistance from friend or family member, or with
    Velcro strap)
Walking (with or without assistive device such as walker, cane, or ankle
    foot brace)
Swimming
Recumbent stationary bicycle
Recumbent stepper
Modified rowing machine

Depending on your level of weakness, you may be able to use a treadmill with or without assistance. If you choose to purchase a treadmill, you should select one that allows users to operate the treadmill at slower speeds, with the slowest setting .5 mph or less. Some stroke survivors also use rowing machines, occasionally with modifications, to get their cardiovascular exercise. Any of these options are reasonable, and if you use more than one of these machines, you are *cross-training*, which is a good idea. Cross-training means doing different types of exercise at different times; this helps to improve your overall fitness while avoiding overuse injuries. Table 16.3 lists cardiovascular options for people with mild limitations after a stroke.

Minimal to No Functional Limitations

If your limitations after your stroke are minimal to none, your cardiovascular exercise options are endless—walking, jogging, bike riding, singles tennis, swimming, basketball, golf, ice hockey, and soccer, to name a few. If you had a favorite activity prior to your stroke, continue that activity if you can. If you did not exercise regularly before your stroke, try different options and pick the one (or several, if you want to cross-train) that you enjoy most. You are more likely to exercise regularly if you enjoy the activity. Table 16.4 lists cardiovascular exercise options for someone with minimal to no functional limitations after a stroke. The possibilities are limited only by any other medical conditions you may have.

Table 16.4. **Cardiovascular Exercise Options for People with Minimal to No Functional Limitations**

Aerobics	Jogging
Badminton	Jumping rope
Basketball	Rowing machine
Bicycling	Soccer
Climbing stairs	Squash
Cross-country skiing	Stairmaster
Dancing	Swimming
Elliptical trainer	Tennis (singles)
Hiking	Walking (in the mall, on a treadmill,
Ice hockey	around the neighborhood)

The Risks of Exercise

As with most things in life, there are benefits and risks to exercise. In most instances, the benefits of exercise far outweigh the risks. People in certain situations, however, must avoid exercise altogether. Even for people without any known health problems, there are risks to exercising. It is important to familiarize yourself with these risks.

Injury is an obvious risk of exercise. A "pulled" muscle or sprained ankle may occur during almost any exercise, but these injuries can occur during everyday activities as well. Stretching prior to exercise helps reduce the risk of injury. This warm-up period should be about ten minutes long and should ideally include a five-minute period of stretching and a five-minute period of participating in your physical activity of choice at a reduced intensity. For example, if you are using the recumbent bicycle, after stretching for five minutes you should start out by bicycling at a very slow or reduced speed for five minutes. The cool-down period, after exercise, is just as important as the warm-up period. After exercising at the target intensity, it is a good idea to slow down and reduce the intensity for at least five minutes before stopping entirely. This slow down gives your body time to readjust: time for the blood to leave the muscles and rejoin the circulation, time for the heart rate to gradually slow, and time for the muscles to relax. Five minutes of stretching after exercising will help to reduce your chances of having an injury and will increase your overall flexibility.

Another important point to consider is that there are certain medical conditions that must be addressed before someone can begin to exercise regularly. If you have one of these medical conditions, you should definitely not begin to exercise without a long and careful discussion with your doctor. If you develop one of these problems, you should stop exercising and consult with your physician. If you have one of these medical problems, an expert medical opinion is needed before starting (or resuming) an exercise program. These medical conditions include

> unstable angina (chest pain that comes on at rest);
> angina with exertion (chest pain with activity such as walking up stairs);
> severe heart failure with symptoms of shortness of breath;
> active infection such as pneumonia or an infected knee joint;
> a recent blood clot in the vessels of your leg, lung, or brain;
> heart rhythm problems (cardiac arrhythmias) such as atrial fibrillation that is not well controlled;
> extremely high blood pressure (systolic >200 and diastolic >100);
> uncontrolled diabetes with high blood sugar; and
> dizziness or fainting episodes that put you at risk for a serious injury.

Any exercise becomes risky if you experience symptoms such as chest pain, shortness of breath, or extreme exhaustion. If you or someone you love experiences these symptoms, the exercise should be stopped right away. Contact your physician promptly for any of these symptoms. *If you develop new chest pains, call 9-1-1 immediately.*

The Stroke Savvy Exercise Plan

The Surgeon General recommends that "Americans accumulate at least 30 minutes (adults) or 60 minutes (children) of moderate physical activity most days of the week. More may be needed to prevent weight gain, to lose weight, or to maintain weight loss" (www.surgeongeneral.gov/topics/obesity/calltoaction/fact_glance.htm). The American Heart Association has similar recommendations: thirty to sixty minutes of physical activity most days of the week for adults.

Exercise can be so important and such a powerful treatment that we believe it should be discussed with all stroke patients. A prescription for an exercise program has four basic parts:

Type   Intensity   Duration   Frequency

We explain this program in detail in this section.

Table 16.5. **Heart Rate Calculations**

Age	Maximum Heart Rate	Target Heart Rate
20	220 – 20 = 200	60% – 75% of 200 = 120 – 150
30	220 – 30 = 190	60% – 75% of 190 = 114 – 143
40	220 – 40 = 180	60% – 75% of 180 = 108 – 135
50	220 – 50 = 170	60% – 75% of 170 = 102 – 128
60	220 – 60 = 160	60% – 75% of 160 = 96 – 120

Cardiovascular Exercise

As we mentioned earlier, there are different types of exercise, but the one that is most important for preventing a second stroke is cardiovascular exercise (also known as aerobic exercise). When you talk with your doctor about a cardiovascular exercise plan that's right for you, the first questions to address are: What kinds of exercise do you want to do and what kinds are you able to do? As we discussed earlier, your exercise options will depend on any limitations or weakness you have as a result of your stroke. Pick a type of exercise that is not only feasible for you but that you will find enjoyable or even fun. Your choice may change as your strength and endurance increase. Of course, you can pick more than one type of exercise and rotate through the week.

Intensity of exercise. In addition to the type of exercise that's right for you, talk with your physician about the appropriate intensity of the activity before you begin your program. Three ways are commonly used to monitor the intensity of your exercise. One way is to monitor your heart rate during the activity. Heart rate increases during exercise, and (generally) the faster your heart rate, the harder you are exercising. A target heart rate is often chosen relative to the predicted maximum heart rate for someone your age. In general, for healthy individuals without any underlying illnesses, the maximum heart rate a person can achieve with exercise is estimated by taking the number 220 and subtracting his age. Thus, a 50-year-old man has a maximum predicted heart rate of 170 beats per minute. Target exercise heart rates are typically selected to be between 50 and 85 percent of your age-predicted maximum heart rate. (Refer to Table 16.5 for specific examples.) This method of estimating maximum heart rate and selecting an exercise intensity has proven less useful for people over age 60, as the calculated number is often too low and does not allow for adequate ex-

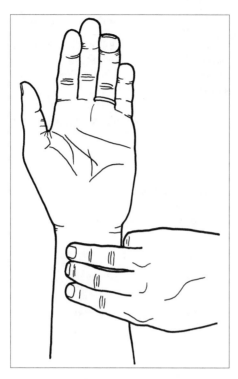

Figure 16.3. Taking your pulse. The pulse can be measured by placing two or three fingers over the artery on the wrist known as the "radial artery." This artery is located on the same side of the wrist as the thumb. The number of pulsations counted in one minute is the heart rate.

ercise intensity. Also, if you are taking medications such as beta-blockers that affect your heart rate, this heart rate calculation will not be useful for monitoring your exercise intensity.

To use your heart rate to monitor the intensity of your activity, you need to be comfortable taking your pulse. You may check either the radial artery in your wrist or the carotid artery in your neck. (Only check one side of your neck at a time, because putting pressure on both the left and right carotid artery at the same time could diminish or stop blood flow to the brain and cause fainting.) Although the wrist is a safe and easy option, some people may have difficulty finding the pulse there, since it is a small artery. Figure 16.3 shows where to find the radial artery on your wrist. You may also want to consider purchasing a heart-rate monitor, a device that goes around your chest and provides an electronic read-out of your heart rate.

Table 16.6. The Borg Rating of Perceived Exertion Scale

Instructions: During the work we want you to rate your perception of exertion, i.e., how heavy and strenuous the exercise feels to you and how tired you are. The perception of exertion is mainly felt as strain and fatigue in your muscles and as breathlessness or aches in the chest.

Use this scale from 6 to 20, where 6 means "No exertion at all" and 20 means "Maximal exertion."

9	Very light. As for a healthy person taking a short walk at his or her own pace.
13	Somewhat hard. It still feels OK to continue.
15	It is hard and tiring, but continuing is not terribly difficult.
17	Very hard. It is very strenuous. You can still go on, but you really have to push yourself and you are very tired.
19	An extremely strenuous level. For most people this is the most strenuous exercise they have ever experienced.

Try to appraise your feeling of exertion and fatigue as spontaneously and as honestly as possible, without thinking about what the actual physical load is. Try not to underestimate, nor to overestimate. It is your own feeling of effort and exertion that is important, not how it compares to other people's. Look at the scale and the expressions and then give a number. You can equally well use even as odd numbers.

Number Value	Exertion Level
6	No exertion at all
7	
8	Extremely light
9	Very light
10	
11	Light
12	

(continued)

Table 16.6. The Borg Rating of Perceived Exertion Scale, *continued*

13	Somewhat hard
14	
15	Hard (heavy)
16	
17	Very hard
18	
19	Extremely hard
20	Maximal exertion

© Gunnar Borg, 1970, 1985, 1994, 1998. Reprinted with permission.

Using target heart rate as a way to quantify your exercise intensity is helpful, but it is not recommended for everyone. You may be over 60 years old, or you may have a medical condition or be taking medications that preclude the use of these maximal and target heart rate calculations. In these circumstances, some physicians recommend using a different measure of exercise intensity that involves your own perceived level of exertion.

Using self-rated exertion to measure the intensity of exercise is, by definition, subjective. Most people intuitively use this type of monitoring, even if they are also using the target heart rate method. We recommend that most people exercise at a somewhat hard or moderate level. At this level you feel like you are working hard but you don't feel that you can't continue.

In determining your level of perceived exertion, take into consideration many different factors such as your heart rate, breathing rate, amount of sweat, and muscle fatigue. A specific scale for measuring this activity level, called the Borg Scale of Perceived Exertion, is used in most cardiac rehabilitation programs around the country. The goal is to reach a somewhat hard level, in between light and hard, which correlates to a number value of 12 to 14 on this scale. Table 16.6 presents the full scale.

Speak to your physician specifically about your recommended level of intensity for exercise. If you have coronary artery disease or a heart rhythm problem (cardiac arrhythmia such as atrial fibrillation or ventricular tachycardia), it is not safe for you to use maximal and target heart rate calculations. You will probably need to take a stress test before your cardiologist can determine a safe exercise level for you. This stress test will allow your cardiologist to determine your own target heart rate for exercise. (For more information, see the section at the end of this chapter titled "What If I Have Coronary Artery Disease?")

Duration of exercise. How long each exercise session should last will vary depending on your particular circumstances (the limitations you have after your stroke, your previous exercise history, and your current medical condition). If exercise is new to you or you have weakness that makes exercise difficult, we recommend aiming for ten minutes or so to start. If you can only do five minutes at one time, that's fine. Just do another five minutes at a different time that day. Even though the formal recommendations for adults are thirty minutes a day, if you do any exercise at all, even five minutes, it will help. You will find that your endurance improves the more you exercise. It may be a bit frustrating in the beginning, but we urge you to stick with it.

For seasoned exercisers with minimal limitations and no cardiac problems, your physician may recommend thirty to sixty minutes as your initial goal. The recommendation will depend on your medical condition after your stroke. Regardless of physical limitations and medical condition, everyone starting an exercise program should plan to start slowly and gradually increase the intensity and duration of exercise over time. Setting unrealistic initial goals when beginning an exercise program may be hazardous to your health, cause muscle strains, and result in frustration when you do not achieve these goals. "Slow and steady" is the only way to win this race.

Frequency of exercise. Exercise as many days as you reasonably can. If this is your first experience with regular exercise, start with a goal of at least three days each week, and work up to a goal of five to seven days a week. Remember, the Surgeon General recommends exercising "most days of the week." For anyone, regardless of age or risk factors, it is very important to start slowly and gradually build up the amount of exercise you perform. If you are not in shape, remember that it took you many years to get out of shape—this situation can't be reversed in one week. Moreover, if you have had a stroke, you will need to build your endurance back up to your baseline and then increase your activity level to the point where you can tolerate exercising regularly.

Table 16.7 provides a suggested schedule for gradually increasing your cardiovascular exercise. Your medical circumstances may dictate a more gradual or different program.

Resistance Training

Lifting weights and working on Nautilus machines are examples of resistance training. Resistance training with weights has been shown to increase muscle mass and strength. Increased strength can translate into improved functional ability, more independence, fewer falls, and improved perfor-

Table 16.7. **A Proposed Schedule for Gradually Ramping Up Your Aerobic Exercise Program**

Weeks 1–2	10 minutes of low-intensity exercise three times per week
Week 3	Add a fourth exercise session to your weekly schedule.
Week 4	Increase your schedule to five exercise sessions per week.
Week 5	Increase your workout to 15 minutes for each session.
Week 6	Increase your workout to 20 minutes for each session.
Week 7	Increase your workout to 25 minutes.
Week 8	Increase to 30 minutes.
Week 9	Increase to 35 minutes.
Week 10	Increase to 40 minutes.
Week 11	Increase to 45 minutes.
Weeks 12–18	Increase the intensity of your workout gradually until you achieve your target exercise intensity.
Week 19 and beyond	Keep up the good work!

mance in activities. Talk with your doctor about resistance training to see if it is recommended in your specific situation.

Intensity. Pick a weight that you can use comfortably for the exercise. For example, if you are exercising your biceps muscle by elbow flexion, pick a weight and try to perform fifteen biceps curls with it. If that is too easy, try the next weight up. If you can only complete six repetitions comfortably and you cannot make it to ten, then you need to start with a lighter weight.

Duration. Perform ten to fifteen repetitions of the weight lifting exercise (a specific number of repetitions is called a *set*). Work eight to ten different parts of your body each time you exercise, such as your arms, shoulders, chest, trunk, back, hips, legs, and ankles. Rest your muscles for fifteen seconds between each set of repetitions.

Frequency. Weight lifting resistance training is recommended two times a week. Resistance training should not be done on consecutive days, because the muscles need forty-eight hours to recover.

Stretching Exercises

Stretching increases flexibility and decreases the risk of injury. It can also increase range of motion of a joint, allowing more extensive and more comfortable movement at that joint. Stretching is one exercise that we all should do, no matter what our current limitations or medical condition. Stretching exercises are particularly useful if you are experiencing weakness and stiff-ness in one or more limbs after a stroke. You may want to speak to your doc-tor about which exercises he or she recommends in your specific situation.

Intensity. Stretch a given muscle to the point of discomfort but not severe pain. If you do not feel any discomfort at all, the stretch is not affecting the muscle.

Duration. Stretches should be held for thirty seconds. The old-fashioned "bouncing" type of stretching has been shown to be less effective, and may cause injury.

Frequency. Performing stretching before and after each aerobic activity is beneficial for the muscles. Performing stretching exercises every morning or evening, even if you do not plan to perform aerobic activity, is beneficial to the muscles as well. The more you stretch, the more flexible you will be. The more flexible you are, the more comfortably you are able to perform activities.

Table 16.8 summarizes the recommended duration, intensity, and fre-quency for cardiovascular exercise, resistance training, and stretching.

What If I Have Coronary Artery Disease?

If you have coronary artery disease (CAD), it is very important to exercise. Exercise can help lower your LDL and raise your HDL, changes that could significantly alter the interior of your arteries and help to reduce plaque formation. Exercise also helps with weight control, and being overweight is a risk factor for CAD (as well as for hypertension and diabetes).

You should not exercise if you have chest pain with physical activity, or chest pain at rest. In fact, you may be concerned about exerting yourself for fear that you will experience chest pain. If you have had a heart attack and you have CAD, chances are that you have had a stress test, which means that your heart has been evaluated with an EKG before, during, and after exercise. These tests will tell your cardiologist if it is safe for you to exercise; if it is safe, these tests will help your cardiologist guide you with your exercise prescription. The stress test will provide the information your cardiologist needs to determine a suitable target heart rate specifically for your exercise sessions. It may be best for you to start exercise under careful supervision in a cardiac rehabilitation program with nurses and therapists guiding you.

We need to stress that each person's case is individual. We cannot make generalizations for an exercise prescription for CAD patients. Speak with your cardiologist about the details but keep in mind the guidelines offered

Table 16.8. Recommended Duration, Intensity, and Frequency of Three Types of Exercise

Type	Intensity	Duration	Frequency
Cardiovascular	Moderate to somewhat hard perceived exertion (on Borg Scale)	30–60 minutes	5 days each week
Resistance training of 8–10 different parts of the body	Submaximal weight	10–15 repetitions	2 days each week
Flexibility	To point of discomfort	30 seconds per stretch	7 days each week

here. Use this information to spark questions and conversation about exercise with your physician.

What If I Have High Blood Pressure?

If you have high blood pressure, it needs to be under control before you take part in an exercise program. Do not exercise if your blood pressure is greater than 200 systolic or 100 diastolic. Once your blood pressure is in a reasonable range, perhaps through a combination of medications and a low-salt diet, then you should be able to safely exercise.

Monitoring your blood pressure before and after exercise may be helpful. You can do this at home with an inexpensive blood pressure monitor (available in drugstores, medical equipment stores, and online at various Internet sites). The automatic monitors are extremely easy to use. If you have a large upper arm, be sure to get the large cuff, as a cuff that is too small can give you an inaccurate reading. As we discussed earlier, you can also monitor your level of exercise intensity by checking your pulse as you exercise. This is a good idea for anyone, but it is especially important if you have CAD or hypertension. If you have difficulty finding your pulse, monitor your perceived level of exertion with the Borg Perceived Exertion Scale. Again, most people should be exercising at a moderate to somewhat hard

Table 16.9. **Strategies to Avoid Too High or Too Low Blood Sugar during and after Exercise**

Strategy	Diabetes Type I
Adjustments to the insulin	Take insulin at least 1 hour before exercise regimen
	If less than 1 hour before exercise, take insulin in nonexercising part of body (e.g., avoid injecting insulin into the leg before bicycling)
	Decrease dose of both short- and intermediate-acting insulin before exercise
	Alter daily insulin schedule
Meals and supplemental snacks	Eat a meal 1–3 hours before exercise and check to see if blood glucose is in safe range before exercise
	Take carbohydrate snacks or beverages at least every 30 minutes if exercise is vigorous or of long duration
	Increase food intake for up to 24 hours after exercise to avoid late-onset post-exercise hypoglycemia
Self-monitoring of blood glucose and urine ketones	Monitor blood glucose before, during, and after exercise to determine the need for and effect of changes in insulin dosage or eating schedule
	Delay exercise if blood glucose is less than 100mg/dL or if it is greater than 250mg/dL and ketones are present
Determination of unique metabolic responses	Learn how your glucose responds to different types, intensities, and conditions of exercise
	Determine effects of exercise at different times of the day on blood glucose response

Strategy	Diabetes Type II
Adjustments to the insulin regimen	Hypoglycemia is rare in Type II, but more likely for people taking insulin or sulfonylurea. May need to reduce dose
Meals and supplemental snacks	If taking insulin or sulfonylurea, may need supplemental carbohydrate snacks or beverages

(continued)

Table 16.9. Strategies to Avoid Too High or Too Low Blood Sugar during and after Exercise, *continued*

Strategy	Diabetes Type II
Self-monitoring of blood glucose and urine ketones	Not required
Determination of unique metabolic response	Not required

Sources: Adapted from Edward S. Horton, M.D., "Diabetes Mellitus," in *Exercise in Rehabilitation Medicine,* ed. Walter R. Frontera, D. M. Dawson, and D. M. Slovik (Champaign, Ill.: Human Kinetics, 1999), reprinted with permission; and J. F. Bean, A. Vera, and W. R. Frontera, "Benefits of Exercise for Community Dwelling Older Adults," *The Archives of Physical Medicine and Rehabilitation* 85, no. 7 (July 2004): 31–42, reprinted with permission of the American Congress of Rehabilitation Medicine and the American Academy of Physical Medicine and Rehabilitation.

level of intensity. The good news for people with high blood pressure is that with regular exercise and weight loss, blood pressure may be reduced and need for medication may decrease or even be eliminated.

What If I Have Diabetes?

If you have diabetes, it is important to get your blood sugar under control before you start an exercise program. Also, you must be on a stable medication regimen and should be following an appropriate diet. Just as insulin works to clear the bloodstream of glucose, exercise uses available glucose as energy, taking it out of the bloodstream. Your doctor might suggest to you that one way to get your blood sugar under better control is to exercise regularly. As long as your doctor is monitoring the situation, it should be safe for you to begin. In order to avoid having too low of a blood sugar level during exercise (called *hypoglycemia*), it is important to time your exercise according to when you eat and when you take your medications. Table 16.9 offers strategies for controlling your blood glucose during and after exercise. You may be able to take less medication to control your diabetes as you increase your activity. Some people with Type II diabetes who exercise regularly are even able to stop taking diabetes medication entirely.

What If I Am Overweight and Have Difficulty Walking?

How can you exercise if you have trouble walking? The swimming pool may be the best place for you to start exercising, because movement is much easier in the pool. You can walk in the water or do water aerobics (knee bends, leg lifts, arm circles). If the pool is not an option for you, you can start by doing stationary exercises while stabilizing yourself as needed. For example, you can bend your knee and lift it up twenty times, bend at the waist twenty times, or sit in a chair and do twenty leg lifts. Once you start to shed a few pounds, you might be surprised how quickly you can make walking and other cardiovascular activities a part of your exercise routine.

Why Don't People Exercise Regularly?

If exercise is so wonderful, why aren't more people doing it? There are several reasons, but in most cases these barriers can be overcome when someone is committed to exercise as a major improvement in their lifestyle. The barriers to exercise include:

- *Exercise is too time-consuming.* Time is a precious commodity in contemporary culture, and exercise is inherently time-consuming. Unlike many other activities, such as preparing a meal or cleaning a carpet, there are no labor-saving devices to allow someone to exercise in less time. Some people deal with the time demands of exercise by reevaluating their priorities and recognizing that thirty minutes of exercise may be more important than other activities on which they currently spend time.
- *I can't get to the gym.* The availability and convenience of a place to exercise and exercise equipment is a significant issue for many people. Many types of exercise do not require a gym, however. Walking is excellent exercise and can be done anywhere. Stationary exercise bicycles can be purchased inexpensively and provide an indoor option at home when the weather is unsuitable for outdoor activities. While a bit more expensive, home treadmills are another excellent option.
- *Exercise is boring.* Any repetitive activity can be boring, but exercise can easily be varied and made more interesting to prevent this. As we have mentioned, cross-training (varying your exercise routine so that you don't always do the same exercise), has multiple advantages. Other approaches include outdoor activities, such as walking, which are inher-

ently more varied than indoor exercise. You may find that you enjoy the social aspect of joining an exercise group at a gym. Almost any exercise can be done with a buddy, and getting a buddy is one way that many people overcome the monotony of exercising. Finally, you can combine exercise with activities that you like to do, such as watching television, listening to the radio, reading, or chatting on the telephone (using a speaker phone or telephone headset is best, so your hands are free). You may find that you are less bored if you do something to entertain yourself while you exercise.

* *Exercise is sweaty, painful, and unpleasant.* Exercise may cause you to sweat, but it shouldn't be painful or unpleasant. The trick is finding an exercise program that you enjoy and that you can look forward to, rather than viewing exercise as a chore.

Exercise has many important health benefits, but be sure to check with your physician prior to starting any exercise program. If you have a medical condition (such as unstable angina, uncontrolled high blood pressure, uncontrolled diabetes, congestive heart failure, or infection) that precludes exercise, the most important thing for you is to control that condition. If your doctor recommends that you start making exercise a part of your daily routine, you are on your way to reaping all the rewards. These include: weight loss, stress reduction, higher HDL and lower LDL levels, lower blood pressure, slower heart rate, and maybe even better sleep and mood. Making exercise a part of your life is the key. Make it fun. Pick an activity that you enjoy and stick with it. Soon you will start to see a difference in your body and your outlook, and most importantly, you will reduce your risk of having a stroke.

Chapter 17

● ●

How Smoking, Alcohol, and Illegal Drugs Affect Stroke Risk

As you develop a plan for stroke prevention, you need to consider the role that habits such as tobacco or alcohol use may play in your risk of having a stroke. These habits form over time and tend to become part of our everyday routine. Changing them can be hard but is important as you strive to reduce your risk of having a stroke.

Tobacco

How does tobacco affect stroke prevention and health? Are cigarettes, cigars, and pipes equally risky? What about chewing tobacco? How bad is secondhand smoke? Because smoking cigarettes is the most common and most dangerous form of tobacco use, we will focus on this topic. However, all forms of tobacco are harmful to health when used regularly. Smokeless tobacco (snuff and chewing tobacco) appears to be much less risky with regard to stroke than smoking, but it carries other health risks, such as oral cancer and periodontal disease.

Risks of Tobacco

While many people are somewhat aware that smoking is bad for their over-all health, most don't realize that smoking is the single largest preventable cause of death and disease in the United States. *Smoking is one of the top two treatable risk factors for stroke.* (The other is high blood pressure.) If you are a smoker or are regularly exposed to secondhand smoke, you owe it to yourself to take action.

How does smoking contribute to causing a stroke? Tobacco smoke is a complicated mixture of chemicals, and more than one chemical contained within smoke may contribute to the risk of developing a stroke. The nicotine in cigarettes (and other forms of tobacco) can raise blood pressure and heart rate by releasing large amounts of a hormone called *epinephrine* from the adrenal gland. This epinephrine causes the blood vessels to constrict, creating high blood pressure in the arteries. Chronic smoking also increases the number of red blood cells in a given amount of blood (the *hematocrit*) and the stickiness, or *viscosity*, of the blood, making it more likely to form clots and create a thrombotic stroke. For women who are taking estrogen (such as in birth control pills or for menopause), smoking greatly increases the risk of clotting and stroke. If you are a smoker who has had a stroke, one of the most significant steps you can take to prevent a recurrent stroke is to quit smoking.

Other chemical toxins in cigarettes damage the *endothelial cells* in the arteries, paving the way for atherosclerosis. Atherosclerosis causes blockages within the blood vessels, potentially leading to a stroke.

If stroke prevention alone isn't enough to motivate you to quit smoking, consider some of the other problems that smoking can cause:

Lung cancer
Bladder cancer
Bronchitis and emphysema
Stomach ulcers
Bad breath
Premature wrinkles

Quitting Smoking

Why is it so hard to quit smoking? Most physicians would argue that smoking is an addiction and should be considered a treatable medical condition rather than simply a bad habit. There are now medical treatments that can help overcome this addiction.

The "active ingredient" in tobacco smoke is nicotine, a chemical that provides feelings of calm and pleasure. Nicotine is absorbed very quickly through the lungs into the bloodstream and reaches the brain in seconds. Each puff of a cigarette provides a small nicotine "rush" that leads people to want to repeat the experience. Over time, smokers need the nicotine just to feel normal, and they continue smoking largely to avoid the unpleasant feelings of nicotine withdrawal. Nicotine withdrawal triggers feelings of restlessness, anxiety, and craving in most smokers.

Some individuals are capable of discontinuing their smoking through "willpower" alone. Somehow these individuals can tolerate and control the cravings that occur and the feelings of restlessness that are common among people withdrawing from nicotine. Most individuals, however, despite strong motivation and sincere efforts, cannot break free of this addiction by simply stopping "cold turkey." They require help.

Three main treatment strategies are available to assist with smoking cessation, and they can be used in combination to improve their effectiveness. They are: (1) behavioral training programs, (2) nicotine replacements, and (3) bupropion (Zyban or Wellbutrin), a medication that reduces the craving for tobacco.

Behavioral training works to change the psychological behaviors that sustain smoking addiction. As people smoke over many years, smoking becomes a part of their normal behavior; the "habit" of smoking is one of the reasons it is difficult to quit smoking. Certain settings or situations become linked in a person's mind to smoking, such as going to a bar or watching a ball game on television. These situations act as *triggers* for smoking, much as the smell of fried chicken might be a trigger for a craving for fried chicken wings. By learning behavioral techniques, individuals can increase their control over their own response to triggers in their environment that would normally lead them to reach for a cigarette. Combining behavioral training with medication to reduce the cravings for tobacco is a particularly effective strategy.

Nicotine replacements come in various forms, but all share the goal of reducing the cravings for tobacco by replacing the primary addictive ingredient with a safer form that is not smoked. Once this replacement has been accomplished, the goal is gradually to reduce the amount of nicotine used to allow the body to readjust to living without this chemical. Nicotine replacements include lozenges, gums, inhalers, nasal sprays, and skin patches. While nicotine can cause temporary rises in blood pressure, it appears safe for short-term use as an aid to smoking cessation. People must not smoke while using a nicotine replacement (for example, a nicotine patch), because smoking can provide a "double dose" of nicotine and cause more serious elevations in blood pressure.

Bupropion (Zyban or Wellbutrin) was originally developed as an antidepressant medication, and it is still used to treat depression. But patients using this medication to treat depression also noted that it seemed to help reduce the cravings associated with nicotine withdrawal. Scientific tests have now shown that bupropion is effective in helping smokers quit.

A key aspect of successful smoking cessation is to avoid environments and situations that may trigger relapse. As with alcoholism, it may be best for former smokers to consider themselves "recovering" smokers for the indefinite future. A smoke-free environment at home and work are critical for success. A person attempting to discontinue smoking will rarely succeed if they are living with an active smoker. Discarding all cigarettes in the house (and car, pocketbook, desk drawer, etc.) to avoid an impulsive decision to resume smoking is essential. Avoiding smoke-filled clubs or bars, and activities or locations associated with smoking, can help prevent a renewed craving. These cravings can occur for many years after smoking cessation, and are ingrained in the brain to some extent. A person who has successfully completed withdrawal from tobacco and weaned off nicotine replacements is not protected from tobacco cravings in the future.

Many people successfully quit smoking only after several attempts: relapse of smoking is common among those who quit. A relapse should be dealt with openly and constructively and should not be seen as a failure. The only reasonable approach is to stop smoking again and redouble your efforts to prevent a relapse. Family members and friends can be influential in encouraging the smoker to stop smoking again. The health risks of smoking and the risk of a stroke are just too consequential to accept any other alternative.

Alcohol

Alcohol has been a component of human diets since before the beginning of recorded history, and it is part of many social activities and gatherings throughout the world. Many people consider alcohol use to be a normal part of living. If alcohol is used in small quantities, this may be an accurate perception, but when used in larger amounts, alcohol can be dangerous.

Risks of Alcohol

Alcohol has a variety of effects on the body and the brain that may affect your risk of having a stroke. Unlike many other risk factors for stroke that increase the risk of a blood vessel blockage (a cerebral infarct), alcohol is more of a risk factor for developing bleeding within the brain (a cerebral hemorrhage). This increase in the risk of bleeding within the brain may be due to alcohol-induced brief elevations of blood pressure that can cause a blood vessel to burst.

Alcohol can also be an indirect contributor to the risk of developing a cerebral infarct, primarily through increasing other risk factors. Chronic alcohol use can be a factor in developing high blood pressure, a major risk factor for stroke. It can contribute to obesity (alcohol is quite high in calories) and can cause atrial fibrillation in the heart (see Chapter 8).

Alcohol causes many problems, both medical and social. Alcoholism can lead to depression, family and social disruption, car accidents, and job loss, and can increase the risk of suicide. Medical conditions that can be caused or worsened by alcohol use include

liver disease,
inflammation of the pancreas,
stomach ulcers and inflammation,
heart muscle damage,
high blood pressure,
obesity,
vitamin deficiencies,
memory loss and dementia,
nerve damage,
muscle damage, and
cancer.

Can alcohol be good for you? You may have heard that limited alcohol use can protect you against heart disease. There is some truth to this, as small amounts of alcohol do help to increase the "good" cholesterol (HDL) and lower the "bad" cholesterol (LDL). The American Heart Association acknowledges that limited amounts of alcohol use may reduce the risk of heart disease, but the AHA does not advise individuals who are not presently using alcohol regularly to begin. Moreover, certain risks of alcohol appear to be greater in stroke survivors, so the risks of regular alcohol intake outweigh the benefits for these people. Many stroke survivors take medications that reduce blood clotting, such as aspirin or Coumadin, and the combination of these medications and alcohol can lead to an increase in bleeding from the stomach and other bleeding complications.

How Much Alcohol Is "Safe"?

We recommend that people who have had a stroke in the past, especially if they also have a history of high blood pressure (hypertension), limit their alcohol intake to *no more than one drink per day*. In many cases, even this level of usage may be hazardous. Discuss the risks of alcohol with your physician before resuming even modest alcohol use after a stroke or TIA.

How is a "drink" defined? People use varying amounts of alcoholic beverages in each drink. The medical definition of a "standard" drink used by the American Heart Association is that it should contain no more than half an ounce of pure alcohol. This translates into a twelve-ounce beer or a four-ounce glass of wine. For 80 proof spirits, a drink consists of one and a half ounces of liquor. For 100 proof spirits, the portion is smaller, and a drink consists of one ounce of liquor.

How much alcohol is safe to drink depends on the perspective. Many definitions of excessive alcohol use focus on its effects on social functioning and symptoms of dependence (needing a drink). While these are valid definitions for many people, stroke survivors need to use a stricter standard. Even small amounts of alcohol may be dangerous in combination with your medical condition and/or medications. If you are considering resuming "social" drinking, discuss the specific amounts with your physician.

How Much Alcohol Is Too Much?

What if you are using too much alcohol? The first step in dealing with excessive alcohol use is to recognize this as a problem. Many people think of alcohol use as falling into one of two categories: normal ("social") use or alcoholism. The fact is, there is a broad spectrum of alcohol use, and even use that may not interfere with daily functioning (working, taking care of a family) may be medically problematic. Are you drinking too much? *If you are drinking more than one drink a day on average, your drinking may be having a negative impact on your health.* Some stroke survivors should avoid alcohol altogether, because of potential adverse interactions with their medications. A frank discussion with your physician of your actual alcohol use is a good place to help determine if you are endangering your health through drinking. Keep in mind that most people don't accurately report how much alcohol they drink. Be honest with your doctor, so she can do her best to help you recover and prevent a stroke in the future.

Quitting or Controlling Drinking

Once you have determined that you need to cut back on your alcohol use, the next step is to create a plan. For occasional alcohol users, the only plan needed may be to make a conscious decision and stick with it. For many others, however, alcohol use has become ingrained in many aspects of their lives, including their social lives. Avoiding situations where others will be drinking is a key step in avoiding temptation. Get rid of alcohol in your house, to eliminate an easy source of accessible alcohol. Find alternative ways to socialize that do not involve alcohol. Let your friends and family know that you need to avoid alcohol use for health reasons.

Some people cannot control their alcohol use on their own. They have become dependent on alcohol, and they need to enlist major supports to deal with this problem. Alcoholics Anonymous and similar groups provide a support network of people contending with the same issues. If you or a loved one is drinking excessively, reach out and get help.

In summary, if you do not already drink alcohol regularly, do not start. The benefit that small amounts of alcohol might provide with regard to an increased HDL can be attained in many other ways, such as exercise, that avoid the dangerous side effects of alcohol.

If you already drink alcohol regularly, you need to be honest with yourself about the amount you drink and discuss this issue with your physician. Even if your doctor feels that it is safe for you to drink small amounts of alcohol, we do not recommend drinking more than one drink per day. Most stroke survivors take aspirin, Plavix, or Coumadin, or have a history of cerebral hemorrhage. *In these situations, we advise against regular alcohol consumption* because of the increased risk of bleeding or of a second cerebral hemorrhage.

Illicit Drug Use

The risk of having a stroke is probably the last thing on anyone's mind when they consider whether or not to use cocaine or other illicit drugs. But some of these drugs can cause stroke, and we need to help alert stroke survivors to this lesser-known risk of using drugs.

Cocaine

Cocaine is a powerful stimulant that has been used recreationally for many years, its popularity waxing and waning over time. Cocaine is a *vasoconstrictor*—it causes the blood vessels to constrict and become narrower. It also causes temporary numbness when applied to certain areas of the body (for example, the tissues in the mouth and throat). Cocaine is sometimes used in certain types of surgery, combining its numbing effects with its blood vessel narrowing effects to good purpose.

Cocaine can reduce the flow of blood to the brain, however. It also increases the level of a substance in the blood known as *norepinephrine,* leading to blood vessel constriction, increased heart rate, and increased blood pressure. The sudden increase of blood pressure that results from cocaine use can cause bleeding within the brain due to the rupture of blood vessel walls. *Using cocaine even once can result in a cerebral hemorrhage without any warning.*

Cocaine can cause the blood vessels to constrict so severely that the blood supply to a part of the body becomes too low to keep the cells alive. If the constricted blood vessel is one that supplies the brain, the person may have a stroke; if the blood vessel supplies the heart, the person may have a heart attack. Cocaine can cause both ischemic and hemorrhagic strokes.

Finally, chronic cocaine use can cause inflammation of the blood vessels supplying the brain—the condition known as *cerebral vasculitis*. The inflammation causes the blood vessels to become narrowed and therefore more likely to develop blockages. These blockages can cause ischemic strokes, which can develop at any time, even on a day when a person is not using cocaine.

Amphetamines

Amphetamines are stimulant medications that increase alertness, reduce appetite, and may help focus attention. Amphetamines have some legitimate medical uses, and are sometimes prescribed for the treatment of attention deficit hyperactivity disorder (ADHD) or certain sleep disorders, including narcolepsy. Amphetamines and related medications, such as methylphenidate (Ritalin), are sometimes prescribed for stroke survivors in low doses to help improve attention.

Unfortunately, amphetamines are also popular drugs of abuse, and are taken illegally by people trying to feel energetic, stay awake, or lose weight. Illegal amphetamines are often known as "speed," though there are other common street names for these medications. Amphetamines have many potential side effects, including increasing blood pressure, heart rhythm disturbances, palpitations, and chest pain. Amphetamine abuse has been associated with both hemorrhagic and ischemic strokes as well as with cerebral blood vessel inflammation.

Lysergic Acid Diethylamide (LSD) and Other Hallucinogens

LSD and related drugs, such as mescaline and phencyclidine (PCP, angel dust), cause hallucinations. These hallucinations can cause agitation and sudden blood pressure elevation, leading to cerebral hemorrhage.

Why You Need to Avoid Using Illicit Drugs

The bottom line is that illicit drug use can lead to a stroke, even in someone who is using a drug for the very first time, as well as in people who have been using these drugs regularly without apparently suffering any ill effects. Experimenting with illicit drugs can be very dangerous. We strongly advise any stroke survivor to avoid any illicit drug use. For people with re-current drug use, we urge prompt treatment. A full discussion of treatment for drug addiction is beyond the scope of this book. An important first step is to recognize that these drugs can affect your health and can lead to an-other stroke. If you have a drug problem, get help. Begin by talking to your doctor and also enlist the support of trusted friends, family, or clergy.

Part V

LOOKING TO THE FUTURE

Chapter 18

Research on the Horizon

Medicine has been practiced for thousands of years, beginning with, among other approaches, the use of naturally available remedies. In a sense, medical research has a similarly long history. Trial and error use of various berries, barks, and leaves to alleviate symptoms could be considered a primitive form of medical research.

Research has grown more and more sophisticated as we have learned more about the biological processes of the body. The discovery of DNA, for example, opened the door to uncovering genetic factors that may influence the risk of having a stroke. Our understanding of how stroke-causing blood clots form points us in the direction of new medications to prevent these clots from developing. In this chapter we describe how medical research is conducted and how to make sense of research results that are reported in the media. We also provide a snapshot of selected areas of active research on stroke.

How Research Is Conducted

Researchers have developed research design guidelines to ensure reliable results. Understanding how studies are conducted can help you interpret the results of medical research and carry on a meaningful dialogue with your physician when making decisions about your medical treatment options.

Not all research studies are created equal. Their goals vary widely. Some studies provide only preliminary evidence but stimulate new ideas and bring about additional in-depth research. Others are designed to test a new treatment or other medical theory.

Research conducted early in the development of a new treatment is designed to explore the new treatment rather than to prove that it works. The purpose is to assess the safety of the treatment, the range of safe dosages, and so on. Some preliminary studies are performed to generate theories, rather than to prove them. An example of this type of study is a study looking at the relationship between a vitamin level in the blood and the risk of stroke. If a lower level of the vitamin is found in people who have strokes, scientists may hypothesize that this vitamin protects against stroke. To test this theory, however, would require a second study in which people at risk for stroke are divided into two groups, one group receiving extra vitamins and the other not receiving them.

Many studies of possible treatments involve the use of placebos. Placebos are fake treatments (like sugar pills) that are believed not to have any effect on the medical condition being studied. The purpose of placebos is to prevent bias from affecting results. For example, suppose that, in a study of treatment for a painful condition, half of the subjects take a pill containing pain-relief medication, and half of the subjects take a pill that looks identical to the "real" pill but contains only sugar. Subjects receiving the "real" pill may feel better even though the medication isn't having any effect, because they *expect* to feel better when they are having treatment. This is known as the *placebo effect*. The subjects taking the placebo treatment (the sugar pills) are expected to experience the same psychological benefits as those taking the "real" pills, and they, too, may feel better. If the study medication works, then the people taking the "real" pills will have *greater* improvement in symptoms than those receiving the placebo medicine.

Making Sense of Research

Research is often misunderstood and mistrusted by the public, who expect a definite answer that doesn't change over time. People are often confused and frustrated by new research results that seem to contradict old results. Doctors may recommend certain treatments based on the available research one year, and then recommend entirely different treatments the next year. There is no doubt that medicine is dynamic and that our advice changes as we learn new information.

Unfortunately, a single research study rarely provides a definitive answer. Rather, research studies gradually chip away at a problem by testing various theories. Over time, the repeated experiments gradually produce a picture that is stable and generally accepted as correct. Sometimes a new study will overturn the status quo by showing that previously accepted ideas were based on false assumptions and misinterpretations of research results. Such a dramatic and sudden shift in medical practice can be disconcerting.

It is common for physicians to jump ahead of the methodical and often slow-paced research on a health condition and try to extrapolate from preliminary studies. A recent prominent example of this approach was the drastic shift in the use of hormone replacement therapy (estrogen) for women after menopause. Based on preliminary research, women taking these medications seemed to have a lower risk of a variety of health conditions when compared with women who were not taking hormone replacement therapy. Since there are many factors influencing decisions to take these medications, this research observation should have been viewed somewhat skeptically by practicing physicians. For example, women who took hormone replacement therapy generally were wealthier and better educated than women who did not. Because financial resources and education are predictors of better health, it may well be that these women had a lower incidence of disease because of other factors, not because of their hormone use. This sampling defect became clear when larger, more definitive studies "randomized" women (assigned them at random) to receive either hormone replacement or sugar pills. In these studies, the two groups of women were very similar in terms of education, wealth, and other factors that might influence health outcomes. In fact, the only significant difference between them was that one group took hormone replacement treatment and one group did not. When the results of these studies were revealed, it became clear that the hormone therapy increased the risk of getting sick, rather than preventing it. Overnight, prescriptions for hormone replacement drugs fell dramatically, and they remain at a much lower level today than before these studies.

Similar issues face doctors regarding the use of vitamins to prevent stroke, and the use of C-reactive protein to predict stroke risk. Both of these proposed innovations are still in early phases of investigation, and definite answers are likely to be years away. Because stroke survivors and doctors need to make health care decisions now, however, they often need to work with incomplete information. Many important stroke treatment questions being asked today won't be answered definitively for another five or ten years. It is important for you and your doctor to have open discussions about these uncertain areas, so that you can make the best choices for you personally.

Finding Out about Research

Most people learn of new medical research from their physician or from the media. Many local television newscasts have a daily segment on health care and provide a quick sound bite about the latest study results. Even health care providers may first learn about an important research study in the popular media—some doctors joke that the "*New York Times* Journal of Medicine" is a good source of information.

When you hear about a research study of interest, take the initiative to learn more. Consider obtaining a summary of the article. A few medical journals (for example, the *Annals of Internal Medicine*) now post brief summaries of articles written for the lay public on their websites. In other cases, only the more technical summary of an article (known as an abstract) is available, but the abstract may be worth reviewing. Summaries of virtually all research studies published are available on a free government website known as "Pubmed" (see the Resources section of this book).

Make certain to discuss the research with your physician. Research must be considered in a broader context, which your doctor can help provide. Are this study's results consistent with prior research results? Does the study appear to have been well designed? Do the results apply to your situation?

New Methods of Assessing Stroke Risk

Homocysteine

Homocysteine is a chemical that occurs naturally in the human body. Interest in homocysteine as a possible risk factor for stroke was sparked by the observation a number of years ago of people with dramatically elevated levels of this chemical. These individuals suffer from a genetic disorder that interferes with normal metabolism and causes homocysteine to build up to high levels in the body. They have a very high risk of heart disease and stroke, often succumbing to these conditions while still in their thirties. Based on this observation, scientists suspected that even individuals with more modest elevations in their level of homocysteine might be at increased risk for stroke.

Some physicians are using the simple blood test for measuring homocysteine to assess their patients' risk for stroke or heart disease. In patients with high levels of homocysteine, levels can be lowered with the vitamins folate, pyridoxine (vitamin B_6), and vitamin B_{12}.

Research on homocysteine is in an intermediate phase. Initial studies suggested that people with elevated levels are at higher risk of stroke than those with lower levels. Since homocysteine levels can be changed using vitamin supplements, the real question for many people is whether changing the homocysteine level changes their risk of stroke. A recent study, known as the VISP (Vitamins in Stroke Prevention) study, failed to find evidence that taking vitamins lowered stroke risk for people who had already had a stroke.

Does this mean that vitamins are useless for stroke prevention? Not necessarily. It is still quite possible that certain populations (for example, people with markedly elevated homocysteine levels) might benefit from reducing their level of homocysteine, or that larger doses of the vitamins used might be more effective. Should stroke survivors take vitamins in an attempt to reduce their risk of stroke? At present, most physicians would not recommend this as a routine measure, though the risks of taking these vitamins are quite low. A discussion with your physician may be appropriate.

C-Reactive Protein

C-reactive protein is a chemical in the bloodstream that is normally produced by the body as part of its response to inflammation. Scientists have found evidence of an elevated risk of heart disease and stroke in people with inflammation, and they have found in some studies that C-reactive protein levels can be used to help predict the risk of having a future stroke or heart attack. C-reactive protein can be measured using a simple blood test.

Unfortunately, no treatments have been established to lower the level of C-reactive protein. Even if such treatments are developed, it is not clear that lowering the level of C-reactive protein would affect the risk of stroke and heart disease. At the present time, some physicians use C-reactive protein levels as an additional technique to help determine a person's overall risk of stroke. If the risk is found to be high, aggressive lifestyle and medical treatments are advisable, such as improving diet, smoking cessation, and using cholesterol-lowering medications.

At the moment, knowing their C-reactive protein levels is probably of limited use for most stroke survivors. Stroke survivors are clearly at an increased risk of having a second stroke, and should take maximum action to reduce their risk factors and minimize their future risk. An elevated C-reactive protein level shouldn't change their behavior with regard to risk reduction, and a low level shouldn't give them false comfort.

In the future, research will likely clarify the underlying reasons for the apparent relationship between C-reactive protein levels and the risk of stroke and heart attack. This understanding should lead to new treatments directed specifically at reducing this risk.

Emerging Treatments for Stroke Prevention

Diet

Research on the role of diet in preventing stroke is ongoing—and often confusing. Many studies are done by identifying differences in the risk of stroke in different groups of people. These *cross-sectional studies* may be done at a single point in time and may involve questionnaires regarding food and drink intake in the past. They are important as a first step in identifying dietary factors that might contribute to stroke prevention, but they are not the final word on these questions. An example of this type of study might be a research study that found that people who drank red wine regularly had a lower risk of stroke than people who drank beer, or who didn't drink at all. While many might seize on this result as a reason to run to the wine cellar, the reality would inevitably be more complex. What other factors might have influenced this low risk of stroke? Perhaps people who drink red wine are also inclined to eat more asparagus, or to exercise more frequently. While scientists attempt to record and account for as many factors as possible, there is no guarantee in a study like this that they have not missed a key factor that is the *real* reason why certain people have a lower risk of stroke.

Another important challenge in this type of research is *recall bias.* People are often asked to recall their typical intake of a food over a long period of time, and they may not be able to accurately remember what they ate. Their responses may reflect what people would like to have eaten or they may reflect their assumptions about which foods are healthy. Unless the person kept a log of what they have actually eaten, it is hard to know if their report is accurate.

From the point of view of the stroke survivor, this type of study, though often highly touted by the media, should be viewed cautiously, and may not be a good basis for changing your diet. When you learn of a new study suggesting that you change your diet, discuss it with your doctor. Is the research definitive, or is it intended to develop a new theory? Are there other studies that corroborate this new research report? Don't jump to conclusions.

Another way of studying the relationship between diet and the risk of stroke is a *cohort study.* In a cohort study, a group of people are enrolled in the study and carefully observed over time. The subjects record their diet or other behaviors of interest to the researchers, and a careful medical record is kept through the years. A cohort study is similar to a cross-sectional study in some ways, but it has two advantages: (1) more accurate recording of diet and other risk factors and (2) more accurate recording of strokes, TIAs, or other medical problems over the course of the study. These studies are logistically challenging and expensive to run, so there aren't many of them. The Framingham study (mentioned in Chapter 1) is a famous cohort study that is ongoing and that has provided many insights into stroke risk factors.

While cohort studies are extremely useful, they still don't answer the most important question: *Will my risk of stroke be reduced if I change my diet (or other behavior)?* Cohort studies, too, can be influenced by unmeasured differences in behavior or risk factors that make it seem as if the measured factor is the one that is causing the difference in stroke rates. For example, let's assume a study was looking at alcohol use and the risk of lung cancer. Let's also assume that people who drink alcohol regularly are more likely to smoke. People in this study who drank might be found to have a higher rate of lung cancer, but the risk would be caused by the smoking, not by the drinking. If the researchers failed to ask about cigarette use, they might mistakenly conclude that drinking alcohol causes lung cancer. Studies of this type are prone to influence by factors that are not known to be risk factors or that were not adequately measured.

The definitive study is an *intervention study,* in which a group of people are randomly divided into two or more groups and encouraged to change their diets or modify some other behavior. These studies are also logistically challenging, since the researchers must monitor the diet or other behavior of the participants closely for a number of years. Even when these studies are carefully done, they do not always provide the final answer to a question. For example, as mentioned above, a recent study of vitamins for preventing stroke, the VISP study, failed to show a clear benefit to using vitamins. Despite this outcome, some researchers speculate that a study that lasts longer, uses higher vitamin doses, or includes a larger number of participants might yet show the value of this treatment.

We recommend the following overall guidelines for thinking about studies of diet for stroke prevention:

Don't be too quick to change your diet based on a news report or magazine article about a certain food or diet. Instead, discuss any changes you are considering with your physician at your next visit.

Be wary of fad diets that suggest that a single food or vitamin is the "answer" for preventing stroke. No research has ever suggested that the route to health is through any single food.

Don't ignore well-established guidelines in favor of the newest preliminary scientific report. Advice to increase fresh fruits and vegetables, control overall caloric intake, and eat more whole-grain foods is unlikely to be invalidated by a single study suggesting that a particular food is beneficial for stroke prevention.

Don't let research distract you from taking action against the biggest and most well-understood risk factors. Even if drinking red wine or eating almonds were proved to reduce the risk of stroke somewhat, this would not change the fact that smoking cessation and blood pressure control are extraordinarily important for prevention of stroke.

Find out about official guidelines. The American Stroke Association and other organizations periodically publish guidelines on particular aspects of stroke prevention. These guidelines are based on a measured and thoughtful consideration of the overall scientific evidence, rather than focusing on a single scientific report. Relying on these "official" guidelines will keep you up to date in stroke prevention, so you won't feel the need to jump at each new tidbit of research that is publicized in the news media.

Research in Medical and Surgical Treatments for Stroke Prevention

The treatment of blockages in the arteries to the brain continues to be studied, with several promising approaches. The use of wire mesh stents to hold partially blocked blood vessels open is likely to become more widespread in coming years, as these devices and techniques are refined. New surgical techniques to reduce the risk of stroke resulting from blood vessel blockages are also being developed.

A variety of different medications are under development for use in stroke prevention. Improvements are being sought in safety, efficacy, and convenience for these important treatments. A new oral anticoagulant (blood thinner) medication, ximelgatran, is under study as a possible replacement for Coumadin. This medication has the potential to be easier to regulate, and may not require the frequent blood tests that Coumadin requires. While studies have not yet focused on ximelgatran and stroke, this agent may ultimately join the list of options for stroke prevention.

Research in Treatment of Acute Stroke

The advent of medications that dissolve blood clots ("clotbusters") when stroke first occurs has opened a new chapter in stroke research. These clot-dissolving medications can only be used in a small percentage of stroke victims because of time limitations and other factors. Research is ongoing to find safer, more effective, and more flexible treatments for acute stroke, and research on clot-dissolving medications continues. The use of catheters to direct the medication more specifically to the area of the clot is one promising technique. Other researchers are studying the use of mechanical devices to physically remove blood clots. Current clot-busting medications can only be used in the first three hours after a stroke, so finding treatments that can be used beyond the three-hour limitation is another research priority.

Other areas being studied include reducing the degree of damage from stroke using cooling of the brain, more precisely controlling blood pressure in someone having a stroke, and stabilizing blood sugar in people with diabetes and stroke. Various chemicals have been studied in an attempt to find *neuroprotectant* medications that can reduce the injury to brain cells from stroke.

Research in Restoring Lost Abilities after Stroke

Exercise Treatments

Research over the past several years has provided evidence that exercise can influence the process of stroke recovery. The brain has the ability to "rewire" itself to some degree, and exercise stimulates this rewiring. While there are limits to the brain's ability to rewire itself in response to damage, this capability has generated considerable interest in exercise as a treatment after stroke. Most current research on how best to exercise to optimize recovery after stroke has focused on the recovery of movement. Several promising approaches are being studied.

Constraint-induced movement therapy. In this technique, the stroke survivor's unaffected arm is placed in a restraining sling for up to six hours per day for a two-week period, preventing him from using it and forcing the weak arm to exercise. This program, which has been tested in a number of small studies, appears to help increase the functional use of the affected arm. Various modifications of this technique are also being tested, though these have not yet been shown to be as effective. A larger study of constraint-induced movement therapy, known as the EXCITE study, is in progress at this time. Results of this study are expected within the next few months and should provide a definitive answer regarding the value of this therapy.

In the meantime, some centers are now offering constraint-induced movement therapy programs for interested stroke survivors. These programs vary in how closely they adhere to the original protocol; it is not known whether the variations affect the value of the treatment.

Robotic rehabilitation. A number of centers are testing both upper- and lower-limb robots for exercise training purposes after stroke. These robots more closely resemble health club exercise machines than the humanoid robots seen in movies. They provide assistance with movement and may help with the recovery of motor function. Much more research is needed before the value of this treatment approach becomes clear and we know which devices and training programs are most effective.

Virtual reality training. *Virtual reality* consists of a computer-generated display that mimics the real world. Many computer games provide a basic virtual reality environment, where activities appear to take place in an artificial world. Some virtual reality systems use special screens mounted on goggles, so the user feels as if she is really inside the computer-generated scene. Scientists have been interested in using virtual reality for rehabilitation to allow stroke survivors to practice activities in a safe environment, with the computer acting as a trainer. Preliminary studies have been conducted to determine whether this treatment is effective in restoring or improving movement after stroke, but only limited data are available thus far.

Partial weight-supported treadmill training. Partial weight-supported treadmill training is a technique to help reestablish walking after stroke. In this technique, the stroke survivor is placed in a supportive harness to reduce the amount of weight he needs to support with his legs. He then uses a treadmill to practice normal walking movements. This technique appears promising but is labor intensive, typically requiring two physical therapists and considerable time to set up. Some centers are exploring the use of electromechanical or robotic gait trainer devices to accomplish the same goals in a more efficient manner. These devices mechanically assist the stroke survivor to move his legs. Research on the use of gait-training robots is ongoing.

Medications

The simplest treatment for stroke recovery would be a pill to help the brain recover. A number of medications have been studied to see if they might help the brain enhance its own natural recovery process.

Amphetamines. There is some preliminary evidence that the use of amphetamine and related medications within the first few weeks after stroke may help the brain recover. Other research studies have found conflicting evidence, suggesting that these medications do not help recovery. Larger studies are in progress to test these medications to determine if they should be routinely used to facilitate recovery after stroke. At the present time amphetamines are not generally used to treat stroke, although they are sometimes used to treat other problems in stroke survivors, such as difficulty staying alert or paying attention.

Growth factors. Growth factors are chemicals naturally produced by the body that instruct cells to grow and multiply. These chemicals are essential in developing the normal connections within the brain. As scientists identify and can produce larger quantities of them, it is hoped that these chemicals may be useful in stimulating a damaged brain to form new connections. Only limited human studies of growth factors have been conducted, and no growth factors are currently in use for treatment of stroke.

Stem cells. Stem cells (and related cells known as *precursor cells*) are normally present in various parts of the body and are the reserve source of new cells to replace those lost through aging, illness, or injury. Human embryos have large numbers of stem cells, while adults have fewer stem cells. The use of embryonic stem cells has generated considerable ethical and political debate, since obtaining these cells for research purposes requires the destruction of a human embryo. The U.S. government has restricted federal funding for this type of research in response to these concerns. In spite of these limitations, research using both embryonic and adult human stem cells continues in this country and around the world.

Small numbers of stem cells have recently been identified in the adult human brain. Scientists are trying to determine if these cells can be stimulated to effectively repair injuries caused by stroke. Most of the research in this area has taken place in animals; human studies are still in the earliest stages.

Consider Participating in Clinical Research

Some stroke survivors may be offered an opportunity to participate in research studies of stroke prevention techniques. Participating in a research study may provide patients with early access to new treatments. Sometimes participating in a research study is the only way to obtain new treatments before they become widely available. It can also be a chance to improve the health of future stroke survivors.

If you have the opportunity to participate in such a study, you should carefully consider all aspects of participation so you can make a fully informed decision. Research studies are designed to answer a research question, and participants may or may not personally benefit from a study. Some research studies carry significant risks, and you should understand the risks thoroughly before agreeing to participate. Here are some key questions to ask:

What is the purpose of the research study?

Will I receive a medication or other treatment in this study, or does this study focus on testing or monitoring stroke survivors?

If there is a medication or treatment involved, is it available outside of this study?

How large a time commitment is required for this study?

What are the risks of being in this study? Are there any possible benefits to me?

Will the results of the study be monitored during the course of the study? If so, will I be notified if the early results show that one of the treatments is better than the other?

Is there any compensation for my time? For my travel expenses and parking?

How can I find out the results of this study?

Participants in research are better protected now than ever before. Researchers are required to thoroughly discuss the risks and benefits of participation with a potential subject of a study before a participant enrolls. A detailed consent form should be provided (and reviewed carefully) that explains the participant's role in the study and gives contact information to use if questions come up. Researchers with larger or riskier studies are required to monitor the safety of the study while it is in progress. If participants are found to be exposed to unexpected hazards, or if one of the studied treatments is found to be clearly superior to the other, the study must be terminated, and participants must be informed. Researchers are required to protect the privacy of the subjects in the study, so that their family members, employers, insurers, or other individuals do not receive information about the patient that they are not entitled to receive.

Participating in research may provide early access to new medications or treatments, but with the significant possibility that these treatments may not prove useful in the end.

We live in a time of rapid change in medical science, which creates unique challenges for people trying to reduce their risk of a stroke. The answers you receive from your doctor today may be different than the ones you received three months ago. How are you to know what to do?

Recognize that despite the advances, medicine will always be an imperfect and evolving science. Rarely do doctors have definite answers to complex medical problems. Your best defense against uncertainty is a vigorous offense. Educate yourself and participate in your own health care decisions. Discuss research studies you have learned about with your physician, and remember to ask him about new treatments that may have become available for stroke prevention.

• •

Chapter 19

Prevent Another Stroke by Taking Charge

As we noted earlier, medicine does not stand still. It keeps changing as we learn more about how to stay healthy and how to recover from injury and illness. Medicine in the twenty-first century is vastly improved over medicine in the past. No one wants to be sick, of course, but if you have had a stroke, you may be reassured by knowing that our skills for helping you to recover and to prevent another stroke are better than they have ever been. We still have a long way to go, but consider how far we have come since the days of King Charles II of England, who had a stroke in 1685. Charles was bled, his head was shaved and blistered, he was given an enema containing antimony, sacred bitters, and rock salt, among other ingredients, a plaster that included pigeon dung was applied to his feet, and he was given forty drops of an extract containing human skull. How awful this must have been for him! Needless to say, the king's treatment sealed his fate, and he died.

Even in the more recent past, doctors understood so little about how to heal that most sick people were better off without medical attention. President James Garfield was shot at a Washington, D.C., train station on July 2, 1881. His doctor arrived on the scene almost immediately and used an unsterilized probe to try to locate the bullet. The instrument slid down his wound away from the bullet and shattered his ribs. The doctor then stuck his unwashed hand into the wound, causing a serious infection. Doctors spent the next eighty days compounding the original medical errors, and President Garfield finally succumbed to what historians now believe were complications from the treatment, rather than the initial injury.

Today we have proven effective treatments for many serious medical conditions. The medical and scientific communities increasingly have worked toward basing treatments on evidence gained from rigorous studies. This approach, known as *evidence-based medicine,* includes a wide variety of medical treatments as well as preventive treatments.

We know that a stroke suddenly changes your life, and that you may feel as if you have lost control over your future. In this book we have provided information about what causes a stroke and how you can reduce your risk of having one. In this chapter, we want to pull this information together into an action plan to help you regain control of your destiny. We want to put you in charge of your own life as much as possible.

One thing we know for certain is that stroke prevention relies heavily on the patient's effort. We want to help you organize and prioritize the major steps needed to prevent stroke. You have taken an important step by reading this book. What else do you need to do? *Develop an action plan.*

Developing Your Action Plan

Your action plan will have three major components:

1. Educating yourself
2. Improving your lifestyle
3. Taking care of yourself medically

Step 1: Get Informed

Understanding the "hows" and "whys" of stroke will help you motivate yourself to take steps to improve your lifestyle and reduce your risk of stroke. As we said, reading this book is a great way to become knowledgeable about stroke. But you want to be sure to discuss your medical history and unique issues with your physician, because excellent medical advice is critical to your success.

The very first thing you need to do, therefore, is team up with your doctor and discuss what each of you will be doing to help prevent a stroke (or another stroke) from occurring. This teamwork will be most effective if you schedule a doctor's visit specifically to discuss how you can reduce your risk of stroke. If you find that you do not receive enough information and guidance from your primary care physician, request a referral to a neurologist or other physician specializing in stroke, and get additional information from that specialist.

Once you have the necessary information, you need to boil it down into a short list of actions that can help you reduce your risk of stroke. The most common action items are discussed here, but there may very well be issues specific to your situation that come out of your discussion with your doctor. Obviously, some of the actions you identify will be harder to accomplish than

Step 1 Checklist

✓ Identify a physician you trust and with whom you can communicate.

✓ Write down questions to ask your physician.

✓ Discuss stroke prevention with your physician and come up with a specific list of things you need to do.

others. It may be easy to take a medication once a day, while changing your diet or exercise habits may be harder. You should know that you have the power to change your situation, however, and that a great time to form new habits is right after a serious illness. If you are worried about having another stroke, use your concern to motivate yourself in a positive direction.

Step 2: Adopt a Healthy Lifestyle

Doctors tend to give short shrift to lifestyle modifications, in large part because physicians are pessimistic about their ability to influence their patients' behaviors. Most doctors find that prescribing medications is a more expedient way to accomplish the desired medical goal. It is often easier to prescribe a medication to reduce blood pressure, for example, than to convince stroke survivors to increase their exercise levels and improve their diets.

If you or a loved one has had a stroke, however, we encourage you to take the second step and make an enormous effort to incorporate lifestyle changes in diet and exercise into your recovery plan. The information you have gathered should help you identify a number of ways to reduce your risk of stroke through diet and exercise. Making these changes will also greatly reduce your risk of developing other serious medical conditions.

Good health is more than the absence of disease. Improving your lifestyle actually makes you healthier, rather than merely treating illness. The benefits are multiple and synergistic: an improved lifestyle can improve your mood, energy levels, and sense of well-being.

Step 2 Checklist

✓ Stop smoking.

✓ Lose excess weight.

✓ Improve your diet.

✓ Exercise regularly.

✓ Avoid alcohol completely or drink in moderation.

✓ Never use illicit drugs.

Step 3 Checklist

✓ Control your blood pressure.

✓ Control your diabetes.

✓ Control your cholesterol.

✓ Take your stroke-prevention medications reliably.

Step 3: Follow Your Doctor's Advice

Studies reveal that many patients do not comply with their doctor's advice, or they only partially comply. There are a number of reasons for noncompliance. Some people do not understand what their doctor wants them to do, some are not sure how to take their medications or forget to take their medications on schedule, and some don't understand how the treatment will benefit them. If you have had a stroke, *you must get good medical advice and you must follow your doctor's recommendations.* Your doctor can only help you if the two of you work together on a stroke prevention plan.

The third step is to identify your medical conditions that require good management to reduce the risk of stroke. A number of very common medical conditions contribute to the risk of stroke. While you may not be able to eliminate the increased risk that comes with these conditions, you can substantially reduce it. You and your physician are partners in accomplishing this goal. You can enhance your role in this partnership by developing a checklist of goals as well as an action plan for carrying out these goals. If you can't do something that your doctor recommends, talk to him about it. Your doctor may well be able to offer you another solution that is equally effective.

Putting the Plan into Action

You have informed yourself about the causes of stroke and developed an action plan of steps you need to take to reduce your risk of stroke. But how can you actually make these changes in your life?

Stop Smoking

If you smoke, the single most important action you can take to reduce your risk of stroke is to stop smoking. Effective treatment programs are available (see Chapter 17). Enlist the help of family members. Avoid situations where other people will be smoking as well as situations that you associate with smoking.

Don't accept smoking among your family members or other people you spend time with. Remind them that they are endangering not only their own health, but yours as well. Some people have the peculiar notion that smoking is a "right," and that you shouldn't interfere with other people's rights. A close review of the U.S. Constitution reveals no mention of a right to smoke. Don't let smokers infringe upon your "right" to clean air (admittedly, this right is not listed in the Constitution either, but you don't have to mention that).

Improve Your Diet

Everyone talks about "eating right," but what does this dictum actually mean? Even more importantly, how can you start eating right when the world is full of delicious fattening foods? The Stroke Savvy Diet is easy to describe (see Chapter 15) but not always easy to stick to. Unfortunately, temptation is woven into our environment in ways we often fail to recognize. Here is a typical scenario that can contribute to a bad diet:

Jim Smith wakes up on Monday morning and realizes that he needs to get to the office early to finish preparing a presentation. He skips breakfast at home, stopping by the drive-thru donut shop for a coffee with cream (extra light, with two sugars). The coffee shop is offering samples of their new breakfast muffins, so Jim accepts a free muffin and munches it on the way to work.

Jim works until 12:30 p.m., until he has only thirty minutes before his presentation. He runs across the street from his office to a fast food restaurant and picks up a burger, fries, and a soda. As he is ordering, the clerk suggests that he might like to "supersize" the fries and soda for only another 55 cents. Jim can't resist a bargain. After Jim finishes his supersized lunch, he resumes work for the afternoon. Then he joins the late afternoon goodbye party for a co-worker who is retiring, where he finds himself holding a large piece of cake. He's not that hungry but the cake looks good, and he eats most of it.

When Jim arrives at home at 6:30 p.m., he is tired from a long day at work. His wife is working an evening shift at the hospital, so he is responsible for dinner. He quickly makes some fast-cooking white rice and finishes up last night's beef stew with the rice. He would enjoy a salad but is too tired to begin cutting up vegetables.

At around 11:30 p.m. Jim's wife returns home from the hospital and sits down at the kitchen counter. She and Jim enjoy bowls of ice cream as they catch up on their busy days. Jim puts a tablespoon of hot fudge sauce on his portion. Jim's diet is atrocious, yet he feels there is little he can do about it. He would like to "eat right" but doesn't feel he has the time to do so. Moreover, he feels that certain social situations, such as the party at work, don't leave him any other choice but to eat unhealthy foods.

Is Jim right? What can he do? Consider a different version of Jim's day, with a more appropriate diet that still works with his lifestyle:

Jim realizes that he won't have time for breakfast at home, so he grabs a low-fat yogurt from the refrigerator on his way out the door. When he stops for his coffee, he requests skim milk rather than cream. He declines the free muffin, remembering that he has brought yogurt for breakfast.

When lunch comes, Jim walks half a block to the grocery store. He is in a rush, so he grabs a premade salad from the produce department and a small foil package of tuna fish to crumble over the salad. He discards the high-fat dressing enclosed with his salad and uses a low-fat vinaigrette dressing he keeps in the office refrigerator instead.

When his co-worker's retirement celebration comes, he declines the cake but swipes one of the large strawberries used for garnish. He finds a bottle of sparkling water to enjoy instead of drinking soda.

Dinner includes some of last night's grilled chicken breasts and some whole-grain toast. He slices up a tomato and grabs some prewashed lettuce from the refrigerator to enhance his sandwich.

When his wife comes home, they enjoy small portions of low-fat frozen yogurt together. He skips the hot fudge sauce and enjoys the frozen yogurt just the same.

As this second scenario illustrates, changing your diet is not accomplished with a single decision or act. Rather, it requires a *series of choices and actions each day.* Improving your diet requires a lifestyle change. The Stroke Savvy Diet described in Chapter 15 can help.

Exercise

Sometimes exercise seems like the weather: everybody talks about it but nobody does anything about it. Exercising regularly seems impossibly daunting to many people. Moreover, many people who have had strokes have physical limitations that make exercise more difficult. Chapter 16 describes a Stroke Savvy Exercise Program for people with all different levels of physical ability. This program will help stroke survivors begin and continue a program of regular exercise to help reduce the risk of another stroke.

How often should I exercise? This question is at the center of ongoing research in medicine and the "ideal" answer to this question is still evolving, but we advise you to exercise no fewer than three times per week for thirty minutes at a time. An exercise routine of five to seven times per week for forty-five minutes to an hour is preferable. There is no harm in increasing the length of time you exercise beyond this level, although the additional benefits in terms of stroke prevention are likely to be small.

Lower Your Blood Pressure

The first step in taking charge of your blood pressure is to become more aware of it. Anyone can learn to check their own blood pressure at home. Purchase an automatic blood pressure machine (available in every drugstore) to monitor your blood pressure. Keeping a log of blood pressure readings can help you and your physician understand the variation in your blood pressure and optimize your treatment. It can also help you see the benefits of your lifestyle changes, as you see your blood pressure gradually coming down. If you are on blood pressure medications, you can see whether or not they are working and help your doctor make decisions regarding changing your dose or medication. After all, your physician can't make the right decision regarding your medication unless he or she has a clear picture of your blood pressure readings.

Ask your physician about once-daily medications. One of the major reasons people do not take their medications is that they forget. It is hard to remember to take a medication two, three, or four times a day. If a once-a-day option exists for your blood pressure medication, you may find that you can take your medication more reliably and control your blood pressure better.

Be honest with your physician about medication costs. Many Americans lack prescription plans, or they have high co-pays for certain types of medications. Let your physician know if you are having difficulty affording the medications prescribed. There are many low-cost alternative medications available for the treatment of high blood pressure. Make certain to ask for generic alternatives, which are as effective and substantially cheaper than brand name drugs. Also inform your doctor if you are experiencing any side effects, such as difficulty sustaining an erection. You should tell your doctor about any side effect that is bothering you or that will make you less likely to take your medication regularly.

Control Your Diabetes

Virtually everyone with diabetes who has had a stroke should be checking their blood sugar at home. If a stroke survivor can't personally check her blood sugar due to physical or other limitations, a family member should periodically check her sugar for her. Knowledge is power, and knowledge of blood sugar provides the power to control your diabetes. It also allows you to see the immediate benefits of altering your diet or of exercising.

Don't accept elevated blood sugar readings—make it your job, not your doctor's job, to control your diabetes. Gain an understanding of what factors exacerbate your diabetes. If certain snack foods are responsible, you owe it to yourself to stop eating them. Only you can control your diet. Make sure you aren't your own worst enemy.

Ask your physician about your overall level of diabetic control. Your physician is probably monitoring a blood test known as *hemoglobin-A-1-C*, a test that provides an overall "average" of your diabetes control. Establish a target level for this test with your physician, and monitor your progress. Don't forget that diabetes isn't only about diet and medication; exercise and weight loss can help your diabetes come under control as well.

Monitor Cholesterol

What does your cholesterol test say? What is your LDL level? HDL? After reading this book you know how important the answers to these questions are. Knowledge of your health is the first step in controlling your medical destiny. Tracking your progress in lowering your cholesterol level is an essential part of risk reduction.

You should establish a target cholesterol level with your physician, and then track your progress toward this goal. If you are using diet and exercise to try to lower your cholesterol, are they working sufficiently? Are you complying with your diet? If you are taking medication to lower your cholesterol, are you receiving a sufficient dose to reach your objective?

Take Stroke Prevention Medication

Are you taking aspirin, Plavix, Coumadin, or another medication to prevent stroke? If so, are you taking it consistently? If you understand the purpose of these medications, you will be more likely to take them reliably as prescribed to help reduce your risk of stroke.

The rewards of restructuring your life are many. You can reduce the risk of stroke, control other medical problems, reduce the risk of heart and vascular disease, and improve your fitness and energy levels. Illness is a profound motivator: use your experience with stroke as motivation to learn what you need to do to help prevent another stroke and to improve your overall health.

One of the questions our patients ask us most often is, "What is my prognosis?" This is a difficult question to answer even if we know the patient well. While we can't tell you what your prognosis is, we can assure you that your prognosis stands an excellent chance of being significantly better if you follow the advice in this book.

Resources

This list contains information on a variety of public and private resources. Inclusion in this list does not imply endorsement of any service or product.

Books

After Stroke, by David M. Hinds, foreword by Peter Morris
Thorsons Publishing, 2000
ISBN: 0-722-53885-5
Available at local bookstores and online booksellers

The Diving Bell and the Butterfly: A Memoir of Life in Death, by Jean-Dominique Bauby, translated by Jeremy Leggatt
A first-person account of living with "locked in" syndrome
Vintage Books, 1998
ISBN: 0-375-70121-4
Available at local bookstores and online booksellers

My Stroke of Luck, by Kirk Douglas
Memoir by the well-known actor about his stroke and recovery
William Morrow, 2002
ISBN: 0-060-00929-2
Available at local bookstores and online booksellers

My Year Off: Recovering Life after a Stroke, by Robert McCrum
Broadway Books, 1999
ISBN: 0-767-90400-1
Available at local bookstores and online booksellers

The New American Heart Association Cookbook, 25th anniversary edition
A heart and stroke healthy cookbook
Random House, 2001
ISBN: 0-609-80890-7
Available at local bookstores and online booksellers

Non-Chew Cookbook, by J. Randy Wilson
Cookbook for individuals with chewing and swallowing disorders. Sample recipes are posted on the book's website.
Wilson Publishing, 1986
P.O. Box 912464
Sherman, TX 75091
1-800-843-2409
www.nonchewcookbook.com
Available at local bookstores or online booksellers

One-Handed in a Two-Handed World, 2nd edition, by Tommye-Karen Mayer
Practical guide to managing with only one functional hand
PrinceGallison Press, 2000
ISBN: 0-965-28051-9
Available at local bookstores and online booksellers

Stroke and the Family, by Joel Stein, M.D.
Guide for stroke survivors and their families that focuses on living with the physical and emotional consequences of stroke
Harvard University Press, 2004
ISBN: 0-674-01667-X
Available at local bookstores and online booksellers

Stroke: Your Complete Exercise Guide, by Neil F. Gordon
Guide to exercise after stroke
Human Kinetics, 1993
ISBN: 0-873-22428-0
Available at local bookstores and online booksellers

Your Mother Has Suffered a Slight Stroke, by Kathleen Bosworth
A daughter's account of her mother's stroke and its effect on her family
Publish America, 2001
ISBN: 1-588-51288-6
Available at local bookstores and online booksellers

Cerebral Amyloid Angiopathy

Cerebral Amyloid Angiopathy Website
Website devoted to cerebral amyloid angiopathy research and education
www.angiopathy.org

Diabetes

American Diabetes Association
Provides support and education for people with diabetes. The website addresses topics such as prevention, nutrition, weight loss, exercise, and research.
www.diabetes.org

The Johns Hopkins Guide to Diabetes: For Today and Tomorrow, by Christopher D. Saudek, Richard R. Rubin, and Cynthia S. Shump
Guide to living with diabetes
Johns Hopkins University Press, 1997
ISBN: 0-8018-6657-X
Available at local bookstores and online booksellers

Driving

Association for Driver Rehabilitation Specialists (ADED)
For professional driver rehabilitation instructors
711 S. Vienna Street
Ruston, LA 71270
phone: (318) 257-5055 or 1-800-290-2344
fax: (318) 255-4175
www.driver-ed.org

Equipment

Abledata
Federally funded resource with information on rehabilitation equipment and assistive technology aids
8630 Fenton Street, Suite 930
Silver Spring, MD 20910
(301) 608-8997; or 1-800-227-0216 (8:00 a.m.–5:30 p.m. EST)
TTY (301) 608-8912
fax: (301) 608-8958
www.abledata.com

Nautilus, Inc.
Commercial vendor that supplies exercise equipment such as treadmills and stationary bicycles
16400 SE Nautilus Drive
Vancouver, WA 98683
1-800-728-4799
www.nautilus.com

Sammons Preston Rolyan
Commercial vendor with an extensive catalogue of devices to assist with living at home with a disability
270 Remington Boulevard, Suite C
Bolingbrook, IL 60440
1-800-323-5547
email: customersupport@sammonspreston.com
www.sammonspreston.com

Exercise

The President's Council on Physical Fitness and Sports
U.S. government website promoting exercise and sports for health
www.fitness.gov/

United States Department of Health and Human Services
The Surgeon General's Call to Action to Prevent and Decrease Overweight and Obesity is documented in this website.
www.surgeongeneral.gov/topics/obesity/

Healthy Lifestyle

HealthierUS.gov
U.S. government website promoting healthier living. Addresses diet, exercise, smoking cessation, and other aspects of a healthy lifestyle
www.healthierus.gov/

Heart Disease

American Heart Association
Organization dedicated to helping people with heart disease. The website contains information on cholesterol, high blood pressure, arrhythmias, and congestive heart failure. It also provides healthy lifestyle tips, including diet and exercise recommendations.
www.americanheart.org

Medical Information

Medicine Plus Health Information
A free service sponsored by the National Library of Medicine and the National Institutes of Health, providing information about health conditions and medications, a health encyclopedia and glossary with pictures, diagrams, and health news
www.nlm.nih.gov/

Pubmed
Free service sponsored by the National Library of Medicine that provides a searchable database of medical literature. Abstracts of many articles are available online, and links to full text of some articles are available. While this resource is primarily intended for health professionals, it provides a wealth of information for individuals seeking to research specific medical topics.
www.pubmed.gov

Mental Health Resources

American Psychiatric Association
1000 Wilson Boulevard, Suite 1825
Arlington, VA 22209-3901
1-888-35-PSYCH
www.psych.org

American Psychological Association
750 First Street, NE
Washington, DC 20002-4242
1-800-374-2721
www.apa.org

National Association of Social Workers
750 First Street, NE, Suite 700
Washington, DC 20002-4241
(202) 408-8600
www.socialworkers.org

Nutrition and Diet

Basic Nutrition and Diet Therapy, by Sue Rodwell Williams
A textbook for the study of nutrition, this book explains the basics of carbohy-
drates, fats, and proteins. It also discusses body mass index and energy expendi-
ture.
Mosby, 2000
ISBN: 03-23-00569-1
Available at local bookstores and online booksellers

Calorie Counter
Calorie counter titled "Your Game Plan for Preventing Type 2 Diabetes," put together by The National Institute of Health and the Centers for Disease Control and
Prevention, the National Diabetes Education Program, and the U.S. Department
of Health and Human Services
www.ndep.nih.gov/diabetes/pubs/GP_FatCal.pdf

The Complete Book of Food Counts, by Corinne T. Netzer
Pocket guide to food counts that lists calories, fat, cholesterol, fiber, and sodium
for a wide variety of foods
Dell, 2003
ISBN: 0-440-22564-7
Available at local bookstores and online booksellers

Coumadin/Vitamin K
Pharmaceutical company website from the makers of Coumadin, includes a list of
the vitamin K content of common foods
www.coumadin.com

TheDietDiary.com
This website can be used to estimate your daily energy expenditure.
www.thedietdiary.com/diet/nutrition/RestingEnergy.html

Food and Nutrition Information Center
U.S. government sponsored website with information on healthy diets
www.nal.usda.gov/fnic/

HealthStatus.com
Health Status Internet Assessments provides various calculators, including one that estimates calories burned during different activities and exercises.
www.healthstatus.com/calculate/cbc

National Heart, Lung, and Blood Institute
As part the institute's obesity education initiative, this website educates people about aiming for a healthy weight and provides a body mass index (BMI) calculator.
www.nhlbisupport.com/bmi/bmicalc.htm

Nutrition.gov
A U.S. government website providing information regarding nutrition and diets
www.nutrition.gov/

The TFactor 2000 Fat Gram Counter, by Jamie Pope and Martin Katahn
A pocket guide to food counts that lists calories, cholesterol, sodium, fiber and fat, including saturated fat, for a wide variety of foods
W.W. Norton and Company, 1994
ISBN: 0-393-30655-0
Available at local bookstores and online booksellers

U.S. Food Pyramid
Government website providing information about healthy diets. Features include customized diet recommendations
www.mypyramid.gov

Professional and Consumer Organizations

American Academy of Physical Medicine and Rehabilitation
The professional organization of physicians specializing in physical medicine and rehabilitation. Includes a directory of specialists in this field
330 North Wabash Avenue, Suite 2500
Chicago, IL 60611-3604
(312) 464-9700
email: info@aapmr.org
fax: (312) 461-0227
www.aapmr.org

American Chronic Pain Association
An organization devoted to support and education for people with chronic pain and their caregivers
P.O. Box 850
Rocklin, CA 95677
phone: 1-800-533-3231
fax: (916) 632-3208
email: acpa@pacbell.net
www.theacpa.org

American Neurological Association
Organization of physicians specializing in neurology
5841 Cedar Lake Road, Suite 204
Minneapolis, MN 55416
(952) 545-6284
fax: (952) 545-6073
www.aneuroa.org

American Occupational Therapy Association
National organization of occupational therapists
4720 Montgomery Lane
P.O. Box 31220
Bethesda, MD 20824-1220
(301) 652-2682; or 1-800-377-8555
fax: (301) 652-7711
www.aota.org

American Pain Society
A national organization of professionals who treat or study pain
4700 West Lake Avenue
Glenview, IL 60025
(847) 375-4715
email: info@ampainsoc.org
www.ampainsoc.org

American Physical Therapy Association
National organization of physical therapists
1111 North Fairfax Street
Alexandria, VA 22314
(703) 684-APTA (2782); or 1-800-999-APTA (2782)
TDD: (703) 683-6748
fax: (703) 684-7343
www.apta.org

American Society of Neurorehabilitation
Physician organization devoted to the rehabilitation of stroke and other neurological disorders
5841 Cedar Lake Road, Suite 204
Minneapolis, MN 55416
(952) 545-6324
fax: (952) 545-6073
www.asnr.com

American Speech Language and Hearing Association
National organization of speech language pathologists and audiologists
10801 Rockville Pike
Rockville, MD 20852
Voice/TTY: 1-800-638-8255 (8:30 a.m.–5:00 p.m. EST)
email: actioncenter@asha.org
www.asha.org

American Stroke Association (a division of the American Heart Association)
National organization devoted to the prevention and treatment of stroke
National Center
7272 Greenville Avenue
Dallas, TX 75231
1-888-4-STROKE or 1-888-478-7653
www.strokeassociation.org

American Therapeutic Recreation Association
National organization for recreation therapists
1414 Prince Street, Suite 204
Alexandria, VA 22314
(703) 683-9420
fax: (703) 683-9431
www.atra-tr.org

Association of Rehabilitation Nurses
National organization of nurses specializing in rehabilitation
4700 W. Lake Avenue
Glenview, IL 60025-1485
(847) 375-4710; or 1-800-229-7530
fax: (877) 734-9384
email: info@rehabnurse.org
www.rehabnurse.org

Easter Seals
National organization providing services to individuals with disabilities
230 West Monroe Street, Suite 1800
(312) 726-6200; or 1-800-221-6827
TTY: (312) 726-4258
fax: (312) 726-1494
www.easterseals.org

Family Caregiver Alliance
Organization focusing on the needs of caregivers
150 Montgomery Street, Suite 1100
San Francisco, CA 94104
(415) 434-3388; or 1-800-445-8106
fax: (415) 434-3508
email: info@caregivers.org
www.caregiver.org

Heart and Stroke Association of Canada
Canadian organization for the prevention and treatment of heart disease and
stroke
www.heartandstroke.ca

National Aphasia Association
Organization devoted to individuals with aphasia and their families
1-800-922-4622
email: naa@aphasia.org
www.aphasia.org

National Family Caregiver Association
Organization devoted to the needs of caregivers
10400 Connecticut Avenue, Suite 500
Kensington, MD 20895-3944
1-800-896-3650
fax: (301) 942-2302
email: info@thefamilycaregiver.org
www.nfcacares.org

The National Pain Foundation
A nonprofit organization devoted to providing education and support for individuals with chronic pain
300 E. Hampden Avenue, Suite 100
Englewood, CO 80113
email: aardrup@nationalpainfoundation.org
www.painconnection.org

National Stroke Association
Organization devoted to the prevention and treatment of stroke
9707 E. Easter Lane
Englewood, CO 80112
1-800-STROKES
fax: (303) 649-1328
www.stroke.org

Rehabilitation Engineering and Assistive Technology Society of North America (RESNA)
Professional organization devoted to the use of technology to improve independence for individuals with disability
1700 N. Moore Street, Suite 1540
Arlington, VA 22209-1903
(703) 524-6686
TTY: (703) 524-6639
fax: (703) 524-6630
www.resna.org

Rosalynn Carter Institute for Caregiving
Organization devoted to caregiver issues
800 Wheatley Street
Americus, GA 31709
(229) 928-1234
fax: (229) 931-2663
email: rci@rci.gsw.edu
www.rci.gsw.edu

The Stroke Association (United Kingdom)
A British organization providing support and information for stroke survivors and their caregivers
Stroke House
240 City Road
London, United Kingdom
EC1V 2PR
Telephone the Stroke Information Service on 020 7566 0330, or local rate number (from U.K.) 0845 30 33 100.
email: info@stroke.org.uk
www.stroke.org.uk

Wellspouse Association
Association of spousal caregivers
63 West Main Street, Suite H
Freehold, NJ 07728
1-800-838-0879
fax: (732) 577-8644
www.wellspouse.org

Rehabilitation and Community Resources

Commission on Accreditation of Rehabilitation Facilities (CARF)
Nonprofit organization that accredits rehabilitation hospitals and other facilities
4891 E. Grant Road
Tucson, AZ 85712
voice/TTY: (520) 325-1044
fax: (520) 318-1129
www.carf.org

Council of State Administrators of Vocational Rehabilitation (CSAVR)
4733 Bethesda Avenue, Suite 330
Bethesda, MD 20814
(301) 654-8414
www.rehabnetwork.org

Department of Justice: Americans with Disabilities Act (ADA) Website
United States Department of Justice website with information regarding the ADA
1-800-514-0301
TDD: 1-800-514-0383
www.usdoj.gov/crt/ada/adahom1.htm

Elder Services
The eldercare locator is run by the U.S. Administration on Aging and provides
links to a wide variety of state and local resources for older individuals.
1-800-677-1116
www.eldercare.gov

Home Care Website
A U.S. government Center for Medicare and Medicaid Services (CMS) website
with information on home health care agencies
www.medicare.gov/HHCompare/home.asp

National Council on Disability
A U.S. government council that advises the government on disability issues
1331 F Street, NW, Suite 850
Washington, DC 20004
(202) 272-2004
TTY: (202) 272-2074
fax: (202) 272-2022
www.ncd.gov

National Rehabilitation Information Center (NARIC)
U.S. government–supported information center on disability and rehabilitation.
4200 Forbes Boulevard., Suite 202
Lanham, MD 20706
(301) 459-5900; or 1-800-346-2742
email: naricinfo@heitechservices.com
www.naric.com

Office of Special Education and Rehabilitative Services (OSERS)
The Office of Special Education and Rehabilitation (OSERS), within the U.S. Department of Education, provides information and resources about vocational training and returning to work for the disabled.
400 Maryland Avenue, SW
Washington, DC 20202
(202) 245-7468
www.ed.gov/about/offices/list/osers/index.html

Skilled Nursing Facilities Website
U.S. government Center for Medicare and Medicaid Services (CMS) website with information on skilled nursing facilities
www.medicare.gov/LongTermCare/Static/NursingHome

Vocational Rehabilitation Programs
Provides contact information for the federally supported vocational rehabilitation programs in each state
www.jan.wvu.edu/sbses/vocrehab.htm

Research Resources

Centerwatch
Website listing clinical trials nationwide
www.centerwatch.com

Clinical Research Network
Website about clinical research at several Harvard-affiliated hospitals in the Boston area
crnet.mgh.harvard.edu/home/home.asp

NIH Clinical Trials Database
NIH-sponsored website providing information about ongoing clinical trials
www.clinicaltrials.gov

RehabTrials.org
Website sponsored by the Kessler Medical Rehabilitation Research and Education Corporation, providing a listing of rehabilitation research studies
www.rehabtrials.org

Stroke Trials Directory
National directory of ongoing stroke research clinical studies. Sponsored by the
Internet Stroke Center at Washington University in St. Louis, the American Stroke
Association, and the National Institutes of Health
www.strokecenter.org/trials

Sex and Intimacy

Sex Information and Education Council of the United States
130 West 42nd Street, Suite 350
New York, NY 10036-7802
(212) 819-9770
www.siecus.org

Smoking Cessation

Centers for Disease Control Tobacco Information and Prevention Source
U.S. government website providing information about tobacco risks and resources
for smoking cessation
www.cdc.gov/tobacco/

Quit Net
Smoking cessation website supported by the Boston University School of Public
Health
www.quitnet.com/

Quitworks
Free, phone-based smoking cessation program sponsored by the Massachusetts
Department of Public Health
email: quitworksinfo@jsi.com
1-800-TRYTOSTOP (1-800-879-8678)
fax: (866) 560-9113
www.quitworks.org/

Smokefree.gov
U.S. government website providing resources and support for smoking cessation
www.smokefree.gov/

Try to Stop
Smoking cessation website sponsored by the Massachusetts Department of Public
Health
www.trytostop.org/

Sports and Leisure Activities

Access Sport America
Organization devoted to making windsurfing, kayaking, and other water sports accessible for people with disabilities
119 High Street
Acton, MA 01720
(866) 45-SPORT (77678); or (978) 264-0985
www.accessports.org

Disabled Sports USA
National organization promoting sports for people with disabilities
451 Hungerford Drive, Suite 100
Rockville, MD 20850
(301) 217-0960
fax: (301) 217-0968
www.dsusa.org

North American Riding for the Handicapped Association (NARHA)
Organization promoting horseback riding for people with disabilities
P.O. Box 33150
Denver, CO 80233
(303) 452-1212; or 1-800-369-RIDE (7433)
fax: (303) 252-4610
email: narha@narha.org
www.narha.org

Outdoor Explorations
Organization promoting outdoor activities for people with disabilities and their families
98 Winchester Street
Medford, MA 02155
(781) 395-4999
TTY: (781) 395-4184
fax: (781) 395-4183
email: info@outdoorexp.org
www.outdoorexplorations.org

Stroke Information

The Internet Stroke Center
Web resource sponsored by Washington University in Saint Louis, providing information about stroke, with links to directory of stroke research studies and other resources
www.strokecenter.org

Notes

Chapter 1. Understanding Stroke and Its Consequences

1. S. C. Johnston, D. R. Gress, W. S. Browner, and S. Sidney, "Short-term prognosis after emergency department diagnosis of TIA," *Journal of the American Medical Association* 284 (2000): 2901–2906.

2. W. Holland, ed., *Stroke: Past, Present, and Future* (New York: Oxford University Press, 2000), pp. 3, 128.

3. *Heart Disease and Stroke Statistics: 2003 Update* (Dallas: American Heart Association, 2002), p. 15.

Chapter 2. How Strokes Affect Our Brains and Bodies

1. V. Hachinski, "Stalin's last years: delusions or dementia?" *European Journal of Neurology* 6 (1999): 129.

2. Ibid.

3. I. K. Smith, "Different strokes: the misdiagnosis of a former president's illness shows the importance of recognizing symptoms," *Time*, August 14, 2003, p. 86.

4. S. Sontag, *Illness as Metaphor and AIDS and Its Metaphors* (New York: St. Martin's, 1989), p. 3.

Chapter 4. Minimizing Early Post-Stroke Disability and Complications

1. E. N. Babcock, *When Life Becomes Precious: The Essential Guide for Patients, Loved Ones, and Friends of Those Facing Serious Illnesses* (New York: Bantam Books, 2002), p. 13.

2. B. Rollin, *First, You Cry* (New York: HarperCollins, 2000), pp. 102–103.

3. K. Duff, *The Alchemy of Illness* (New York: Crown, 1993), p. xii.

Chapter 5. Maximizing Recovery from a Stroke

1. R. W. Gifford, "FDR and hypertension: if we'd only known then what we know now," *Geriatrics* 51 (1996): 29–32.

2. B. Rollin, *Last Wish* (New York: Perseus, 1998), p. 122.

Chapter 6. Post-Stroke Medical and Social Issues

1. F. X. Brickfield and L. R. Pyenson, "The impact of stroke on world leaders," *Military Medicine* 166 (2001): 231–232.

Chapter 8. Heart and Blood Vessel Conditions and Stroke

1. Bill Cosby, *I Am What I Ate . . . and I'm Frightened!!! and Other Digressions from the Doctor of Comedy* (New York: Harper Entertainment, 2003), p. xxiii.

Chapter 11. Other Causes of Stroke

1. J. E. Rossouw et al., "Risks and benefits of estrogen plus progestin in healthy postmenopausal women: principal results from the Women's Health Initiative randomized controlled trial," *Journal of the American Medical Association* 288 (2002): 321–333.

2. G. L. Anderson et al., "Effects of conjugated equine estrogen in postmeno-pausal women with hysterectomy: the Women's Health Initiative randomized con-trolled trial," *Journal of the American Medical Association* 291 (2004): 1701–1712.

Chapter 12. Genetics and Stroke

1. S. Bak et al., "Genetic liability in stroke: a long-term follow-up study of Danish twins," *Stroke* 33 (2002): 769–774.

2. S. Gretarsdottir et al., "Localization of a susceptibility gene for common forms of stroke to 5q12," *American Journal of Human Genetics* 70 (2002): 593–603.

3. F. Cipollone et al., "A polymorphism in the cyclooxygenase 2 gene as an inherited protective factor against myocardial infarction and stroke," *Journal of the American Medical Association* 291 (2004): 2221–2228.

Chapter 15. Diet and Stroke

1. S. R. Williams, *Basic Nutrition and Diet Therapy* (St. Louis: Mosby, 2001), chapter 5.

2. C. T. Netzer, *The Complete Book of Food Counts* (New York: Dell, 2003); J. Pope and M. Katahn, *The T-Factor 2000 Fat Gram Counter* (New York: W. W. Norton, 1989).

3. L. J. Appel et al., "A Clinical Trial of the Effects of Dietary Patterns on Blood Pressure," *New England Journal of Medicine,* 1997 (336): 1117–1124.
Acarbose (Precose), 153

Index